Visual Perception

Visual Perception
A Clinical Orientation

Third Edition

Steven H. Schwartz, OD, PhD
State College of Optometry
State University of New York
New York, New York

McGraw-Hill
Medical Publishing Division

New York Chicago San Francisco Lisbon
London Madrid Mexico City Milan New Delhi
San Juan Seoul Singapore Sydney Toronto

The **McGraw·Hill** Companies

Visual Perception: A Clinical Orientation, Third Edition

5 6 7 8 9 0   DOC/DOC   0 9 8 7

ISBN 0-07-141187-9

This book was set in Garamond by Deirdre Sheean and Paul Scozzari of McGraw-Hill Professional's Hightstown, NJ, composition unit.
The editors were Darlene Cooke and Andrea Seils.
The production supervisor was Sherri Souffrance.
Project management was provided by Jennsin Services.
RR Donnelley was printer and binder.
This book was printed on acid-free paper.

Library of Congress Cataloging-in-Publication Data

Visual perception: a clinical orientation/ edited by Steven H. Schwartz.— 3rd ed.
    p. ; cm.
  Rev. ed. of: Visual perception / Steven H. Schwartz. 2nd ed. c1999.
  Includes bibliographical references and index.
  ISBN 0-07-141187-9
  1. Vision. 2. Visual perception. 3. Vision disorders. I. Schwartz, Steven H. II. Schwartz, Steven H. Visual perception.
  [DNLM: 1. Visual Perception. 2. Vision. WW 105 V83411 2004]
 QP475.S38   2004
 612.8'4—dc22

                                    2003061474

Contents

Foreword

*If we believed that we must try to find out what is not known, we
should be better and braver and less idle than if we believed that
what we do not know is impossible to find out and that we need not
even try.*

—Socrates, *The Meno*

The core of any profession is its basis in scientific knowledge, and for those in the
eye and vision care professions, we are indeed fortunate that our core is so rich
and deep and broad. Vision science draws its facts and its theories from a wide
range of sources—physics, optics, anatomy, physiology, biochemistry, psychology,
and cognitive neurosciences. Although much of our core knowledge traces back
to Leonardo da Vinci, Thomas Young, Helmholtz, Hering, and Wheatstone, vision
science is a dynamic field, and our current knowledge also owes a great debt to
more recent contributions by such modern workers as Granit, Wald, Hubel and
Wiesel, Enroth-Cugell and Robson, and Nathans. Over the more than 20 years
since Cornsweet's excellent book on the topic, there has been an explosion in our
knowledge and understanding of visual neurophysiology, genetics, development
and aging, and many other key aspects of visual function.

Although there are many books dealing with aspects of visual science in great
depth, there are few books written on the topic with a view to the clinical importance of the topic for those in the eye and vision care professions. In this book,
Dr. Steven Schwartz has, I believe, succeeded in covering a broad range of subjects in visual science and in bringing home the clinical relevance of each section to the reader.

No single volume can address all of visual science; however, *Visual Perception:
A Clinical Orientation* covers an extraordinarily broad range of clinically important
topics, including color vision and its defects, spatial vision, temporal aspects of
vision, psychophysics, physiology, and development and aging. The third edition
incorporates new material on extrastriate visual processing, motion perception, and
the molecular genetics of color vision—all rapidly developing areas. Doctor Schwartz
has a keen understanding of both the fundamental aspects of vision and their

clinical implications, and his unique approach, which brings the science and its applications together, will make this book a very popular one in teaching visual science to optometry students.

Doctor Schwartz has a real skill for explaining difficult concepts in very simple (but technically accurate) terms. Moreover, this book goes well beyond the basics, including information from anatomy to perception, and always highlights the clinical implications. Throughout the book, Dr. Schwartz manages to convey much of the excitement of important new developments, while providing the reader with suitable caution as to what aspects of the unfolding stories are still controversial.

Doctor Schwartz displays a real empathy for his readers. For example, in Chapter 5, "Color Vision," after accurately describing the very difficult concepts related to the CIE system, Dr. Schwartz assures readers by telling them, "If you are having difficulty understanding this system, do not feel alone." This is a nice touch, and Dr. Schwartz goes on to provide helpful suggestions for gaining deeper understanding. The discussion questions (and the "hints") are also likely to be helpful to both teachers of vision science and to the students using the book.

In summary, this book represents a comprehensive text on visual science, providing fundamental concepts in an engaging and interesting style. This information does not exist in any other single volume, and the close links forged between the basic knowledge and the clinical applications make the book particularly appealing for optometric and ophthalmologic students, faculty, and researchers.

Dennis M. Levi, OD, PhD
University of California, Berkeley
April, 2004

Preface

A patient presenting with incipient cataracts complains of a marked reduction in vision. When we measure visual acuity, however, we find little or no reduction. How do we explain this apparent lack of consistency between the patient's symptoms and the near-normal acuity? On the basis of our knowledge of visual perception, how do we best treat this patient?

Eye care professionals routinely diagnose and treat conditions that have profound effects on visual perception. But how well do we understand the fundamentals of visual perception and their application to clinical practice? My experience tells me that the rich body of knowledge developed in recent decades regarding visual perception is not fully utilized in routine clinical practice.

Although there are several fine textbooks on visual perception that address vision and its physiological basis, none are written for the eye care professional. This text covers those essentials of monocular visual perception on which successful clinical practice is predicated, with a strong emphasis on physiologically based models. A patient may present with a perceptual complaint, but the precipitating condition affects the structures of the visual system. Clinically useful models of visual perception link perception with anatomy and physiology.

In addition to providing a basic science background, each chapter discusses the clinical relevance and application of the material. Clinical information is presented in such a manner that beginning clinicians and other readers (e.g., graduate students and experimental psychologists) will benefit from the discussions.

The third edition has been expanded to include certain of the myriad advances in visual perception that have occurred in recent years. Virtually all chapters have been substantially updated to include new information. New figures and photomicrographs have been added, and many of the original figures have been modified. The book now includes over 250 diagrams and photographs. As in prior editions, an effort has been made to present complex and sophisticated concepts in a manner that is concise, comprehensible, and clinically relevant, while maintaining an appropriate degree of scientific rigor.

Self-assessment questions are presented at the conclusion of many chapters, with answers given at the end of the book. These questions are intended to develop and reinforce key concepts. This new edition also includes 162 multiple-choice questions, divided into three practice examinations. The questions are of varying levels of difficulty and should prove useful to the reader for determining his of her mastery of the material. Answers are provided.

Acknowledgments

The data and models presented in this book result from the hard work of many scientists and clinicians, and it is to them that I owe my deepest gratitude. My president, Norman Haffner of SUNY State College of Optometry, and editor, Darlene Cooke of McGraw-Hill, were supportive throughout the duration of this project. Special appreciation goes to Lenge Hong, who provided encouragement and forbearance through yet another book. Below are listed those individuals who generously reviewed or provided feedback on this or earlier editions.

Michael C. Barris, PhD
Fredonia, New York

Mike Fendick, OD, PhD
College of Optometry
Nova Southeastern University
Fort Lauderdale, Florida

Peter F. Hitchcock, PhD
W. K. Kellogg Eye Center
University of Michigan
Ann Arbor, Michigan

Jeff Hovis, OD, PhD
School of Optometry
University of Waterloo
Waterloo, Ontario

Ralph J. Jensen, PhD
Center for Innovative Visual
   Rehabilitation
Boston VA Medical Center
Boston, Massachusetts

David Lee, OD, PhD
Illinois College of Optometry
Chicago, Illinois

Dennis M. Levi, OD, PhD
School of Optometry
University of California
Berkeley, California

Michael S. Loop, PhD
School of Optometry/The Medical
   Center
University of Alabama at Birmingham
Birmingham, Alabama

Joel Pokorny, PhD
The University of Chicago
Chicago, Illinois

Jeff Rabin, OD, PhD
College of Optometry
Pacific University
Forest Grove, Oregon

Alan Riezman, OD
VA Pacific Islands Healthcare System
Honolulu, Hawaii

Thomas O. Salmon, OD, PhD
College of Optometry
Northeastern State University
Tahlequah, Oklahoma

Scott B. Steinman, OD, PhD
Southern College of Optometry
Memphis, Tennessee

Dean Yager, PhD
State College of Optometry
State University of New York
New York, New York

Robert L. Yolton, OD, PhD
College of Optometry
Pacific University
Forest Grove, Oregon

Visual Perception

1

Experimental
Approaches

The visual system extracts information from the environment, transforming it into a neural code that results in perception. This information includes chromaticity, movement, detail, form, and depth. Diseases of the visual system can disrupt this process, leading to muted or incorrect perceptions. By understanding the mechanisms that underlie visual perception,[1] the clinician is better able to recognize and diagnose disease that may otherwise be undetectable.

The data presented in this book were obtained through anatomical, neurophysiological, psychophysical, and imaging experiments. To understand the utility of these approaches, conceptualize the visual system as a novel and complex electronic machine with operations that we wish to understand. How would we go about understanding such a device?

The machine could be opened and its structure determined. Diagrams would be made that illustrate the locations of various components and their interconnections. As with anatomical studies, structure is determined with the expectation that it will provide insight regarding operations.

We would want to ascertain the function of the individual components that constitute the device. Electronic probes could be used to record activity from various elements and circuits. Similar to electrophysiological methodology, local circuits are studied to determine how information is processed.

---

1. Just as there are numerous approaches to the study of visual perception, there are myriad definitions. For this book, we define *visual perception* as the conscious expression of activity within the neural structures of the visual system.

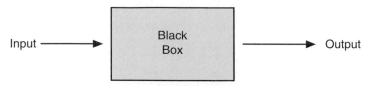

Figure 1–1. Psychophysical approaches may treat the visual system as a black box. A precisely specified input is presented to the system and the output is determined. From the input–output relationship, the operational characteristics of the system are determined.

The capabilities of the intact device could be determined by treating it as a black box (Fig. 1–1). Information would be fed into the black box (data could be entered using the device's keyboard and its various dials and switches) and the output determined. This is analogous to psychophysical methodology.

All of the preceding approaches are necessary to formulate clinically useful models of visual perception. The anatomy must be known to determine the flow of information. Neurophysiological investigations allow us to understand the processing of information at various levels. And psychophysical studies provide insight regarding the visual system's capabilities and operating strategies.

A newer experimental approach that does not readily lend itself to the machine analogy is brain imaging, where metabolic activity is observed in an alert subject while he or she performs a specified task. For instance, metabolic activity could be assessed while a subject views a moving target. The areas of the brain that exhibit the most activity (compared to the baseline activity measured when the subject views a stationary target) are presumably involved in processing motion information.

The data and models presented in this book are derived from these basic experimental approaches. Direct clinical applications, however, typically take the form of psychophysical procedures because such procedures are noninvasive. The text emphasizes this approach.

Introductory Concepts

The information in this chapter is intended for those readers who do not have training in ocular anatomy and physiology and the physics of light. It presents introductory background material critical to the study of visual perception and information processing.

VERY BASIC OCULAR ANATOMY

Three Ocular Layers: Sclera, Uvea, and Retina

Figure 2–1 shows a horizontal cross-section of the human eye. At birth, the average eye has an **axial length** (cornea to retina) of 17 mm, and grows to an average length of 25.4 mm (1 in.) in the adult.

The eye consists of three concentric layers. The outermost is the sclera, the middle is the uvea, and the innermost is the retina.

The sclera is the white portion of the eye that is apparent on gross observation. It consists largely of collagen and provides support and protection for the internal elements of the eye. The sclera is continuous with the cornea, which is the transparent tissue at the most anterior aspect of the eye.

The highly vascularized uvea consists of the iris, ciliary body, and choroid. Within the **iris** are the sphincter iridis and the dilator pupillae muscles that control the

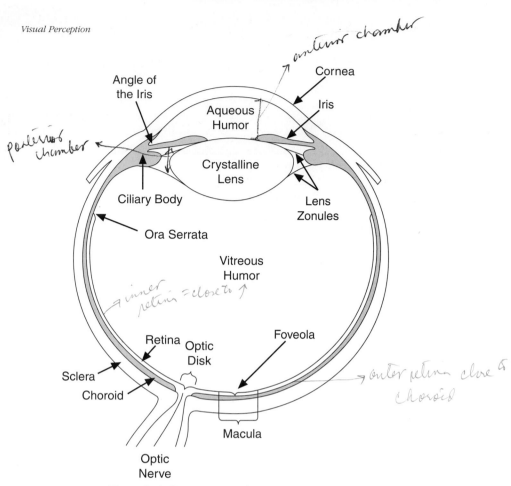

Figure 2–1. Cross-section of the human eye.

diameter of the pupil, thereby helping to regulate the amount of light that enters the eye. The **ciliary body** contains the ciliary muscle, which focuses the crystalline lens for near vision—a process referred to as **accommodation.** It is also the source of the **aqueous humor**, a liquid substance that provides nourishment to certain eye structures, including the cornea and crystalline lens. The blood supply for the outer retina comes from the **choroid,** which is continuous with the ciliary body.

The **retina** is the innermost tissue layer of the eye. It is an exceedingly complex, multilayered neural element that is only 0.2 mm thick. The eye's optical elements focus images on the retina, which then begins the thorny task of analyzing these images.

Ocular Anatomy: Anterior to Posterior

The most anterior aspect of the eye is the **cornea,** a transparent structure that provides approximately two thirds of the refractive power (focusing power) of the eye. Whereas the eye's total refractive power is about 60 diopters, the cornea's power is 40 diopters (Millodot, 1982). Mismatches between the refractive power of the cornea and the axial length of the eye are responsible for most refractive errors.

The aqueous humor is contained within the **anterior** and **posterior chambers** of the eye. (The anterior chamber is bound by the posterior surface of the cornea and the anterior surfaces of the crystalline lens and iris, while the posterior chamber is bound by the posterior surface of the iris and the anterior surface of the vitreous humor.) The aqueous is continuously produced by the ciliary body and drained by the **canal of Schlemm,** which is located in the angle that is formed by the iris and cornea—the **angle of the iris.** The canal of Schlemm runs circumferentially.

The aqueous humor exerts a pressure, referred to as the **intraocular pressure (IOP),** of about 16 mm Hg that helps to maintain the structural integrity of the eye. In certain forms of **glaucoma** the IOP is elevated, presumably leading to retinal damage. Elevated IOPs can result from the overproduction of aqueous, poor drainage of aqueous from the eye, or a combination of these factors.

Posterior to the iris is the **crystalline lens,** which contributes about one third (20 diopters) of the dioptric power of the eye. Through accommodation, the dioptric power of the lens increases, thereby focusing near objects on the retina. Accommodation occurs when the ciliary muscle constricts, releasing tension on the **lens zonules** and allowing the lens to assume a more "natural" position in which its anterior surface bulges forward (Fig. 2–2). The radius of curvature of the anterior lens surface is thereby decreased, increasing the dioptric power of the lens and, consequently, the eye itself.

As we age, the ability to accommodate diminishes, apparently due to reduced elasticity of the crystalline lens. By the time most people are in their middle 40s, their ability to accommodate has diminished to the point where they cannot read without plus lenses, a condition referred to as **presbyopia.**

The crystalline lens becomes less transparent with age, presumably due to the destructive oxidative effects of free radicals. When decreased lens transparency becomes significant and results in a loss of visual acuity, the patient is said to have a **cataract.**[1] During cataract surgery, one of the most common surgical procedures, the lens is removed and replaced with a synthetic lens.

The **vitreous humor** makes up the bulk of the eye volume. It consists largely of collagen and hyaluronic acid and has a gel-like structure. The vitreous provides structural and nutritive support for the retina in addition to creating a dioptrically critical space.

Posterior to the vitreous humor is the retina. It is on this tissue that the visual world is focused. For the study of visual perception, this is the most important ocular tissue.

---

1. Cataracts can be congenital or secondary to aging (senile cataracts), injury, infection, systemic disease (e.g., diabetes), or environmental exposure to ultraviolet radiation.

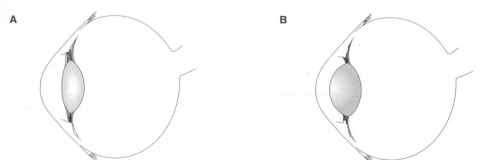

Figure 2–2. A. When the distant objects are viewed, the anterior surface of the crystalline lens is at its flattest, thereby minimizing the lens' refractive power. **B.** When near objects are viewed, the sphincter-like ciliary body constricts; this reduces the tension on the zonules, thereby allowing the anterior surface of the lens to bulge forward. As a result, the dioptric power of the lens is increased. (*From Schwartz, SH.* Geometrical and Visual Optics: A Clinical Introduction. *Copyright 2002. Reprinted by permission of McGraw-Hill, Inc.*)

BASIC RETINAL ANATOMY AND POSTRETINAL PATHWAYS

In some respects, the eye can be considered analogous to a camera. Like a camera, it focuses the world on a light-sensitive element. In the case of a camera, this element is photographic film; for the eye, it is the retina.

This analogy falls apart when we examine the respective roles of camera film and the retina. Film undergoes a chemical reaction in response to the light that falls on it. Shades of black and white are dictated by the intensity distribution of the light. Colors are a bit more complex, but follow the same basic principles. In essence, film acts as a passive receiver of light and simply provides a point-by-point representation of the light distribution falling upon it.

Rather than being a passive receiver of light, the retina is an elaborate neural structure that actively analyzes the image that is focused on it. The signal that is sent to the brain is not merely a point-by-point representation of the retinal image—certain information is highlighted, while other information is disregarded.[2] The information processing that occurs within the retina is discussed extensively in this book.

---

2. Because lower animals have smaller brains, proportionately more visual processing takes place in the retina than is the case for higher animals. For example, the retina of the frog is capable of detecting a bug and triggering the decision to strike it with the frog's tongue (Lettvin et al, 1959). The frog's retina actively analyzes the image that falls upon it, and this analysis serves as a basis for the animal's behavior.

Retinal Layers

Figure 2–3A is a schematic flowchart of retinal processing. The photoreceptors (rods and cones) respond to light, transforming radiant energy into electrical activity, which is transmitted to retinal bipolar cells and then onto retinal ganglion cells. The long axons of the retinal ganglion cells leave the eye, form the second cranial nerve (the optic nerve), and synapse in the dorsal lateral geniculate nucleus (dLGN), a thalamic structure.

This photoreceptor → bipolar cell → ganglion cell arrangement reflects the feed-forward, or **centripetal,** nature of retinal organization. There are also lateral interconnections that provide for the horizontal transmission of retinal information. As indicated in Fig. 2–3, **horizontal** and **amacrine** cells are involved in this lateral integration.

In addition to the feed-forward and lateral interconnections, there is feedback transmission of information. In this pathway, referred to as the **centrifugal pathway,** information is transmitted from the ganglion cell region back toward the photoreceptors by **interplexiform** cells (Lindberg and Fisher, 1986).

Figures 2–3B, 2–4, and 2–5 show cross-sections of the primate retina. Note that light passes through the vitreous and inner layers of the retina, and then hits the photoreceptors, which are located in the outer retina. The inner retinal elements do little to degrade the retinal image because they are somewhat transparent and, as we will learn, laterally displaced in the region of the retina that is associated with the best vision, the fovea.

In the discussion that follows, we examine retinal anatomy going from the outer to the inner layers. The outer retina is composed of those elements proximal to the choroid, whereas the inner retina is comprised of those elements proximal to the vitreous.

The outermost layer of the retina, the **retinal pigment epithelium (RPE),** is not responsive to radiant energy and does not participate in the encoding of visual information. It provides crucial metabolic support, phagocytizing the continuously shed photoreceptor outer segments (Chapter 3) (Young, 1970, 1971). In addition, the darkly pigmented RPE absorbs light photons that are not absorbed by the photoreceptors, thereby reducing light scatter within the eye.

Inner to the RPE are the **photoreceptors.** These cells manifest a very high level of metabolic activity, among the highest in the body. This necessitates their location in the outer retina, close to the choroidal blood supply.

The photoreceptors fall into two groups: **rods** provide nighttime vision and **cones** provide daytime vision. The outermost aspect of a photoreceptor is the **outer segment,** which contains a photopigment that absorbs light, converting it into electrical activity. The outer segments form a distinct retinal layer.

The next retinal layer consists of the **inner segments** of the photoreceptors. This layer contains many of the organelles of these cells, excluding their nuclei.

The **outer limiting membrane,** which is formed by interconnecting processes of Müller cells (retinal glial cells), separates the inner segments of the

Centripetal

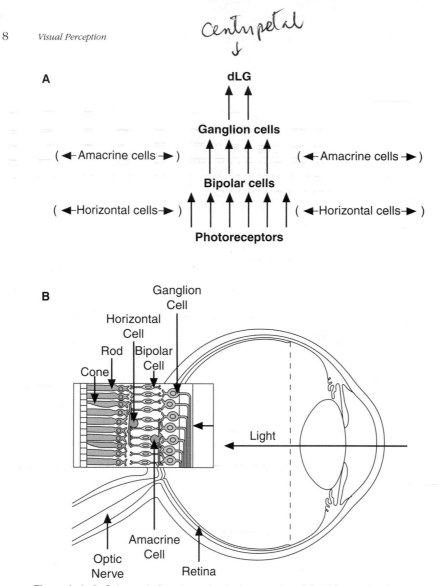

Figure 2–3. A. Schematic flowchart of retinal processing. A feed-forward pathway consists of the photoreceptors → bipolar cells → ganglion cells. The horizontal and
amacrine cells participate in lateral integration within the retina. **B.** Magnified section
of the retina showing that light must pass through the inner retinal layers before it
reaches the photoreceptors. The photoreceptors absorb light quanta and convert this
radiant energy into electrical activity. (*From* Eye, Brain, and Vision *by David H. Hubel,*
© *1988, 1995 by David H. Hubel. Reprinted by permission of Henry Holt & Co., LLC.*)

photoreceptors from their nuclei. Photoreceptor nuclei form a distinct layer,
which is referred to as the **outer nuclear layer (ONL).**

The first retinal synapses occur within the **outer plexiform layer (OPL),**
which consists of the dendrites of the bipolar and horizontal cells, the synaptic
endings of the photoreceptors, and the various synapses among these structures.

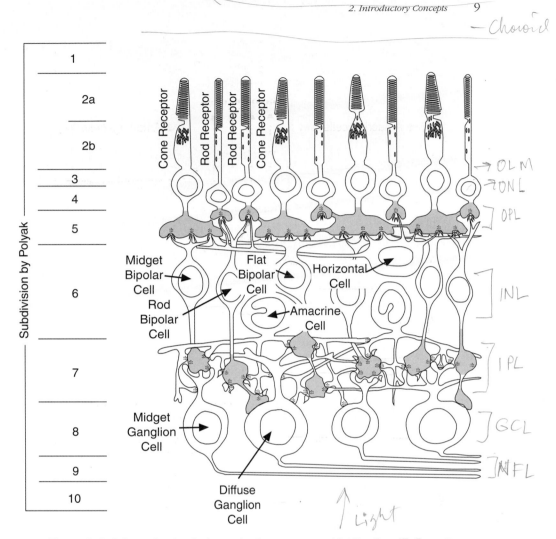

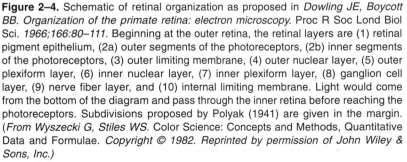

Figure 2–4. Schematic of retinal organization as proposed in *Dowling JE, Boycott BB. Organization of the primate retina: electron microscopy.* Proc R Soc Lond Biol Sci. *1966;166:80–111.* Beginning at the outer retina, the retinal layers are (1) retinal pigment epithelium, (2a) outer segments of the photoreceptors, (2b) inner segments of the photoreceptors, (3) outer limiting membrane, (4) outer nuclear layer, (5) outer plexiform layer, (6) inner nuclear layer, (7) inner plexiform layer, (8) ganglion cell layer, (9) nerve fiber layer, and (10) internal limiting membrane. Light would come from the bottom of the diagram and pass through the inner retina before reaching the photoreceptors. Subdivisions proposed by Polyak (1941) are given in the margin. (*From Wyszecki G, Stiles WS.* Color Science: Concepts and Methods, Quantitative Data and Formulae. *Copyright © 1982. Reprinted by permission of John Wiley & Sons, Inc.*)

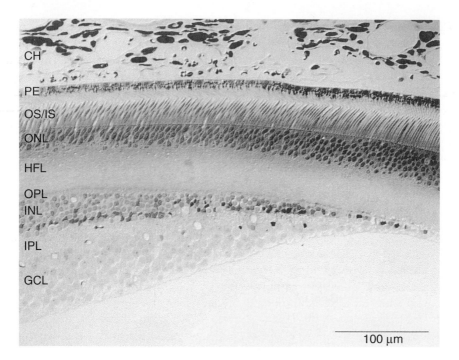

CH

PE

OS/IS

ONL

HFL

OPL
INL

IPL

GCL

100 μm

Figure 2–5. Cross-section of the monkey retina at the slope of the fovea. The labeled layers are the choroid (CH), pigment epithelium (PE), outer/inner segments of the photoreceptors (OS/IS), outer nuclear layer (ONL), Henle nerve fiber layer (HFL), outer plexiform layer (OPL), inner nuclear layer (INL), inner plexiform layer (IPL), and ganglion cell layer (GCL). The Henle fiber layer is constituted of the photoreceptor synaptic processes that extend radially from the foveola. (*Photomicrograph kindly provided by Dr. Heinz Waessle.*)

Inner to the OPL is the **inner nuclear layer (INL).** This layer consists of the cell bodies of the bipolar, horizontal, and amacrine cells.

The second stage of synapses occurs within the **inner plexiform layer (IPL).** Contained within this layer are the various synapses among the bipolar, amacrine, and ganglion cells.

The innermost cell body layer is the **ganglion cell layer.** There are two major classes of ganglion cells. The smaller **midget,** or **parvo (P),** cells comprise about 80 percent of these cells and the larger **parasol,** or **magno (M),** cells about 10 percent (Lennie et al, 1990). In addition to these neurons, there are the less studied, **small bistratified** ganglion cells.

The axons of the ganglion cells constitute the next layer, the **nerve fiber layer.** These axons exit the eye, forming the **optic nerve** (the second cranial nerve), and synapse in the midbrain. Since they are not normally myelinated within the eye, ganglion cell axons do not significantly interfere with vision. They do, however, become myelinated as they leave the eye.

The innermost retinal layer is the **internal limiting membrane.** This membrane acts as an interface between the retina and the vitreous humor.

The preceding description of retinal anatomy is basic and omits many details of both scientific and clinical importance. For instance, there are about 20 different types of amacrine cells. It should be apparent, however, that the complex cellular and synaptic arrangement of the retina points to a high degree of information processing within this structure.

A key feature of retinal organization is lateral interaction. Horizontal and amacrine cells integrate information laterally within the retina, allowing for the processing of visual information across space. This important issue is discussed in detail in Chapters 7 and 12.

Since the diameter of the optic nerve and the number of ganglion cell axons it contains are limited by the structure of the skull, not all information that falls upon the retina is transmitted to the brain proper. Although there are more than 100 million photoreceptors within the retina, there are only 1 million ganglion cells, revealing an extensive degree of neural convergence (Østerberg, 1935; Curcio and Allen, 1990). As information is transmitted through the retina, some is highlighted and encoded, whereas other information is lost.

Optic Disk and Fovea

Figure 2–6A is a photograph of the human retina. It shows the appearance of the normal retina as observed during ophthalmoscopy.[3] The **optic nerve head** (or **optic disk**)—a prominent clinical landmark of the fundus—is constituted of the ganglion cell axons as they leave the eye to form the optic nerve. The whitish appearance of the optic nerve head is due to the myelin sheath that covers these axons as they leave the eye. Normally, the ganglion cell axons do not acquire a myelin sheath before they reach the optic nerve head.

There are no photoreceptors in the optic disk, resulting in a **physiological blind spot** in each eye, located approximately 15 degrees temporal to the point of fixation. The right eye's physiological blind spot can be demonstrated by observing Fig. 2–7A.

Temporal to the optic disk is a highly specialized region of the retina referred to as the **fovea.** (This term has different meanings to clinicians and anatomists, as indicated in Table 2–1.) It is the area of the retina with which you are now reading these words. The fovea subtends a visual angle of about 1.2 degrees,

---

3. The retina and other ocular structures, as seen during ophthalmoscopy, are referred to as the **fundus.**

A

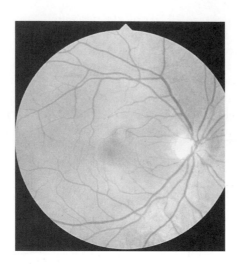

B

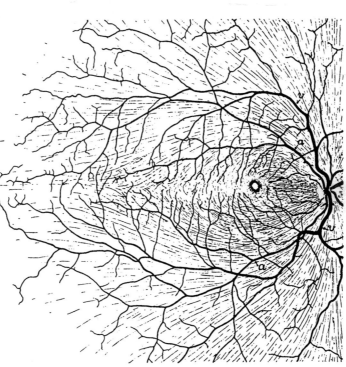

Figure 2–6. A. Photograph of a normal fundus of a right human eye. Vessels that supply the inner retina emerge from the optic nerve head. The avascular fovea is left (temporal) of the optic nerve head. (*Photograph courtesy of Dr. Mohammad Rafieetary.*) **B.** Sketch of the fundus of a rhesus monkey. Note the avascular fovea which is left (temporal) of the optic disk. The striations show the course of the nerve fiber layer. (*From Polyak SL. The Retina. Copyright 1941. Reprinted by permission of the University of Chicago Press.*)

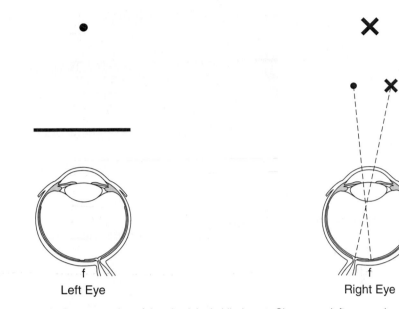

Figure 2–7. A. Demonstration of the physiologic blind spot. Close your left eye and view the dot at a distance of 10 to 12 in. Note that the X disappears. This is because the image of the X falls on the optic disk. **B.** Looking down onto the eyes, it can be seen that the optic disk is nasal to the fovea. This results in the physiologic blind spot being temporal to the fixation point.

twice the angular subtense of the moon (Pirenne, 1967). It provides the basis for highly developed visual acuity (visual resolution).

Observe the E in Fig. 2–8. It is easily resolvable. Yet, while looking at the E, the surrounding letters are not easily resolvable. This is because the image of the E falls on the fovea, while the images of the other letters fall on more peripheral regions of the retina.

A number of anatomical features distinguish the fovea. There are only cones; rods are absent. The packing density of these foveal cones is greater than for any other region of the retina (see Fig. 3–7).

To maximize foveal vision, the neural elements of the inner retina are pushed aside to allow light to fall directly on the photopigment-containing outer segments

TABLE 2-1. DIMENSIONS OF VARIOUS RETINAL LANDMARKS[a]

Anatomical Term	Clinical Term	Diameter (mm)	Diameter (degrees)
Optic nerve head	Optic disk	1.8	5.0
Foveola	Fovea	0.3	1.2
Fovea	Macula	1.8	5.0
Macula	Area centralis	5.8	18.5

[a]Data from Polyak (1941).

F   B

                              E

H   M

Figure 2–8. While fixating the letter E, note that the other letters are not easily resolvable. Visual resolution is most acute in the fovea and less developed in the peripheral retina.

of cones. This pushing aside of retinal elements produces a pit, referred to as the **foveal pit** (Fig. 2–9).

A vascular network covers the retina, except in the fovea, which is avascular (see Fig. 2–6). This adaptation prevents the scattering of light by retinal vessels, maximizing the visual resolution provided by the fovea. Metabolic nourishment for foveal (and nonfoveal) cones is provided by the choroid.

These adaptations—absence of rods, maximal density of cones, pushing aside of inner retinal elements to expose the cone outer segments to light, and absence of retinal vasculature—all contribute to the excellent resolution provided by the fovea. The fovea, although physically small, plays a very large role in visual perception. As discussed in Chapter 14, a disproportionate area of the visual cortex is devoted to processing foveal information, a phenomenon referred to the **cortical magnification** of foveal vision.

Surrounding the fovea is a region of the retina referred to as the **macula lutea**, which contains a nonphotosensitive yellow pigment that is located in the inner retina. This pigment absorbs blue light (maximal absorption is in the region of 460 nm) and may aid vision by reducing light scatter or minimizing the effects of chromatic aberration (Wald, 1945). By absorbing high-energy ultraviolet radi-

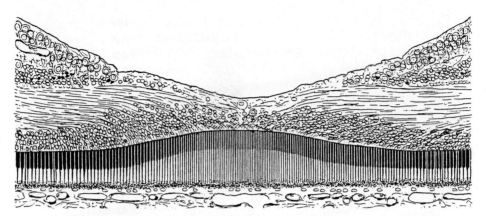

Figure 2–9. Cross-section of the human foveola. Note the pit that is formed by the pushing aside of inner retinal elements. This exposes the photoreceptors directly to light, which would be coming from the top of this diagram. (*From Polyak SL. The Retina. Copyright 1941. Reprinted by permission of the University of Chicago Press.*)

ation, it may also serve to protect the underlying retinal tissue. Studies are underway to determine if dietary supplements that include lutein and zeaxanthin, which are found in the macular pigment, are useful for prophaylaxis and/or treatment of age-related macular degeneration (ARMD), a leading cause of blindness in the elderly (Gale et al, 2003).

Postretinal Pathways

The axons of the retinal ganglion cells leave the eye via the second cranial nerve, the **optic nerve.** The precise course and projection of these nerve fibers are beyond the scope of this text. Rather, discussion is limited to the general path of those fibers that are central to visual perception.

At the **optic chiasm,** ganglion cell fibers from the nasal retina of each eye cross over to join the temporal fibers of the fellow eye to form the **optic tract** (Fig. 2–10). As a result, the fibers constituting the left optic tract carry information regarding the right visual field, and fibers in the right optic tract encode the left visual field.

General schemes of postretinal organization are given in Figs. 2–10 and 2–11. The primary target of the optic tract is the **dorsal lateral geniculate nucleus (dLGN),** a thalamic nucleus. Most, but not all, retinal ganglion cells synapse in this six-layered structure. Layers 2, 3, and 5 receive input from the ipsilateral eye, whereas layers 1, 4, and 6 receive input from the contralateral eye (see Fig. 13–1).

The dLGN is composed of three distinct regions. The dorsal four layers, which are constituted of comparatively small neurons called parvo, or P-cells, are the **parvocellular** layers. Larger neurons, commonly called magno or M-cells, comprise

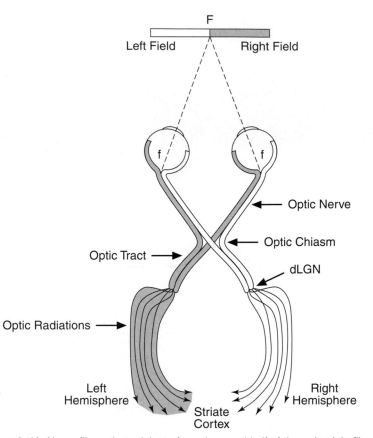

Figure 2–10. Nerve fibers that originate from the nasal half of the retina join fibers from the temporal retina of the fellow eye at the optic chiasm. Consequently, objects in the right half of the visual field are processed in the left cortical hemisphere and objects in the left half of the visual field are processed in the right cortical hemisphere. In this schematic, the foveas (f) are aligned with the fixation point (F).

the two ventral **magnocellular** layers. The layers between the parvocellular and magnocellular layers (interlaminar or intercalated regions) contain very small neurons called **konio** cells. Axons from midget ganglion cells synapse on P-cells in the dLGN to form the **parvo pathway,** while axons from parasol cells synapse on dLGN M-cells to form the **magno pathway.** The konio cells receive projections from the retinal small bistratified ganglion cells, forming what is sometimes labeled the **konio pathway**. The parvo, magno, and konio pathways are referred to as parallel pathways because they each apparently process different aspects of the image that falls upon the retina. As discussed in Chapter 13, the parvo pathway encodes detail and color, while the magno pathway encodes fast movement. The role of the konio pathway is less well understood.

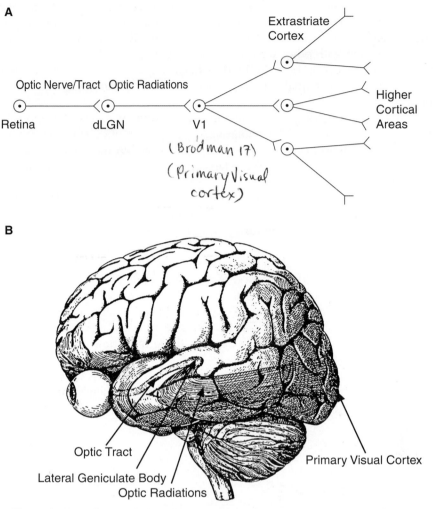

A. Extrastriate Cortex

Optic Nerve/Tract   Optic Radiations

Higher Cortical Areas

Retina   dLGN   V1

(Brodman 17)

(Primary Visual cortex)

B.

Optic Tract

Lateral Geniculate Body

Optic Radiations

Primary Visual Cortex

Figure 2–11. A. Schematic flow diagram of the retinocortical visual pathway. There is a divergence of information within the cortex. **B.** Sketch of the human brain showing the retinocortical visual pathway. The first postretinal synapse is at the dorsal lateral geniculate nucleus (dLGN). The dLGN projects to striate cortex. (*Reprinted with permission from Hubel DH. Eye, Brain, and Vision. New York: Scientific American Library; 1988.*)

The cells of the dLGN send most of their axons to the cerebral cortex, the most highly evolved portion of the brain. This structure consists of two hemispheres, connected by the corpus callosum. The cortical area in which most dLGN axons synapse is **striate visual cortex.** This region is also referred to as visual area 1 (V1), primary visual cortex, and Brodmann area 17. Striate cortex is dominated by foveal input, a phenomenon we have previously referred to as the cortical magnification of foveal vision.

Cells in striate cortex send axons to nearby visual cortical areas, which are collectively called **extrastriate visual cortex.** From this point, axons are sent to a great diversity of higher cortical areas that are involved in the integration of visual information with other senses and memory. Importantly, striate cortex also sends a major projection back to the dLGN. This feedback loop, which in some ways is similar to the retinal centrifugal pathway, may be involved in the gating of information.

The anatomical organization of the cortex is, in some respects, the opposite of that of the retina. Whereas the retina manifests convergence from the photoreceptors to the ganglion cells, there is a divergence within the cortex, with information broadly distributed to a very large number of neurons throughout this structure (see Fig. 2-11A). Information is sent first to areas of extrastriate cortex that are specialized for analyzing attributes such as motion and color, and then to higher centers, which combine visual information with memory and other senses. Higher visual centers, in turn, send information back to striate cortex via backward projections.

The pathway from the retina to the dLGN to striate visual cortex is referred to as the **retinocortical pathway.** While the great majority of retinal ganglion cells contribute to this pathway, a smaller percentage contributes to the **retinotectal pathway.** These axons synapse in the midbrain's superior colliculus (or tectum), bypassing the dLGN. The tectum apparently does not project to the cortex. This pathway appears to be important for encoding eye movements.

This book is concerned with the mechanisms by which visual information is analyzed by the retina and the brain proper. Before we begin this discussion, some basic characteristics of light are reviewed.

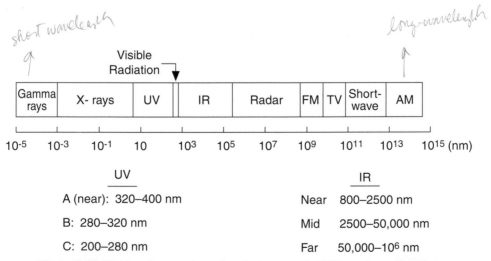

Figure 2–12. The top diagram shows the electromagnetic (EM) spectrum. Note that visible radiation (light) takes up a very small portion of the EM spectrum. Below are common designations for ultraviolet (UV) and infrared (IR) radiation.

ELECTROMAGNETIC SPECTRUM

Humans are capable of detecting only a small portion of the electromagnetic (EM) spectrum (Fig. 2–12). Light, or visible radiation, ranges in wavelength from about 380 to 700 nm [1 nanometer (nm) = 10^{-9} m]. Other wavelengths are not visible, either because the ocular media does not transmit them or because they are not absorbed by the retinal photopigments.

Wavelength and Frequency

The EM spectrum ranges from short-wavelength radiation, such as gamma rays, to long-wavelength radiation, such as AM transmission. Wavelength and frequency of EM radiation are inversely proportional, as indicated by the following relationship (Fig. 2–13):

$$\nu = c/\lambda \qquad\qquad \nu = \dfrac{c}{\lambda}$$

where

ν = frequency of light
c = speed of light (3×10^{8} m/s)
λ = wavelength of light

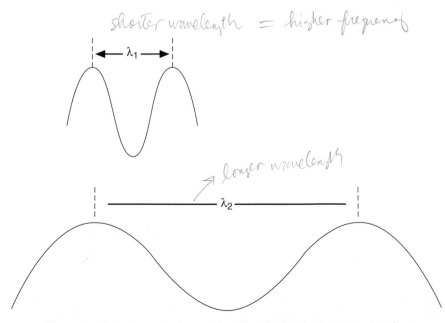

shorter wavelength = higher frequency

longer wavelength

Figure 2–13. λ_1 has a shorter wavelength and a greater frequency than λ_2.

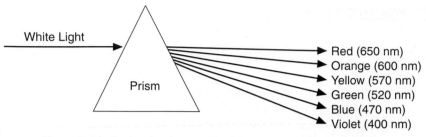

Figure 2–14. A prism breaks up white light into its various components.

The color of light is determined by its wavelength composition. This can be demonstrated by directing white light, which is a mixture of the various wavelengths of light, onto a prism (Fig. 2–14). Because the prism has a different index of refraction for each wavelength, a spectrum of colors produced.

Students traditionally remember the sequence of colors with the acronym **ROY G BIV** (red, orange, yellow, green, blue, indigo, violet). Wavelengths associated with these colors are commonly given in nanometers.

Dual Nature of Light

Up to now, we discussed EM radiation only in terms of its wave nature. It is, however, often convenient to conceptualize it in terms of its quantal nature. In this conceptualization, EM radiation consists of discrete packages of energy called **quanta** or **photons** (Fig. 2–15).

The amount of energy in a quantum of light is given by the following relationship:

$$E = h\nu$$

where

E = energy per quantum
h = Planck's constant (6.626×10^{-37} J/Hz)
ν = frequency

or

$$E = hc/\lambda$$

where

c = speed of light (3×10^{8} m/s)
λ = wavelength

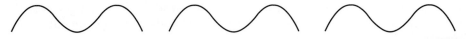

Figure 2–15. Light can be considered as consisting of packets of energy referred to as quanta or photons.

These relationships show that quanta of short wavelengths have more energy than do quanta of longer wavelengths. This is clinically important because high-energy quanta produce more tissue damage when absorbed than do low-energy quanta.

Because of its short wavelength, ultraviolet (UV) radiation contains much energy per quantum (see Fig. 2–12). Consequently, when absorbed by the skin, this radiation can produce substantial cellular damage, including mutations that lead to malignancy. Excessive exposure to UV radiation, as occurs in sunbathing, is a preventable cause of skin carcinoma.

Ultraviolet exposure may damage ocular tissues. Cataract formation is promoted by exposure to UV radiation, and this radiation may also play a role in the development of ARMD. For this reason, it is common for eye care practitioners to recommend spectacles that block UV rays.

TRANSMISSION CHARACTERISTICS OF THE EYE

Atmospheric scatter (for short wavelengths) and absorption eliminate much of the sun's radiation. To protect the sensitive retina upon which EM radiation is focused, the remaining short-wavelength radiation is largely blocked by those ocular elements that precede the retina. Since long-wavelength radiation contains relatively less energy, its blockage is less critical.

The cornea absorbs much of the very short wavelength UV C radiation (<280 nm; see Fig. 2–12) (Pitts, 1974; Lerman, 1980). Consequently, excess ocular exposure to UV C, as may occur when skiing without appropriate sunglasses, can lead to solar keratitis (i.e., corneal inflammation).

The crystalline lens provides most of the protection against UV A and UV B. It can be thought of as a filter that absorbs UV radiation and, thereby, protects the retina. However, this absorption of UV radiation, over many years, damages the lens and can result in cataract formation (Weale, 1983).

During cataract surgery, the crystalline lens is typically replaced with an artificial lens (intraocular lens implant) that contains a UV filter to protect the retina. In those instances where an intraocular lens is not implanted, it is critical that UV protection be provided to the patient. This can be accomplished by including a UV filter in the patient's spectacle lenses.

Because longer wavelengths (>700 nm) contain little energy (compared to shorter wavelengths), their blockage by the ocular media is less critical. Nonetheless, excessive exposure to near-infrared radiation (~1450 nm) can produce a so-called "glass blower's cataract" (Knowles, 1982). Longer wavelength radiation is not visible because it is not absorbed by the retinal photopigments.

SUMMARY

Electromagnetic radiation incident on the eye is focused on the retina. Those wavelengths that may damage the retina are, for the most part, filtered out by the ocular media.

The cornea provides two thirds of the refractive power of the eye, with the crystalline lens providing the remaining power. These tissues are nourished by a complex metabolic system that is dependent on the production of aqueous by the ciliary body and its drainage by the canal of Schlemm.

From a teleologic perspective, the purpose of the eye is to focus an image of the world on the retina. The retina is a multilayered neural structure, approximately 0.2 mm thick, rich in both the varieties of neurons it contains and the various synaptic connections between these neurons. The retina begins the process of analyzing the image that falls upon it. This analysis is an active process whereby visual information is encoded such that it is useful to the higher visual centers. In a very real sense, visual perception begins in the retina, a component of the brain.

Cornea 40 D
Crystalline lens = 20 D
purpose of eye — to focus an image on to the retina
Retina = multi layered neural structure
      = analyzes the image
      = where visual perception begins

The Duplex Retina

The human visual system operates over a remarkably broad range of light levels (Table 3–1). At one extreme, we are able to detect a star on a dark, moonless night, while at the other, we can see a jet flying in the bright midday sky. This constitutes an adaptational range on the order of **10 log units** (Boynton, 1979).

How much of this adaptation is due to changes in the pupil's diameter? Suppose the pupil diameter increases from 3 to 9 mm. By using the formula for the area of a circle, we can calculate the increase in light reaching the retina. For a 3-mm-diameter pupil, we have

$$A = \pi r^2$$
$$A = \pi (1.5)^2$$
$$A = 2.25\pi$$

When the pupil is 9 mm in diameter, the area is

$$A = 20.25\pi$$

The ratio of the pupil area under dim illumination to that under bright illumination is

$$20.25\pi/2.25\pi = 9.0$$

This calculation shows that changes in pupillary area account for only a small portion of adaptation, about 1 log unit out of the 10-log-unit range. The remaining adaptation is due largely to the existence and properties of two classes of retinal photoreceptors, rods and cones.

23

TABLE 3-1. VISIBLE LIGHT INTENSITIES

Stimulus	Luminance (candelas/m²)		
Sun	10^{10}		
	10^{9}	Tissue damage possible	
	10^{8}		
	10^{7}		
100-W bulb filament	10^{6}		
Sunlit paper	10^{5}		
	10^{4}	Photopic vision	
	10^{3}		
This page (normal lighting)	10^{2}		(Optimal acuity)
	10		(Rod saturation)
	1		
Moonlit paper	10^{-1}	Mesopic vision	
	10^{-2}		
Starlit paper	10^{-3}		
	10^{-4}	Scotopic vision	
	10^{-5}		
Threshold light	10^{-6}		

BASIC DISTINCTIONS BETWEEN SCOTOPIC AND PHOTOPIC VISION

Scotopic vision occurs under dim (nighttime) lighting conditions. Exquisite sensitivity to very dim lights, poor visual acuity (20/200 vision), and the absence of color discrimination characterize scotopic vision, which is mediated by rods.

Photopic vision, which occurs under bright (daytime) lighting conditions, shows poor sensitivity to dim lights; however, it is characterized by both excellent visual acuity (20/20) and color discrimination. Cones mediate photopic vision.

The existence of two classes of photoreceptors, each operating under different lighting conditions, leads to what has been referred to as a **duplex retina.** Under twilight **(mesopic)** conditions, both rods and cones contribute to vision.[1]

MORPHOLOGICAL DISTINCTIONS BETWEEN RODS AND CONES

Figure 3–1 displays schematic drawings of rods and cones. Figure 3–2 is a scanning electron micrograph of these two classes of photoreceptors. Note that rods and cones share several features. Both have an outer segment consisting of disk-like

---

1. It is an oversimplification to think that rods and cones always operate independent of each other. Under certain conditions, interactions between rods and cones occur.

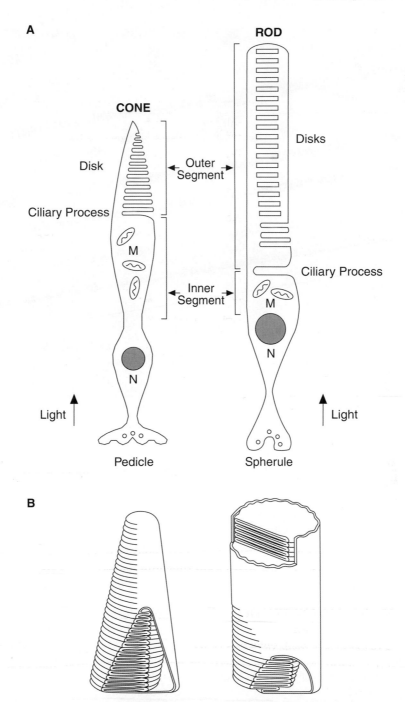

Figure 3–1. A. Schematic drawings of a cone (left) and a rod (right). The nucleus is designated by "N" and the mitochondria by "M." **B.** Schematic drawings of the outer segments of a cone and rod (Young, 1970).

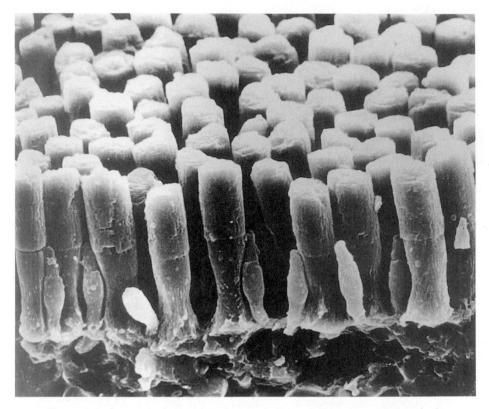

Figure 3–2. Scanning electron micrograph of photoreceptor outer segments in the tiger salamander. The larger outer segments are rods and the smaller are cones. In humans, the rod and cone outer segments are more similar in size. (*This scanning electron micrograph was made by Scott Mittman and Maria T. Maglio, and is reprinted with their permission.*)

structures. Within these disks is a photopigment that absorbs light quanta, initiating those processes that ultimately lead to vision.

The outer segment is connected to the inner segment by a thin ciliary connection. Within the inner segment are cellular organelles, excluding the cell nucleus. The innermost aspects of rods and cones synapse in the outer plexiform layer.

Although there are similarities in the morphology of rods and cones, there are also important differences. Consider the outer segments. True to their respective names, rod outer segments are rod shaped, whereas cone outer segments are cone shaped. The outer segment disks represent infoldings of the cellular membrane. They are generated in the region of the ciliary connection and migrate outward (Young, 1970, 1971). In the rods, these disks break away and become free-floating as they migrate outward (appearing somewhat like a stack of poker chips). The cone disks, as indicated in Fig. 3–1, remain attached to the cone outer segment as they migrate outward—they do not become free-floating.

The disks are continuously produced and shed, and subsequently phagocy-tized by the retinal pigment epithelium (RPE), which lies outer to the rod and cone outer segments (Young, 1971). Rod disks are shed at the rate of about 10 percent per day. Rod disks tend to be shed during the day, and cone disks tend to be shed at night (Young, 1978).

Phagocytosis of photoreceptor disks is essential to maintaining retinal health. In the absence of effective phagocytosis, metabolic waste products collect, thus damaging the rods and cones. This may be the case in **retinitis pigmentosa,** a rod-cone degenerative disease that can result in the progressive loss of vision, with scotopic vision typically affected first (Apple and Rabb, 1991).[2]

Another distinction between rod and cone morphology concerns their synap-tic endings. Rods have a roundish **spherule,** whereas cones have a flat **pedicle** (see Fig. 3–1).

PHOTOPIGMENTS IN RODS AND CONES

The disks of rods and cones contain photosensitive pigments that absorb light quanta, resulting in electrical activity. This is the first step in a sequence of events that ultimately leads to vision.

Rod Photopigment

The photopigment **rhodopsin** is contained within the disks of the rod's outer segment.[3] A disk contains about 10,000 molecules of rhodopsin. Because each rod has about 1000 disks and an eye contains 120 million rods, there are about 10^{15} molecules of rhodopsin per eye (Boynton, 1979). Each molecule of rhodopsin is capable of absorbing one photon of light. The large number of rhodopsin mole-cules provides the eye with a tremendous ability to capture light and contributes to our exquisite sensitivity under nighttime lighting conditions.

Figure 3–3 shows the absorption spectrum for rhodopsin and the manner in which this curve could be generated. A fixed quantity (e.g., 100 quanta) of monochromatic light is incident upon a container of rhodopsin. The ratio of transmitted light to incident light is calculated. This procedure is repeated for many wavelengths (e.g., 400 nm, 401 nm, 402 nm, and so forth) across the spec-trum. The results are plotted as a curve that shows the proportion of light trans-mitted as a function of wavelength (see Fig. 3-3B).

Light quanta that are incident on the rhodopsin, but not transmitted, have been absorbed. Consequently, the absorption curve is the reciprocal of the transmission

---

2. Although there is currently no effective treatment for retinitis pigmentosa, there is considerable ongoing research. Retinal tissue transplantation (adult and embryonic stem cells) and retinal pros-theses hold promise.

3. An older term for *rhodopsin* is *visual purple.*

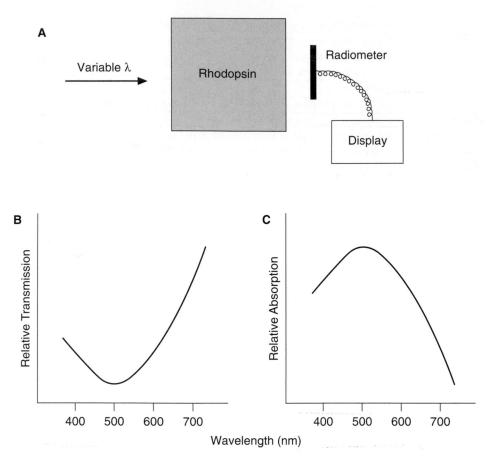

Figure 3–3. **A.** Monochromatic light incident upon a container of rhodopsin. The amount of transmitted light is determined as a function of wavelength. **B.** Transmission curve for rhodopsin **C.** This absorption spectrum for rhodopsin is the reciprocal of the transmission curve.

curve (see Fig. 3–3C). Note that wavelengths in the region of 507 nm are most likely to be absorbed by this photopigment.

A molecule of rhodopsin becomes bleached (i.e., transparent) when it absorbs light. The absorption of only one quantum of light is required to bleach a molecule of rhodopsin (Hecht et al, 1942). When a rhodopsin molecule is in the bleached state, it is not capable of capturing another quantum—it will transmit a quantum of light incident on it. A bleached molecule will spontaneously revert back to the unbleached state. The probability that a molecule of bleached rhodopsin will revert to the unbleached state within a 5-minute period is 0.50 (Rushton, 1965a). Therefore, if a quantity of rhodopsin is bleached, 50 percent of the rhodopsin will recover in 5 minutes. In commonly used terminology, the half-life for rhodopsin regeneration is 5 minutes.

Let us consider the rhodopsin absorption spectrum, which shows the probability of absorption (indicated as log relative absorption on the ordinate) as a function of wavelength, in more detail (see Fig. 3–3C). Quanta of 507 nm have the highest probability of absorption. This is due to quantum mechanics: the rhodopsin molecule and a quantum of 507 nm "fit together" well, thus increasing the probability of absorption.

This does not mean that quanta of other wavelengths cannot be absorbed by the rhodopsin. Other wavelengths are absorbed, but with less probability. To illustrate this point, compare the effects of 1000 quanta of 507 nm and 1000 quanta of 580 nm that are incident on a container of rhodopsin. Assume that the rhodopsin absorption curve gives a probability of 0.20 that a quantum of 507 nm will be absorbed and a probability of 0.10 that a quantum of 580 nm will be absorbed. The 507 nm will bleach 200 rhodopsin molecules, whereas the 580 nm will bleach 100 molecules. (Multiply 1000 quanta by the proportion absorbed at each wavelength.)

If the intensity of the 580-nm light were doubled to 2000 quanta, it would produce the same number of absorptions as does the 1000 quanta of 507 nm. Consequently, 1000 quanta of 507 nm produce the same effect as does 2000 quanta of 580 nm.

Once a quantum of light is absorbed, all information regarding its wavelength is lost, a principle referred to as **univariance.** Whether 580 or 507 nm bleaches a molecule of rhodopsin, the effect is the same. Analogous is a bathroom scale that is designed to make a loud noise when it registers 10 pounds. Although the sound tells us that the scale registers 10 pounds, it does not tell us what is on the scale—it could be 10 pounds of lead or 10 pounds of feathers.

Scotopic Spectral Sensitivity

The ability to detect stimuli under scotopic conditions is determined by the rhodopin absorption curve. This can be demonstrated by measuring a person's scotopic spectral sensitivity (i.e., sensitivity as a function of wavelength). First, we dark-adapt an individual by asking him or her to sit in a dark room for 45 minutes, thereby maximizing the regeneration of the rhodopsin. Subsequently, the minimum amount of energy required for the person to detect stimuli of various wavelengths is determined. The minimum amount of energy required for detection of a stimulus is referred to as the **threshold** for that stimulus.

A curve showing threshold as a function of wavelength and another showing sensitivity as a function of wavelength, both obtained under scotopic conditions, are given in Fig. 3–4. The sensitivity curve is simply the reciprocal of the threshold function. A low threshold indicates high sensitivity. Note that this scotopic spectral sensitivity curve has essentially the same form as the rhodopsin absorption spectrum (Wald, 1945).[4] This similarity in form shows that the human scotopic spectral sensitivity function is determined by the absorption characteristics of rhodopsin.

---

4. The scotopic spectral sensitivity curve may differ slightly from the rhodopsin absorption curve due to absorption by the ocular media.

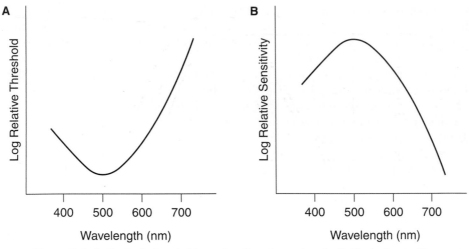

Figure 3–4. A. Scotopic threshold as a function of wavelength. **B.** Scotopic sensitivity as a function of wavelength.

Absolute Sensitivity of Vision

One quantal absorption is sufficient to activate one rod. Ten such activated rods are sufficient to activate a ganglion cell, with the result that the stimulus is detected. However, a stimulus that emits only 10 quanta is not visible because many quanta are either reflected or absorbed by tissue inner to the photoreceptors (preretinal and retinal) or not absorbed by the rhodopsin. Less than 20 percent of the quanta incident on the retina are absorbed by rhodopsin (Hecht et al, 1942). For 10 quantal absorptions to result in detection, they must occur within certain space and time constraints. These constraints reflect the limits of spatial and temporal summation of the visual system, which are discussed in more detail later in this chapter.

Cone Photopigments

In a typical human eye, there are three fundamental cone photopigments, cyanolabe, chlorolabe, and erythrolabe, which show maximal absorption at about 426, 530, and 557 nm, respectively (Fig. 3–5A).[5] Each cone contains only one photopigment.

It is common to speak of three different classes of cones, each containing a different photopigment. The cyanolabe-containing cones are referred to as short

---

5. There are two variants of erythrolabe, with some individuals inheriting a variant that shows maximal absorption at 552 nm, and others manifesting a form that has maximal absorption at 557 nm (Merbs and Nathans, 1992).

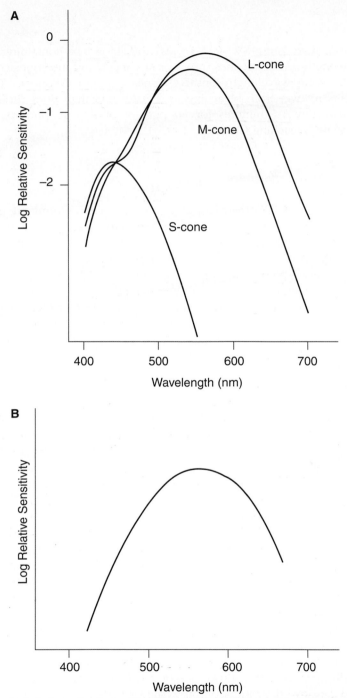

Figure 3–5. A. Approximations of the absorption spectra of cyanolabe (S-cone), chlorolabe (M-cone), and erythrolabe (L-cone) based on the data of Smith and Pokorny, 1975. (*From Boynton RM.* Human Color Vision. *New York: Holt, Rinehart, and Winston; 1979. Reprinted with permission of Dr. Boynton.*) **B.** An approximation of photopic sensitivity as a function of wavelength.

wavelength-sensitive cones (SWS or S-cones), the chlorolabe-containing cones as middle wavelength-sensitive cones (MWS or M-cones), and the cones containing erythrolabe as long wavelength-sensitive cones (LWS or L-cones).[6] The cone photopigments recover from bleaching at a faster rate than does rhodopsin. It takes approximately 1.5 minutes for 50 percent of a cone photopigment to recover following bleaching (Rushton, 1963b).

Photopic Spectral Sensitivity

The photopic spectral sensitivity curve (or function) is determined much the same way as the scotopic function, with the primary difference being that it is measured under brighter lighting conditions. Photopic sensitivity as a function of wavelength is given in Fig. 3–5B. Note that the photopic spectral sensitivity curve shows a single broad peak in the region of **555 nm** (Wald, 1945).

The photopic spectral sensitivity curve apparently represents the addition of M- and L-cone absorption spectra. Absorption of light quanta by either of these cones contributes to this function. Although the issue is not settled, it is thought that S-cones make little, if any, contribution to spectral sensitivity (Cavanagh et al, 1987).

Photochromatic Interval

Figure 3–6 shows scotopic and photopic spectral sensitivity functions plotted on the same graph. Thresholds were determined after the subject underwent dark adaptation, thereby allowing both rhodopsin and the cone photopigments to fully regenerate. The curves represent absolute sensitivity in that each is obtained under conditions that lead to the highest possible sensitivity. Two thresholds are present at each wavelength: a threshold for colorless scotopic vision and a threshold for chromatic photopic vision.

Consider a stimulus of 500 nm as its intensity is slowly increased. It is first detected by the scotopic system and seen as colorless (achromatic). As its intensity is further increased, it is eventually seen as colored (chromatic), thus indicating detection by the photopic system. The difference in sensitivity between scotopic and photopic systems, for a given wavelength, is referred to as the **photochromatic interval (PI).**

Note that the scotopic system is more sensitive than the photopic system at all wavelengths, except in the long-wavelength (red) region of the spectrum. In this area, the photochromatic interval is approximately zero and rods and cones are almost equally sensitive. (Curiously, beyond 650 nm, the photopic system is slightly more sensitive than the scotopic system.)

---

6. The three classes of cones are also improperly (and all too frequently) referred to as blue, green, and red cones. Because the cones are not these colors and do not necessarily signal these colors, this terminology is discouraged.

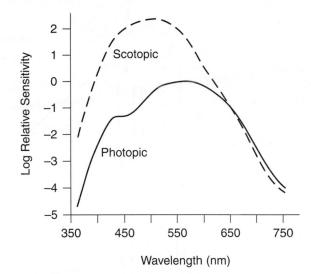

Figure 3–6. Scotopic and photopic spectral sensitivity functions. These functions represent the absolute sensitivities of the two systems. Note that for long wavelengths, the photochromatic interval is close to zero (Wald, 1945).

Purkinje Shift

As lighting conditions change from scotopic to photopic, the wavelength to which we are most sensitive increases from 507 to 555 nm. This is the basis for the **Purkinje shift,** the relative increase in the brightness of longer wavelength stimuli as lighting conditions change from scotopic to photopic.

Consider an example. A dark-adapted individual views an array of monochromatic stimuli (400 to 650 nm) that each emits the same number of quanta. These stimuli are very dim, ensuring that they are detected only by the scotopic system. Due to the absorption spectrum of rhodopsin, the 507-nm stimulus is brightest. Next, the intensity of each stimulus is increased by the same amount so that they are all detected by the photopic system.[7] Which stimulus is now the brightest? Since the photopic spectral sensitivity peaks at 555 nm, the stimulus of this wavelength is brightest.

RETINAL DISTRIBUTION OF PHOTORECEPTORS

The human retina contains approximately 120 million rods and 6 million cones. Rods are most densely packed at about 20 degrees from the fovea, where they reach a peak density of about 150,000 rods/mm^2 (Fig. 3-7). There are no rods

---

7. By increasing equally the intensity of all the stimuli, they will each continue to emit equal number of quanta.

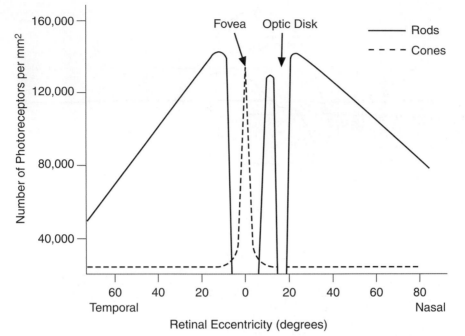

Figure 3–7. Retinal distribution of rods and M- and L-cones (Østerberg, 1935).

in the fovea, which results in the inability to see a small, dim object, such as a star, when it is foveally fixated under scotopic conditions. Looking slightly to the side of a faint star increases its visibility. Whereas the number of retinal cones may remain stable as the eye ages, the number of rods decreases (Curcio et al, 2000).

The distribution of cones is very different from that of rods. Cones are most concentrated in the fovea where their density is 150,000/mm^2, the same as the peak density of rods. Note that although the density of cones is substantially reduced outside of the fovea, they are present throughout the retina (Fig. 3-8). Only a small percentage of the total number of retinal cones are located in the fovea (Boynton, 1979). The ratio of L- to M-cones varies from person to person and has been found to range from 1:1 to 3:1 (Roorda and Williams, 1999).

S-cones show a different retinal distribution than other cones. Not only are S-cones considerably less numerous than either M- or L-cones, constituting about 5 to 10 percent of the cone population, they are not found in the human fovea (Curcio et al, 1991; Roorda et al 2001). Their peak density lies just outside the fovea, accounting for the inability to see very small, centrally fixated blue objects.

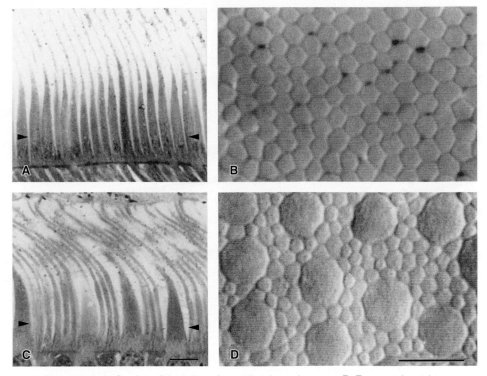

Figure 3-8. A. Section of the human fovea showing only cones. **B.** Face-on view taken at the level indicated by the arrows in A. All cells are cones. **C.** Section through the retinal near periphery. **D.** Face-on view taken at the level indicated by the arrows in C. The smaller, more numerous cells are rods and the larger cells are cones. Extrafoveal cones tend to be larger than those in the fovea. (*Photomicrograph kindly provided by Dr. Christine Curcio. Curcio CA et al, Human photoreceptor topography.* J Comp Neurol *1990;292:497-523. Reprinted by permission of Dr. Christine Curcio and Wiley-Liss, Inc., a subsidiary of John Wiley & Sons, Inc.*)

DARK ADAPTATION

The Basic Curve

Most of us have had the experience of entering a dark movie theater on a sunny afternoon. Immediately on entering the theater, we are virtually blind. Yet, after several minutes, vision recovers to the point where we can walk down the aisle and find an empty seat. This gradual improvement in vision, after exposure to a bright-adapting light (in this case the sun), is referred to as **dark adaptation.**

Following exposure to an adapting light, rods and cones recover sensitivity at different rates. The dynamics of this recovery are made clear in dark adaptation experiments. Dark adaptation has proven useful in the clinical diagnosis of various retinal disorders.

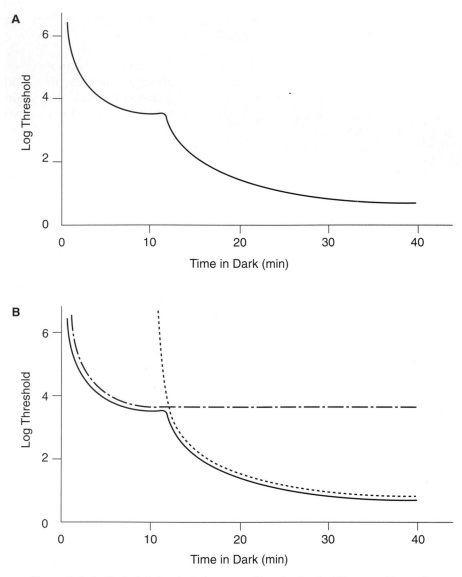

Figure 3–9. A. Typical dark adaptation curve. The stimulus is 420 nm and large. **B.** Dark adaptation curves for a stimulus that is detected by only rods (dots) and a stimulus detected by only cones (dot-dash). A stimulus that is detected by both rods and cones will have the form given by the solid line.

Figure 3–9 is a typical dark adaptation curve. To generate this curve, an individual is exposed to a bright-adapting light that is designed to bleach most of his or her photopigment. The adapting light is then turned off and detection threshold is determined as a function of time for a stimulus flashed against a totally dark background. In this case, the stimulus is large (e.g., 10 degrees) and centrally fixated, with a wavelength of 420 nm. During these experiments, it is important that the room remains perfectly dark and that the individual is not exposed to ambient light.

There are several important features of the dark adaptation curve in Fig. 3–9. Perhaps most obvious is that over a period of about 35 minutes, threshold improves by about 5 log units (i.e., after about 35 minutes in the dark, the person is 100,000 times more light sensitive). Another key feature is its division into two sections, the first showing a rapid reduction in threshold up to about 10 minutes, where the curve plateaus **(cone plateau).** This first section represents photopic thresholds. At about 12 minutes, there is an abrupt change in the slope of the curve, referred to as the **rod-cone break,** that is followed by a slow reduction in threshold out to about 35 minutes, where the curve again plateaus **(rod plateau)** (Hecht et al, 1937, 1942). This second portion of the curve represents scotopic thresholds. The rod–cone break occurs at that point in time when the rods become more sensitive than the cones. Prior to this point, the cones detect the stimulus. After this point, the rods detect it.

The photochromatic interval can be read directly off the dark adapatation curve; it is the difference between the cone plateau, which represents the lowest photopic threshold for a stimulus, and the rod plateau, which represents the lowest scotopic threshold for this same stimulus. For the 10-degree, centrally fixated, 420-nm stimulus used to generate the dark adaptation curve in Fig. 3–9, the photochromatic interval is about 3 log units.

The recovery in sensitivity that occurs during dark adaptation is related to the regeneration of photorcceptor photopigments. As discussed later, however, photopigment regeneration does not fully explain dark adaptation.

Effects of Stimulus Wavelength

The dark adaptation curve given in Fig. 3–9 was obtained with a stimulus of 420 nm. What form does the dark adaptation curve take if the stimulus is 650 nm (Fig. 3-10)? This curve is substantially different: it shows only a cone portion—the rod aspect is missing. This result should not be surprising after reconsidering Fig. 3–6, which shows that the photochromatic interval for a 650 nm is zero. Because the scotopic system is not more sensitive than the photopic system, there is not an obvious rod–cone break (Hecht et al, 1937). In contrast, the photochromatic interval for the 420-nm stimulus is large; consequently, this stimulus produces a dark adaptation curve with a prominent rod–cone break (see Fig. 3–9).

The role of stimulus wavelength in determining the form of a dark adaptation curve is further examined in Fig. 3–11. On the left of this figure are dark adaptation curves for stimuli of 465 and 610 nm; on the right are threshold scotopic and photopic functions. These threshold functions are the reciprocal of the sensitivity curves given in Fig. 3–6.

Consider the 465-nm stimulus. After about 15 minutes of dark adaptation, the cone plateau is reached, representing the lowest threshold (or maximum sen-

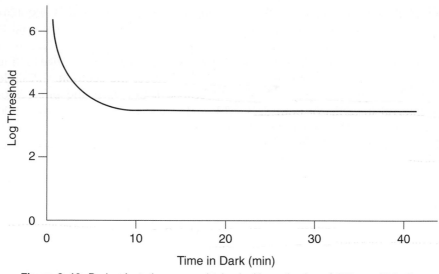

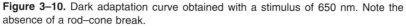

Figure 3–10. Dark adaptation curve obtained with a stimulus of 650 nm. Note the absence of a rod–cone break.

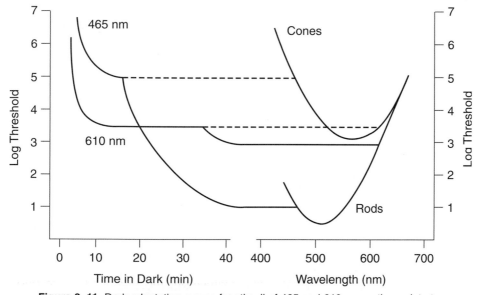

Figure 3–11. Dark adaptation curves for stimuli of 465 and 610 nm as they relate to photopic and scotopic threshold functions.

sitivity) for the photopic system. The dotted line, which extends from this cone plateau and intersects the photopic threshold function at 465 nm, shows that the cone plateau corresponds to a specific point on the photopic threshold function. The rod portion of the dark adaptation curve for 465 nm levels off at about 40 minutes, and has been extended to intersect the scotopic threshold function. This type of analysis is useful because it illustrates the photochromatic interval in terms of both dark adaptation curves and spectral threshold functions. For a dark adaptation curve, the photochromatic interval is the separation of the cone and rod plateaus. When viewing the spectral threshold functions, this same photochromatic interval is the difference between scotopic and photopic thresholds.

Why is the rod-cone break for the 465-nm stimulus more prominent and earlier than for the 610-nm stimulus? Part of the answer relates to the absorption properties of rhodopsin. As illustrated by Fig. 3-3C, the probability that a molecule of rhodopsin will absorb a quantum of 465 nm is relatively high. Therefore, early during dark adaptation, after relatively little rhodopsin has regenerated, the sensitivity of the scotopic system surpasses that of the photopic system. The situation is different for 610 nm. It is considerably less probable that a molecule of rhodopsin will absorb a quantum of 610 nm. Only after a relatively large amount of rhodopsin has regenerated—late during dark adaptation—has the scotopic system recovered to the point where it is more sensitive than the photopic system.

Stimulus Size and Location

It was assumed in the preceding examples that the stimulus was centrally fixed and that its size was such that it covered both the fovea and a portion of the surrounding retina. For example, a 10-degree diameter stimulus would produce the results discussed so far.

Making the stimulus very small, say 0.5 degrees, and confining it to the fovea has a predictable effect: only a cone function is obtained (Fig. 3–12). The absence of a rod function reflects the absence of rods in the fovea.

Physiological Basis of Dark Adaptation

How can we account for the slow recovery in sensitivity that follows exposure to a bright adapting light? During dark adaptation, the regeneration of photopigment increases the probability of quantal absorptions, thereby increasing sensitivity. The **photochemical explanation** of dark adaptation holds that this photopigment regeneration fully explains the recovery of sensitivity that occurs during dark adaptation (Hecht, 1937).

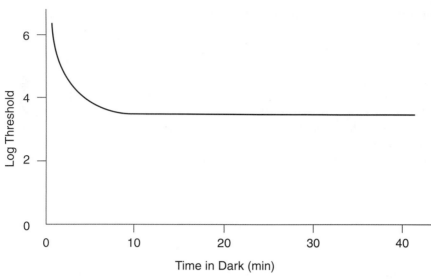

Figure 3–12. Dark adaptation curve for a small stimulus, confined to the fovea. Note the absence of a rod–cone break.

The photochemical explanation is schematically illustrated in Fig. 3–13, which shows rods that have had one half of their rhodopsin bleached. Compared with the unbleached state, there is a 0.50 probability that a quantum of light will be captured by the rhodopsin. Therefore, based purely on photopigment considerations, a 50 percent bleaching is predicted to double the threshold. This is not correct—the threshold increases by a factor of 10^{10}!

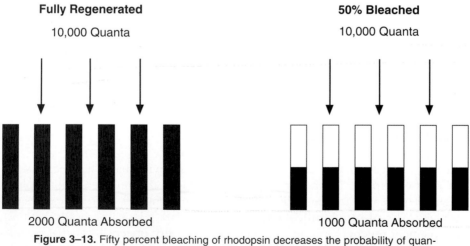

Figure 3–13. Fifty percent bleaching of rhodopsin decreases the probability of quantal absorption by a factor of one half. Yet, the threshold is increased by a factor of 10^{10}.

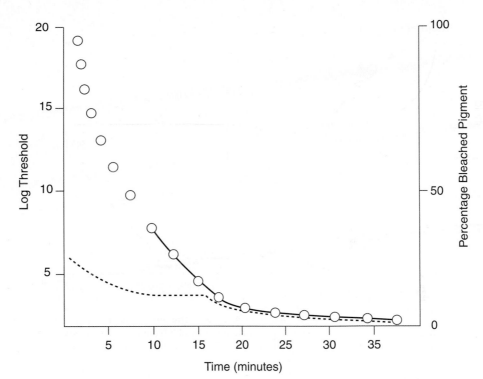

Figure 3–14. Circles show the retinal densitometry results for a rod monochromat subject; solid lines show the thresholds for this subject. The dots show thresholds for a normal subject (Rushton, 1965a).

The open circles in Fig. 3-14 show the recovery of rhodopsin in an individual who has only rods, a **rod monochromat.**[8, 9] The solid lines show the dark adaptation curve for this individual, while the dotted line indicates the dark adaptation curve of a normal individual. It can be seen that bleaching 50 percent of the rhodopsin (right-hand ordinate scale) is expected to increase the threshold by 10 log units, rather than only doubling it, as predicted by the photochemical explanation.[10] Factors other than photopigment regeneration (both receptoral and postreceptoral) apparently contribute to the complex dynamics of dark adaptation (Schnapf and Baylor, 1987).

8. Rod monochromacy is discussed in more detail in Chapter 6.

9. These data were obtained with retinal densitometry. A weak measuring light is shined onto the retina, and the amount of the reflected light is measured (Rushton, 1965a). By comparing the amount of incident light to the amount of reflected light, the proportion of bleached pigment can be determined.

10. Also note that at the rod–cone break, approximately 90 percent of the rhodopsin has regenerated.

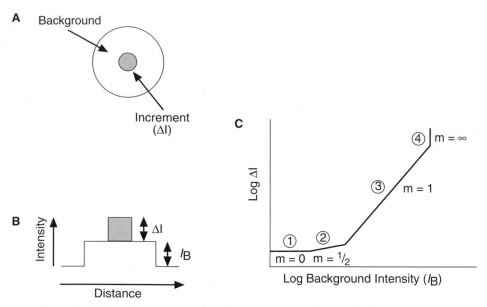

Figure 3–15. To determine a light adaptation curve, an increment, Δ*I,* is presented on a background that has an intensity of *I*B. **A.** Face-on view of the stimulus used in such an experiment. **B.** Intensity profile of this stimulus. **C.** Simplified light adaptation curve. Only the scotopic portion is illustrated.

LIGHT ADAPTATION

When you step outside on a sunny day, the amount of light falling on your retina increases by a factor of several thousand. In spite of this tremendous change in light levels, the appearance of objects remains the same (i.e., a striped shirt looks the same when viewed indoors or outdoors on a sunny day). Within a very brief period—so fleeting that you are unaware of it—your visual system adapts to the changes in illumination levels, a process referred to as **light adaptation.**

Light adaptation may be studied with an **increment threshold** procedure (Fig. 3–15). Threshold is determined for a flash of light—an increment—that is presented on a background of a given intensity.[11] After a threshold has been determined, the background intensity is increased and the threshold measurement is repeated. This procedure is performed for background light levels ranging from darkness to extreme brightness, resulting in a light adaptation curve that shows increment threshold (Δ*I*) as a function of the background adapting (I_B) intensity.

---

11. An increment threshold (Δ*I*) is sometimes referred to as a **just noticeable difference (JND)** or a **difference limen**.

Scotopic Light Adaptation

Figure 3-15C shows the four sections of the scotopic light adaptation function. The explanations for the first two sections are rather technical and they are only briefly touched on in this chapter. Section 1, for which the slope (m) is zero, is that range of light levels where detection is limited by the neural noise inherent within the visual system. The background is practically black, and neural noise produces as much so-called "dark light" as does the background itself[12] (Fechner, 1860; Barlow, 1956).

The second section, having a slope of $\frac{1}{2}$, reflects quantal fluctuations in the background (DeVries, 1943; Rose, 1948). The background is so dim that fluctuations inherent in the light source that produces it play a primary role in determining threshold. This is frequently expressed as the **DeVries–Rose law,** which predicts that ΔI is equal to $(I_{B})^{1/2}$.

The third section, which covers a 4-log-unit range, has a slope of approximately 1, revealing that **Weber's law**[13] is followed (Aguilar and Stiles, 1954; Barlow, 1965; Walraven and Valeton, 1984). As the background brightness is increased, the increment intensity must be increased such that the ratio of the increment intensity (ΔI) to the background intensity (I_{B}) remains constant. This constant ratio, $\Delta I/I_{B}$, is referred to as Weber's fraction or Weber's constant.

The Weber fraction for scotopic vision is approximately 0.14 (Cornsweet, 1970). If the background intensity is 100 units, the increment must have an intensity of 14 units ($\Delta I = 14$) to be detected. If the background is increased to 1000 units, the increment intensity must increase to 140 units ($\Delta I = 140$) to maintain a Weber fraction of 0.14 and thus remain visible. Although the *relative* sensitivity of the visual system (0.14) does not change as the illumination increases, there is a reduction in the *absolute* sensitivity (the threshold goes from 14 to 140 units). This tradeoff between relative and absolute sensitivity is referred to as **sensitivity regulation.**[14]

As discussed in Chapter 7, the ratio of the increment intensity to the background intensity (i.e., relative sensitivity) is referred to as **contrast.** Saying that the visual system follows Weber's law is the same as saying that the threshold contrast remains constant as the illumination changes.

The final section of the scotopic portion of the light adaptation curve, section 4, has a slope of infinity. This indicates that the rods are saturated (Aguilar and Stiles, 1954). At this background illumination, it is not possible for the rods to signal the increment stimulus, no matter how bright it is, because they are overwhelmed by the brightness of the background. On first analysis, you might suppose that

---

12. To experience this "dark light," close your eyes and note that you do not experience pure darkness, but see various visual phenomena.

13. Weber's law is discussed in more detail in Chapter 11.

14. The physiological basis of sensitivity regulation, at the level of the photoreceptor, is beginning to be elucidated. It appears that calcium plays an important role in this process (Fain and Matthews, 1990).

rod saturation occurs when all the rod photopigment has been bleached. In actuality, only about 10 percent of the rhodopsin is bleached at the point of rod saturation (Rushton, 1965a).

The bleaching of rhodopsin molecules results in the closure of sodium channels located in the rod outer segment. This reduces the flow of sodium into the outer segment, leading to rod hyperpolarization.[15] The magnitude of this hyperpolarization is dependent, up to a point, on the intensity of the stimulus. Since the number of sodium channels is finite, the amount of the rod hyperpolarization is limited (Baylor et al, 1984). When approximately 10 percent of the rhodopsin molecules are bleached, all the sodium channels are effectively closed and further bleaching of rhodopsin produces no further hyperpolarization (i.e., the rod is saturated).

Photopic Light Adaptation

Weber's law is also followed under photopic conditions. The Weber fraction is about 0.015, indicating that the photopic system is more sensitive to contrast than the scotopic system (which has a Weber's fraction of about 0.14) (Stiles, 1953). Although the photopic system is more sensitive to contrast than the scotopic system, its absolute sensitivity is less.[16]

SPATIAL RESOLUTION AND SPATIAL SUMMATION

Basic Concepts

Do humans see better under photopic or scotopic conditions? An initial response may be that vision is better under photopic conditions. Certainly, the ability to resolve details is substantially superior (photopic visual acuity is on the order of 20/20, whereas scotopic acuity is about 20/200, a 1-log-unit difference). Moreover, contrast sensitivity is higher under photopic conditions, with a Weber fraction for photopic vision of 0.015 (compared to 0.14 for scotopic vision).

But visual resolution and contrast sensitivity are not the whole story. The ability to *detect* a stimulus is much superior under scotopic conditions. For a 420-nm stimulus to be detected under photopic conditions, it must be 3 log units (1000 times) more intense than is required for detection under scotopic conditions (see Fig. 3-6). While visual resolution and contrast sensitivity are superior under photopic conditions, absolute sensitivity is greater under scotopic conditions. The trade-off between visual resolution and visual sensitivity is, to a large extent, due to the manner in which the rods and cones are connected to the postreceptoral elements of the retina. Rods are connected in such a manner as to sum

---

15. Photoreceptor physiology is discussed in more detail in Chapter 12.

16. A dim stimulus that can be seen under scotopic conditions may not be visible under photopic conditions.

up information over space. This produces great sensitivity, but poor resolution. Cones, on the other hand, manifest connections that maximize visual resolution at the expense of sensitivity.

Figure 3–16 schematically illustrates rod and cone connections to a ganglion cell. (Rods and cones do not actually synapse on a ganglion cell, but this simple

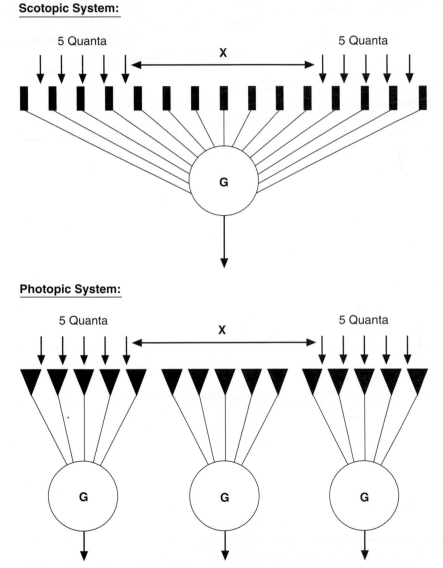

Figure 3–16. Schematic illustrations of scotopic and photopic retinal organization. The scotopic system manifests greater spatial summation than the photopic system. The simplified explanation in the text, which is associated with these diagrams, is best applied to the peripheral retina.

model is useful for instructional purposes.) A major distinction between the scotopic and photopic systems, as depicted by this diagram, is the number of photoreceptors that communicate with a single ganglion cell; many more rods communicate with a ganglion cell than is the case for cones. This illustrates that the scotopic system, to a greater extent than the photopic system, sums up information over space—it manifests greater **spatial summation.**

The following example shows how spatial summation contributes to high scotopic sensitivity. Suppose that for a ganglion cell to signal an event, a total of 10 quanta must be absorbed by the photoreceptors that feed into it, with each photoreceptor absorbing only 1 quantum. Furthermore, assume that these quanta are delivered in two flashes of light, separated by the distance x, and each flash contains 5 quanta. Finally, assume that all the incident quanta are absorbed.[17]

By observation of Fig. 3–16A, it is seen that this stimulus arrangement causes the scotopic system to reach threshold. The two spots of light produce a total of 10 quantal absorptions, and the ganglion cell sums this information to produce a signal that indicates the presence of a single light. It does not signal the presence of two lights; this information is lost due to spatial summation. The scotopic system has excellent sensitivity (a stimulus is seen), yet poor spatial resolution (only one stimulus is seen).

Now consider the situation for the photopic system with the same stimuli (Fig. 3–16B). In these circumstances, no stimulus is seen because the limited spatial summation of the photopic system prevents it from adding up the information contained in both spots of light. A ganglion cell requires 10 quantal absorptions to signal an event, but each of the ganglion cells in this example has input reflecting only 5 absorptions. Therefore, the ganglion cell threshold is not met.

What happens if we double the number of quanta contained in each spot of light. The two ganglion cells, in the photopic case, each reach threshold and signal the presence of a stimulus; consequently, two stimuli are seen. For the scotopic condition, the ganglion cell also reaches threshold; however, because all the rods converge on only one ganglion cell, the two spots of light are not resolved, and one stimulus is seen.

In summary, the scotopic system shows excellent spatial summation. This contributes to its high sensitivity, but results in poor spatial resolution. Consequently, we can see a dim star at night, yet have a scotopic acuity of only 20/200. In contrast, the photopic system shows less spatial summation, resulting in poor sensitivity, but excellent spatial resolution (20/20).

Ricco's Law

Spatial summation classically is demonstrated by the following experiment. An observer is presented with a very small spot of light, and the threshold number

---

17. As we have learned, less than 20 percent of the quanta incident on the retina are absorbed (Hecht et al, 1942).

of quanta necessary to detect this light is determined. The experiment is then repeated with spots of increasing size, resulting in a function like that in Fig. 3–17, which shows the threshold number of quanta required for detection as a function of test spot diameter. These data are for the scotopic system. Note that for stimuli up to 10 minutes of arc in diameter, the total number of quanta necessary for detection is constant (Barlow, 1958). This means that the threshold number of quanta could be delivered in a 1-minute arc test spot or spread out over a larger area, up to 10-minutes arc, the so-called **critical diameter.** The scotopic system manifests total spatial summation for stimuli that fall within the critical diameter.

Total spatial summation is represented mathematically by Ricco's law:

$$IA = K$$

where

I = stimulus intensity (quanta/area)
A = stimulus area
K = constant

The difference in spatial summation between the scotopic and photopic systems is given by a difference in the critical diameters for these two systems. It should not be surprising that the critical diameter of the photopic system is smaller than that for the scotopic system, reflecting the reduced spatial summation capability of the photopic system.

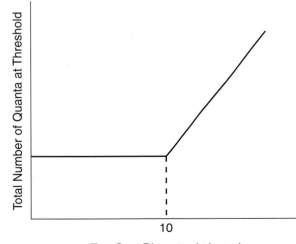

Figure 3–17. Classic expression of Ricco's law regarding spatial summation (scotopic conditions).

TEMPORAL RESOLUTION AND TEMPORAL SUMMATION

Scotopic and photopic vision also demonstrate significant differences in their temporal (time-related) properties. The scotopic system sums up information, over time, to a greater extent than the photopic system. It shows greater temporal summation. The photopic system, however, is better able to distinguish two flashes of light separated by a brief interval in time. It has superior temporal resolution.

Let us examine this in more detail. Figure 3–18A shows two subthreshold pulses of light presented under scotopic conditions. Each pulse of light, by itself, would not be seen. Assume that these pulses are separated by an interpulse interval (IPI) of 120 milliseconds and that the temporal summation (integration) period of the scotopic system is 100 milliseconds. On the basis of this information, it is expected that no stimulus will be seen because the pulses do not both fall within the temporal summation period. If the two subthreshold pulses, however, are separated by 90 milliseconds, they will be summed up to reach threshold; the subject will report seeing a stimulus (see Fig. 3-18B). Since both pulses occur during the temporal summation period, the subject reports only one flash of light, not two.

If the flashes both fall within the temporal integration period, increasing the intensity of the pulses such that they are above threshold (suprathreshold) still does not allow the subject to perceive two flashes of light (see Fig. 3-18C). The scotopic system's high degree of temporal summation limits its ability to resolve distinct temporal events. Only when these two suprathreshold pulses are separated by greater than 100 milliseconds, as indicated in Fig. 3–18D, are two flashes seen.

The photopic system, as indicated in Fig. 3–19A, shows a shorter period of temporal summation. As a consequence, the two subthreshold stimuli are not summed up to reach threshold. They need to be presented closer in time, as indicated in Fig. 3–19B, to produce a percept of a single flash of light.

Although the photopic system demonstrates poor temporal summation, it does manifest superior temporal resolution. As indicated in Fig. 3–19C, two suprathreshold pulses, separated by only 50 milliseconds, are distinguishable as two flashes. The scotopic system, with its high degree of temporal summation, would not be able to resolve these stimuli.

The high degree of temporal summation of the scotopic system is consistent with its greater absolute sensitivity. It sums information over both space (spatial summation) and time (temporal summation) to obtain excellent sensitivity. In contrast, the photopic system shows limited spatial and temporal summation. This, however, provides it with excellent spatial and temporal resolution. It is evident that there is a trade-off between summation and resolution.

Bloch's Law

Bloch's law, the temporal equivalent of Ricco's law, is illustrated in Fig. 3–20. This graph shows that within the so-called **critical duration,** or **critical period,** there is total temporal summation. As long as the threshold number of quanta are

Scotopic System

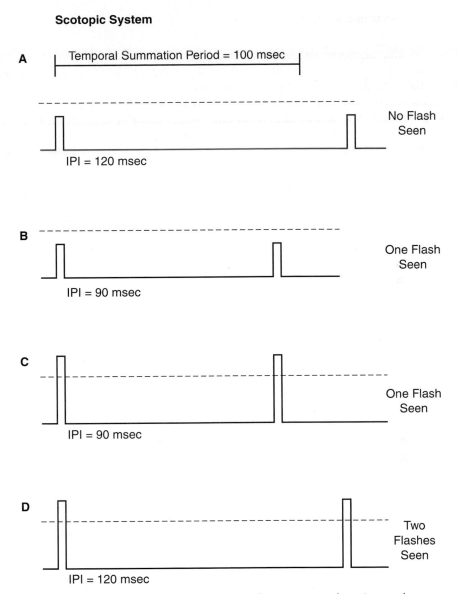

Figure 3–18. Temporal properties of the scotopic system assuming a temporal summation period of 100 milliseconds. The dashed line represents threshold for a single pulse. **A.** Two subthreshold pulses, separated by an interpulse interval (IPI) of 120 milliseconds, do not sum to reach threshold. A stimulus is not perceived. **B.** Two subthreshold pulses, presented within the temporal summation period, result in the perception of a single flash. **C.** Two suprathreshold pulses, presented within the temporal summation period, result in the perception of only a single flash. **D.** Two suprathreshold pulses, presented with an IPI of 120 milliseconds, are perceived as two flashes.

Photopic System

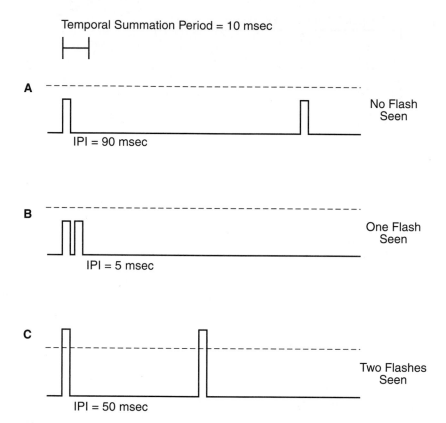

Figure 3–19. Temporal properties of the photopic system assuming a temporal summation period of 10 milliseconds. **A.** Two subthreshold pulses, presented with an interpulse interval of 90 milliseconds, do not sum to reach threshold. **B.** Two subthreshold pulses, presented within the summation period, are summed to reach threshold. **C.** Two suprathreshold pulses, separated by 50 milliseconds, are perceived as two flashes.

delivered within this critical duration, it does not matter how they are delivered. They could be presented in one or more flashes. Of course, multiple flashes presented within this critical duration are not resolved and only one flash is seen.

Bloch's law can be expressed mathematically as follows:

$$It = K$$

where

I = stimulus intensity (quanta/time)
t = stimulus duration
K = constant

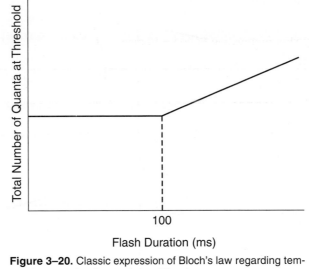

Figure 3–20. Classic expression of Bloch's law regarding temporal summation (scotopic conditions).

Predictably, the scotopic and photopic systems manifest different critical durations. Scotopic vision, with its greater degree of temporal summation, shows a critical duration of about 100 milliseconds, whereas photopic vision manifests a critical duration on the order of 10 to 50 milliseconds (Sperling and Jolliffe, 1965; Krauskopf and Mollon, 1971; Swanson et al, 1987).

STILES–CRAWFORD EFFECT OF THE FIRST KIND

To be maximally effective at bleaching photopigment, a light ray must strike a cone perpendicular to its surface. In comparison, the angle at which a light ray strikes a rod is much less critical.

If an observer is asked to view a point source of light through a pinhole that is centered in front of the pupil, the light rays strike the photoreceptors perpendicular to their surface (Fig. 3–21A). If, however, the pinhole is decentered, as in the bottom diagram, the light rays strike the same photoreceptors at an oblique angle. Under scotopic conditions, the subject notes relatively little difference in brightness, demonstrating that the angle at which light rays are incident on rods is relatively insignificant (Van Loo and Enoch, 1975).

The same experiment repeated under photopic conditions produces a different result. Light rays that strike cones perpendicular to their surface (pinhole centered) are perceived as brighter than those that do not strike perpendicular to the surface (pinhole decentered) (see Fig. 3-21B). This effect, which is strongly manifested by cones, is referred to as the Stiles–Crawford effect of the first kind (Stiles, 1939).[18]

---

18. The Stiles–Crawford effect of the second kind refers to changes in hue and saturation of monochromatic light as the point of entry into the pupil is changed.

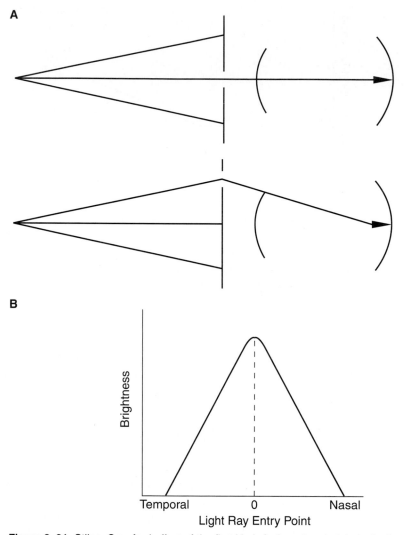

Figure 3–21. Stiles–Crawford effect of the first kind. **A.** A centered pinhole (top) causes the light ray to strike the foveal cone perpendicular to its surface, whereas a decentered pinhole (bottom) causes the ray to strike the cone at an oblique angle. **B.** Under photopic conditions, the centered pinhole produces a brighter image than the decentered pinhole.

The effect is probably due to waveguide properties of the cones (Enoch and Fry, 1958). The physical dimension of a quantum of light is such that it approaches the size of a cone, making critical the angle of entry of a ray of light into the funnel-shaped cone. Any deviation from an orthogonal entry reduces the effectiveness of light rays at bleaching photopigment and, consequently, reduces the perceived brightness of these rays.

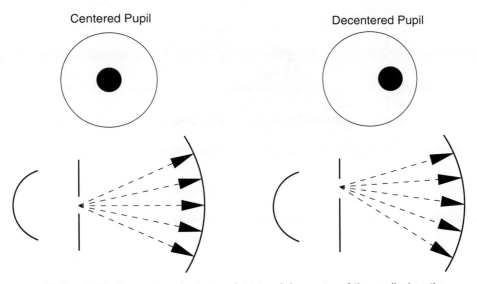

Figure 3–22. The cones migrate to point toward the center of the pupil when the pupil is decentered.

Under normal circumstances, cones point toward the center of the pupil, maximizing their effectiveness. What are the consequences of a chronically decentered pupil, as illustrated in Fig. 3–22?[19] Do the cones point toward the normal pupil position, or do they point toward the location of the decentered pupil? The Stiles–Crawford effect manifested by these eyes is displaced,[20] suggesting that the cones point toward the location of the decentered pupil (Applegate and Bonds, 1981; Enoch and Birch, 1981; Smallman et al, 2001). Taking this a step further, if an adult with a normal Stiles–Crawford effect is fit with a contact lens that has a decentered pupil, the cones eventually point toward it, resulting in a displaced effect. When the contact lens is removed, the cones return to their original state. These results tell us that the cones are mobile and that they orient themselves to light; if the pupil becomes decentered, the cones reorient themselves such that they now point toward the center of the pupil, thereby maximizing their effectiveness in capturing photons of light.

Retinal disease may cause disruption of cone orientation, leading to an abnormal Stiles-Crawford function. The function may be abnormal in areas impacted by disease (e.g., retinal traction), but normal in unaffected areas.

---

19. A decentered pupil can be congenital or secondary to trauma.

20. When the Stiles-Crawford effect is displaced, the maximal sensitivity is no longer at a light entry point of zero (see Fig. 3–21B). .

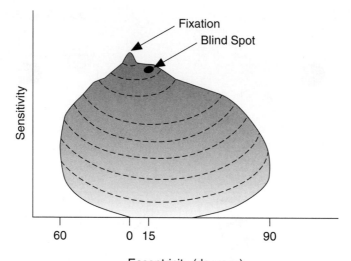

Figure 3–23. Hill of vision obtained under photopic conditions for a right eye. Note the fixation peak for the fovea and the blind spot produced by the optic disk.

CLINICAL CONSIDERATIONS

Visual Field Testing

Visual field testing is a common and important clinical procedure that is critical for the diagnosis and treatment of many neurological diseases of the visual system, including glaucoma. The test involves the determination of increment sensitivity at a large number of retinal locations while the patient views a fixation point. The background is typically photopic, but not overwhelmingly so. The stimulus is an increment (ΔI) flashed on a steady background (I_B), similar to the stimulus used in a light adaptation experiment (see Fig. 3-15A).

Modern visual field devices determine thresholds for a large number of retinal points and compare these values to norms established by the manufacturer of the device. For a healthy visual system, a sensitivity profile similar to that given in Fig. 3–23 is obtained. Sensitivity is greatest centrally and falls off in the periphery of the retina resulting in a profile that looks like a hill, often referred to as the **hill of vision.**

Do the age-related reductions in retinal illumination that are secondary to senile miosis[21] and nuclear sclerosis affect visual field thresholds? The answer is no if the measurements are made at light levels where Weber's law is followed.

21. The pupil diameter decreases and it becomes less responsive to light in the elderly, a condition referred to as senile miosis

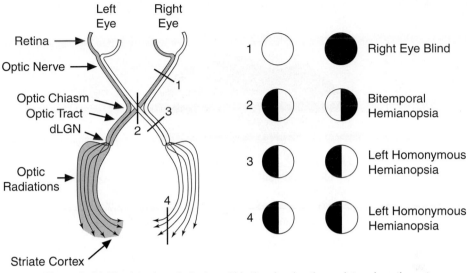

Figure 3–24. The location of a lesion within the visual pathway determines the nature of the field defect.

Since senile miosis and nuclear sclerosis reduce the retinal illumination produced by the increment and background by the same amount, the Weber fraction ($\Delta I / I_B$) remains unchanged.

The location of a lesion within the visual pathway determines the nature of the visual field defect. A simple scheme for classifying such lesions is given in Fig. 3–24. Examples of visual fields as measured clinically are given in Fig. 3–25.

Dark Adaptation

Used in conjunction with the electroretinogram (ERG)[22] and other electrodiagnostic tests, dark adaptation may be useful in the diagnosis of retinitis pigmentosa (RP), congenital stationary night blindness (CSNB),[23] and certain other rod–cone degenerations and diseases (Fig. 3-26). Measurements suitable for clinical applications may be obtained using a commercially produced dark adaptometer such as the Goldmann–Weekers or scotopic sensitivity tester (SST-1) dark adaptometer.

In RP, rods are typically affected prior to the cones. This may lead, early in the disease, to a dark adaptation curve with a rod portion that takes an abnormally long time to level off and/or plateaus at a higher than normal threshold. An abnormal dark adaptation curve is consistent with certain symptoms typical of

---

22. The ERG is discussed in Chapter 16.

23. CSNB is an inherited disorder characterized by rod dysfunction. Visual acuity may be normal or reduced.

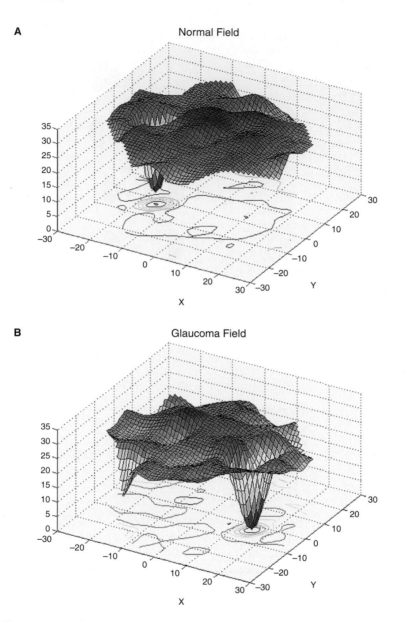

Figure 3–25. Visual field profiles as measured clinically with the Humphrey Visual Field Analyzer. **A.** A normal visual field for a left eye. Note the central foveal peak and the temporal pit, which represents the blind spot. **B.** A visual field for a right eye showing moderate glaucomatous damage. The blind spot is enlarged and there is a reduction in sensitivity in the inferonasal region of the field.(*These visual fields were kindly provided by Humphrey Systems in San Leandro, California.*)

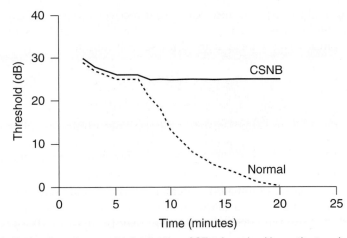

Figure 3–26. Dark adaptation as obtained with a SST-1 for a healthy patient and one with congenital stationary night blindness. Note the elevated rod threshold. (*Figure is courtesy of LKC Technologies, Inc.*)

TABLE 3-2. SUMMARY OF FEATURES OF THE SCOTOPIC AND PHOTOPIC SYSTEMS

Property	Scotopic System	Photopic System
Receptor	Rods	Cones
Outer segment morphology	Free-floating disks	Disks attached to cell membrane
Weber's fraction	0.140	0.015
Photopigment(s) and peak absorption	Rhodopsin (507 nm)	Erythrolabe (552 or 557 nm) Chlorolabe (530 nm) Cyanolabe (426 nm)
Maximal sensitivity of the system	507 nm	555 nm
Chromatic discrimination	Colorblind	Color discrimination
Sensitivity	Very sensitive to dim lights, not to bright lights	Not sensitive to dim lights, but to brighter lights
Spatial resolution (resolution acuity)	Poor (20/200)	Excellent (20/20)
Spatial summation	Excellent	Poor
Temporal resolution (CFF[a])	Poor (20 Hz)	Excellent (70 Hz)
Temporal summation	Excellent	Poor
Contrast sensitivity	Low (0.140)	High (0.015)
Stiles–Crawford effect	Minimal	Yes

[a]Critical flicker fusion

RP, including night blindness and slow visual recovery following exposure to a bright light. The latter is particularly evident following ophthalmoscopy; patients with RP are often visually incapacitated for several minutes.

SUMMARY

Not only do the rods and cones manifest different morphologies, photopigments, and retinal distributions, the postreceptoral organization of the rod system is fundamentally different than that of the cone system (Table 3–2). The result is a duplex retina: a rod-dominated system operates under dim (scotopic) lighting conditions and a cone-dominated system functions under daylight (photopic) conditions. This duplex retina allows us to have usable vision on both a dark evening and a sunny day, even though there may be up to a 10-log-unit difference in the light levels under these two conditions.

Scotopic vision shows extraordinary absolute sensitivity, largely because of its high degree of spatial and temporal summation; however, this high degree of spatial and temporal summation limits scotopic spatial and temporal resolution. Photopic vision, on the other hand, displays substantially greater spatial and temporal resolution, but poorer spatial and temporal summation.

Q Self-Assessment Questions

1. The eyes of a rod monochromat are missing most of their cones, and vision is dominated by rods. **A.** Describe the symptoms you expect a patient who is a rod monochromat to manifest. **B.** What color sunglasses would you recommend for a rod monochromat?

2. Photopic stimuli of 507 and 555 nm are placed side-by-side. An observer is asked to adjust the intensities of these stimuli so that they are equally bright. Their intensities are then reduced by the same amount such that they are detected by the scotopic system. Under these scotopic conditions, which stimulus appears brightest?

3. Which wavelength is most effective at bleaching rhodopsin? Explain.

4. Refer to Fig. 3–11. **A.** After 20 minutes of dark adaptation, what is the color of the 610-nm stimulus at threshold? **B.** Answer the same question for the 465-nm stimulus. Explain.

5. Refer to Fig. 3–11. **A.** After 1 hour of dark adaptation, what is the difference in sensitivity between the rods and cones for a stimulus of 465 nm? **B.** Answer the same question for the 610-nm stimulus.

6. **A.** The cones are exposed to a bright light source that bleaches much of their photopigment. After 3 minutes in the dark, what percentage of the bleached cone photopigment has recovered? **B.** What percentage of the rod photopigment has recovered at the rod–cone break for 610 nm (see Fig. 3–11)?

7. Refer to Fig. 3–9. **A.** What is the rod threshold after about 11 minutes of dark adaptation for a large 420-nm stimulus? **B.** For the same 420-nm stimulus, what is the cone threshold after 20 minutes of dark adaptation? **C.** What is the photochromatic interval for 420 nm?

Q

8. A. Two patches of light are adjacent to each other. The conditions are scotopic. One patch emits light of 507 nm and the other emits light of 620 nm. Both patches produce 40 quanta of light. Which patch is brighter? **B.** A patch of 507 nm and a patch of 620 nm each bleach 30 rhodopsin molecules. Which patch is brighter?

Photometry

4

Photometry, the measurement of light, has numerous clinical applications. Among these are the specification of lighting conditions under which visual tests are performed and the advisement of patients regarding the illumination that should be used for various daily activities. Of related interest is **visual ergonomics,** which is concerned with the design of a safe and comfortable visual environment, particularly the work environment.

PHOTOMETRY AND RADIOMETRY: BASIC CONCEPTS AND UNITS

Radiometry is concerned with the power produced by a source of electromagnetic radiation, irrespective of its effect on vision. In comparison, **photometry** deals with the effect that this radiation has on the visual system. The basis for photometric measurements is the photopic luminosity curve, $V(\lambda)$, which shows that certain wavelengths are more efficient at stimulating the visual system than others (Fig. 4–1).[1]

Let us look at an example. Figure 4–2 shows two stimuli, one of 400 nm and the other of 600 nm. Each produces 10 W of radiant power.[2] Whereas the 400-nm stimulus has a luminous efficiency of zero, the 600-nm stimulus has an efficiency of 0.62. Although radiometrically equal, these two stimuli are photometrically

---

1. Although closely related, luminous efficiency is not the same as brightness. Also note that $V(\lambda)$ has a form that is very similar to the photopic spectral sensitivity function, but is not the same as this function (see Chap. 3).

2. One watt (W) is equal to 1 joule (J) per second.

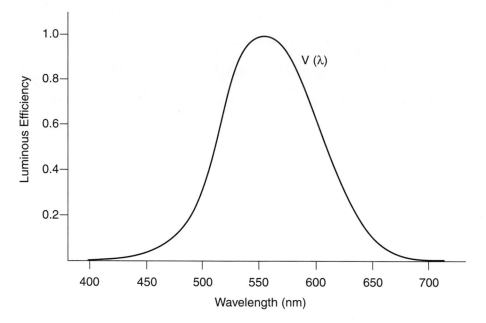

Figure 4–1. Photopic luminosity function, *V*(λ). Luminous efficiency, which is related to brightness, is plotted as a function of wavelength.

different: the 400-nm stimulus is invisible (it produces no light), whereas the 600-nm stimulus is visible.

Lumens and Luminous Power

The basic unit of photometry is the lumen, a measure of **luminous power.**[3] By convention, there are 680 lumens per watt at 555 nm, the peak of the *V*(λ) curve.[4] Other wavelengths are less efficient, producing fewer lumens per watt. For example, at 650 nm there are (0.1)(680 lumens/W), or 68 lumens/W. (The value of 0.1 is the luminous efficiency of 650 nm, and is read off the *V*(λ) curve.)

Let us return to our earlier example, in which patches of 400 and 600 nm each emit 10 W of radiant power (Fig. 4–2). Since the luminous efficiency of 400 nm is zero, this patch emits zero lumens. It has radiant power, but no luminous power. The 600-nm patch produces (0.62)(680 lumens/W)(10 W), or 4216 lumens. This patch, although of the same radiant power as the 400-nm patch, has substantial luminous power. In fact, whereas the 400-nm patch produces no light, the 600-nm patch produces significant light.

---

3. The basic unit of radiometry is the watt, a measure of **radiant power.**

4. There are actually 683 lumens per watt at 555 nm. For convenience, in this text we use the approximation of 680 lumens per watt at 555 nm.

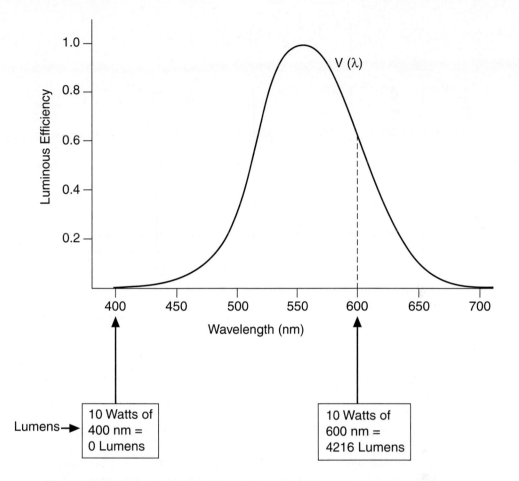

Figure 4–2. A stimulus consisting of 10 watts (power) of 400 nm produces zero lumens of light, whereas a 10-W stimulus of 600 nm produces 4216 lumens. Although both stimuli have the same power, they have different effects on the visual system because of their differing luminous efficiencies.

Luminous power is used to specify the total amount of light that emerges in all directions from a source. Household light bulbs are typically specified by the number of lumens produced.

Abney's Law of Additivity

Most objects emit (or reflect) a mixture of many different wavelengths, not just one wavelength.[5] The luminous power for such a stimulus is determined by cal-

---

5. Stimuli that emit a single wavelength are referred to monochromatic, whereas those that emit a mixture of different wavelengths are sometimes called polychromatic.

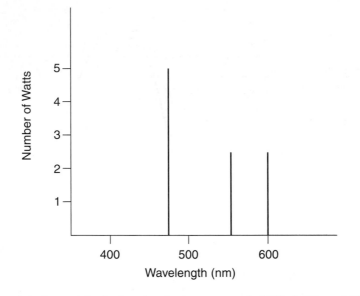

Figure 4–3. Spectral distribution of a stimulus composed of 5 W of 475 nm, 2.5 W of 555 nm, and 2.5 W of 600 nm.

culating the number of lumens produced by each wavelength and then adding these values together. For the simple stimulus depicted in Fig. 4-3, this is done as follows[6]:

5 W of 475 nm:	(0.1) (680 lumens/W) (5 W) = 340 lumens
2.5 W of 555 nm:	(1.0) (680 lumens/W) (2.5 W) = 1700 lumens
2.5 W of 600 nm:	(0.62) (680 lumens/W) (2.5 W) = 1054 lumens
Total =	340 lumens + 1700 lumens + 1054 lumens
Total =	3094 lumens

We can add these different values together because the photometric system is **additive,** a property referred to as **Abney's law of additivity** (Abney, 1913).

Luminous Intensity

Whereas luminous power is a nondirectional measure, luminous intensity refers to the number of lumens produced in a given direction by a point light source. A light bulb may produce a total of 1000 lumens in all directions, but its luminous intensity is specified in one particular direction (Fig. 4–4).

_____

6. Whereas the stimulus depicted in Fig. 4–3 emits light at discrete wavelengths, many stimuli have a continuous spectrum, emitting light at all wavelengths across the visible spectrum (e.g., see Fig. 4–14). For these stimuli, the area under the spectrum is convolved with the $V(\lambda)$ curve to determine the total number of lumens produced.

	Definition	Common Units	Radiometric Equivalent and Units
Luminous Power 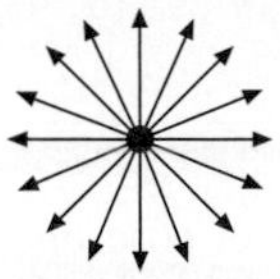	Total light power produced by a source	Lumens	Radiant power (joules/second or watts)
Luminous Intensity 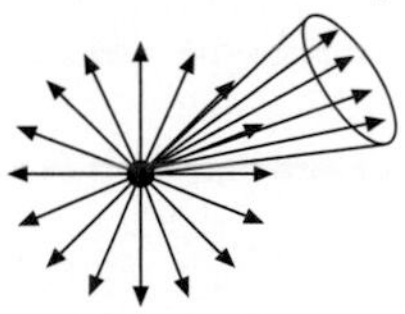	Light power produced in a solid angle by a point source	Lumens/steradian Candelas (1 lumen/steradian = 1 candela)	Radiant intensity (watts/steradian)
Luminance 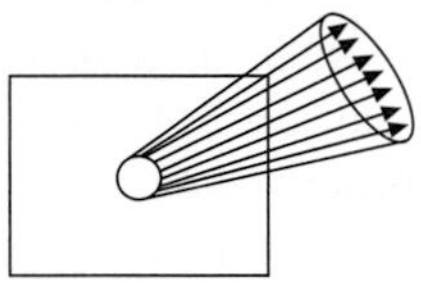	Luminous intensity per unit projected area of an extended source	Candelas/square meter Foot-lamberts	Radiance (watts/steradian/ square meter)
Illuminance 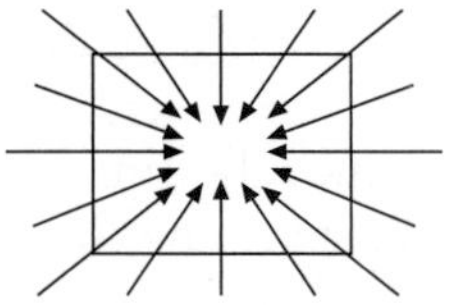	Luminous power falling on a surface	Lumens/square meter Lumens/square foot	Irradiance (watts/ square meter)

Figure 4–4. Various terms, definitions, and units common in photometry and radiometry.

The unit for luminous intensity is the **candela (cd)**, which is defined as one **lumen per steradian.** A steradian (ω or Sr) is a solid angle. It is a conic section of a sphere, defined as (Fig. 4–5):

$$\omega = A/r^2$$

where

      r = radius of the sphere
      A = surface area of sphere subtended

Based on the geometry of a sphere, a 1 cd light source that has equal output in all directions produces a total power of 4π lumens. Consequently, if a uniform point source has an intensity of 10 cd, its total luminous output is expected to be (10 cd)(4π lumens/cd), or 127 lumens.

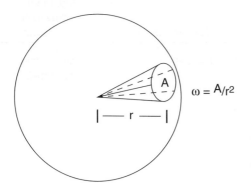

$$\omega = A/r^2$$

Figure 4–5. A steradian, or solid angle, is defined as A/r^2. The symbol ω or the abbreviation *Sr* is typically used to denote a steradian.

Luminance

Luminance quantifies the amount of light coming off a surface, such as a piece of paper, in a specified direction (see Fig. 4–4). The perceptual attribute most clearly associated with luminance (a physical attribute) is brightness. Luminance is given in candelas per projected area of the light source. Common units are **candelas per square meter** (cd/m^2) and **foot-lamberts.**

Both luminance and brightness remain constant as the distance from a surface increases. Why is this so? As the distance increases, the area of the image, either the retinal image or that formed on the sensor of the luminance probe, decreases at the same rate as does the number of candelas contained within the image.[7] Because the ratio of candelas to image surface area remains constant, the luminance and brightness do not change.

Illuminance

Illuminance refers to the luminous power that falls on a surface (see Fig. 4–4). Typical units are **lumens per square meter (lux)** and **lumens per square foot (foot-candles).** Illuminance can be considered analogous to rain: the greater the density of rain drops (lumens), the harder it is raining (the greater the illuminance). Just as the intensity of rain is not affected by the surface on which it falls, illuminance is not affected by the surface on which the light falls.

Lighting standards have been established for certain facilities and activities (Table 4–1). These standards specify the amount of light that should fall upon a

---

7. Geometrical optics explains the decrease in image size. The reduction in the number of candelas is due to the entrance pupil of the eye or luminance probe.

TABLE 4–1.   RECOMMENDED ILLUMINANCE VALUES

Area or activity	Illumination	
	Lux	*Footcandles*
General residential lighting	50–100	5–10
Exhibition hall	100–200	10–20
Elevator	100–200	10–20
Hotel corridor	100–200	10–20
Residential dining room	100–200	10–20
Restroom	100–200	10–20
Library stack	200–500	20–50
Residential reading	200–500	20–50
Industrial packing and labeling (general)	200–500	20–50
Classroom	500–1000	50–100
School science laboratory	500–1000	50–100
Eye surgery	1000–2000	100–200
Clothes fitting area	1000–2000	100–200
Dental procedures	5000–10000	500–1000

Data from Rea (1993).

surface (the illuminance) to provide satisfactory vision. A commercially available illuminance meter can be used to determine if lighting conditions meet industrial standards.

It is easy to confuse luminance and illuminance. Luminance is a property of a surface under a given set of lighting conditions and refers to the light coming off the surface, whereas illuminance refers to the amount of light falling (raining) on a surface. A desk may have the same illumination on its entire surface, but the luminance of the objects on it may vary. The luminance of a white piece of paper on the desk will be greater than that of a black book because the white paper reflects more light.

Photometric Units

A plethora of units are used for luminance and illuminance. Conversions between various units are simple, requiring only a conversion factor (Table 4–2). It should be pointed out that the Système International d'Unités recognizes the metric units of cd/m^2 and lux for luminance and illuminance, respectively. This standardization body does not recognize units such as foot-lamberts and lumens/ft^2, which are based on English measurement units.

TABLE 4–2. CONVERSION FACTORS FOR COMMON UNITS OF ILLUMINANCE AND LUMINANCE[a]

Illuminance Conversion Factors

	Lux (lm/m^2)	Phot	Milliphot	Footcandle	Lumen (per square unit of area)	Abbreviation
1 Lux =	1	10^{-4}	10^{-1}	9.290×10^{-2}	= 1 lm/m^2	[lx]
1 Phot =	10^4	1	10^3	9.290×10^2	= 1 lm/cm^2	[ph]
1 Milliphot =	10	10^{-3}	1	9.290×10^{-1}	= 10^{-3} lm/cm^2	[mph]
1 footcandle =	1.076×10	1.076×10^{-3}	1.076	1	= 1 lm/ft^2	[fcd]

Luminance Conversion Factors

	Nit (cd/m^2)	Stilb	Apostilb	Lambert	Millilambert	Footlambert	Candela ft^{-2}	Candela in^{-2}	Candela (per square unit of area)	Abbreviation
1 Nit =	1	10^{-4}	3.142	3.142×10^{-4}	3.142×10^{-1}	2.919×10^{-1}	9.290×10^{-2}	6.452×10^{-4}	= 1 cd/m^2	[nt]
1 Stilb =	10^4	1	3.142×10^4	3.142×10^3	3.142×10^3	9.919×10^3	9.290×10^2	6.452	= 1 cd/cm^2	[sb]
1 Apostilb =	10^{-1}	10^{-5}	1	10^{-4}	10^{-1}	9.290×10^{-2}	2.957×10^{-2}	2.054×10^{-4}	= $(1/\pi)$ cd/m^2	[asb]
1 Lambert =	3.183×10^3	3.183×10^{-1}	10^4	1	10^3	9.290×10^2	2.957×10^2	2.054	= $(1/\pi)$ cd/cm^2	[L]
1 Millilambert =	3.183	3.183×10^{-4}	10	10^{-3}	1	9.290×10^{-1}	2.957×10^{-1}	2.054×10^{-3}	= 10^{-3} $(1/\pi)$ cd/cm^2	[mL]
1 Footlambert =	3.426	3.426×10^{-4}	1.076×10	1.076×10^{-3}	1.076	1	3.183×10^{-1}	2.210×10^{-3}	= $(1/\pi)$ cd/ft^2	[fL]
1 Candela/ft^2 =	1.076×10	1.076×10^{-3}	3.382×10	3.382×10^{-3}	3.382	3.142	1	6.944×10^{-3}	= 1 cd/ft^2	[cdft^{-2}]
1 Candela/in^2 =	1.550×10^3	1.550×10^{-1}	4.869×10^3	4.869×10^{-1}	4.869×10^2	4.524×10^2	1.44×10^2	1	= 1 cd/in^2	[cdin^{-2}]

Other Equivalent Units

1 equivalent phot	=	1 lambert
1 equivalent lux	=	1 apostilb
1 equivalent footcandle	=	1 footlambert

1 blondel = 1 apostilb

[a]For example, X footlamberts = $X \times 3.426 \times 10^{-4}$ stilbs.
Source: From Wyszecki G, Stiles WS. *Color Science: Concepts and Methods, Quantitative Data and Formulae.* Copyright © 1982. Reprinted by permission of John Wiley & Sons, Inc.

Radiometric Units

The radiometric equivalents of luminous power, luminous intensity, luminance, and illuminance are, respectively, radiant power, radiant intensity, radiance, and irradiance (see Fig. 4–4). These radiometric terms do not take into account the luminous efficiency of the visual system.

COSINE DIFFUSERS

Cosine surfaces, also referred to as **Lambert, perfectly diffusing,** or **matte surfaces**, show the same luminance regardless of the angle at which the luminance is measured. A good example is a piece of nonglossy paper. From whatever angle you view this paper, its brightness is the same, as is its luminance. A **specular surface**, such as a mirror, is not perfectly diffusing because the luminance varies depending on the direction at which it is measured.

It is straightforward to calculate the luminance of a cosine surface if the surface's reflectance factor (a nondimensional unit that ranges from 0 to 1) and illumination are known (Fig. 4–6). The equation for this calculation is

$$L = rE$$

where

L = luminance in foot-lamberts
r = reflectance factor (nondimensional, no units)
E = illumination in foot-candles (lumens/ft^2)

The basis for this relationship is that an illumination of 1 lumen/ft^2, falling on a matte surface with a reflectance factor of 1, produces a luminance of $1/\pi$ cd/ft^2.

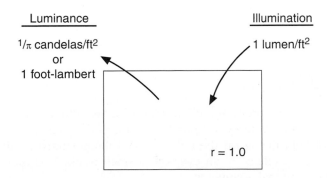

Figure 4–6. A cosine surface with a reflectance factor of 1 has a luminance of 1 foot-lambert when the illumination falling on it is 1 lumen/ft^2.

To avoid the $1/\pi$ factor, 1 foot-lambert is defined as $1/\pi$ cd/ft². Consequently, an illumination of 1 lumen/ft² falling on a surface with $r = 1$ produces a luminance of 1 foot-lambert.

INVERSE SQUARE LAW

As a surface is moved away from a point source, the number of lumens falling on it decreases with the square of the distance, resulting in a decrease in its illumination (Fig. 4–7A.) The inverse square law is expressed as

$$E = I/d^2$$

where

> $E =$ illumination falling on the surface
> $I =$ intensity of the point source
> $d =$ distance from the point source to the surface

This formula assumes that the surface is normal to the light source. If the surface is tilted, as indicated in Fig. 4–7B, fewer lumens fall on it, with a resultant decrease in illumination. The reduction in illumination is proportional to the cosine of angle of tilt of the surface (θ). This cosine law of illumination is

$$E = (I/d^2) \cos \theta$$

or

$$E_2 = E_1 \cos \theta$$

where

> $E_1 =$ illumination falling on the surface when it is normal to the light source
>
> $E_2 =$ illumination falling on the tilted surface

RETINAL ILLUMINATION

Vision scientists often specify stimuli in terms of retinal illumination, which takes into account the area of the eye's pupil. This specification is important because the amount of light falling on the retina (retinal illumination) of an eye with a large pupil is greater than for an eye with a small pupil. This difference could affect the state of retinal adaptation.

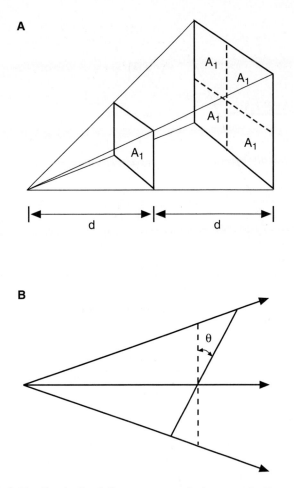

Figure 4–7. A. The illumination falling on an area A_1 decreases by the square of the distance. **B.** The illumination falling on a surface decreases with the cosine of the angle.

The basic unit for retinal illumination is a troland, defined as

$$T = LA$$

where

T = retinal illumination in trolands (td)
L = luminance of the surface that is viewed
A = pupil area

Consequently, if the retinal illumination for an experiment is specified as a given number of trolands, all subjects will have the same amount of light falling on their retinas regardless of pupil diameter.

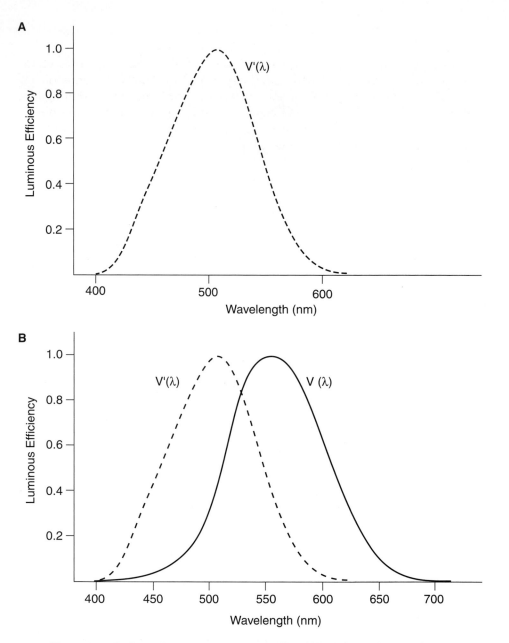

Figure 4–8. A. Scotopic luminosity function, $V'(\lambda)$. **B.** Both the scotopic $V'(\lambda)$ and photopic $V(\lambda)$ luminosity functions plotted on the same coordinates.

SCOTOPIC UNITS

Our discussion of photometry, up to this point, has concerned photopic vision. On occasion, however, it is necessary to specify visual stimuli in terms of scotopic units. For instance, if a stimulus is to be viewed under very dim lighting conditions, where only rods are operative, scotopic units are most appropriate.

The basic unit of scotopic photometry is the **scotopic lumen**, a unit of **scotopic photometric power.** By convention, there are 680 scotopic lumens per watt at 555 nm. The number of scotopic lumens per watt for other wavelengths is determined by the scotopic luminosity function, $V'(\lambda)$, which is given in Fig. 4–8. For example, at 507 nm, the peak of the scotopic luminosity function, the number of scotopic lumens per watt is determined by a proportionality:

$$\frac{\text{luminous efficiency of 555 nm}}{\text{680 scotopic lumens/W}} = \frac{\text{luminous efficiency of 507 nm}}{X \text{ scotopic lumens/W}}$$

$$\frac{0.4}{680} = \frac{1.0}{X}$$

$$X = 1700 \text{ scotopic lumens/W at 507 nm}$$

For 575 nm, the calculation is

$$\frac{0.4}{680} = \frac{0.2}{X}$$

$$X = 340 \text{ scotopic lumens/W at 575 nm}$$

Scotopic lumens can be confusing. It is important to keep in mind that by definition, there are 680 scotopic lumens per watt at 555 nm, the peak of $V(\lambda)$, rather than at 507 nm, the peak of $V'(\lambda)$.

DERIVATION OF THE PHOTOPIC LUMINOSITY FUNCTION

In our discussion of the photopic luminosity function, $V(\lambda)$, the assumption has been made that this function is related to brightness. This is true, but it does not convey the complete story.

If the $V(\lambda)$ function truly represents brightness, it could be determined by a direct brightness matching procedure, as illustrated in Fig. 4–9. One wavelength, say 555 nm, is chosen as a standard, and all other wavelengths (sample wavelengths) are matched to this standard for brightness. The observer adjusts the radiance of a sample wavelength such that its brightness matches the standard. This is done across the spectrum. Such an experiment is challenging for the observer because he or she must match the brightness of two differently colored stimuli. Because it is difficult to ignore color differences, there is much variability in the matches a person makes (Boynton, 1979; Pokorny et al, 1979).

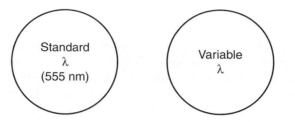

Figure 4–9. Stimulus arrangement for a direct brightness matching experiment. The observer's task is to adjust the radiance of the sample (variable) wavelength such that it matches the brightness of the standard wavelength.

Moreover, the results obtained by direct matching do not follow Abney's law of additivity, seriously limiting their application in photometry.

There are other methods of determining the photopic luminosity function that overcome these problems. Perhaps the most widely known is heterochromatic flicker photometry (HFP) (Wagner and Boynton, 1972). A standard wavelength stimulus, say 555 nm, is temporally exchanged with the sample wavelength stimulus, for example, 650 nm (Fig. 4–10). The rate of flicker is moderate, about 15

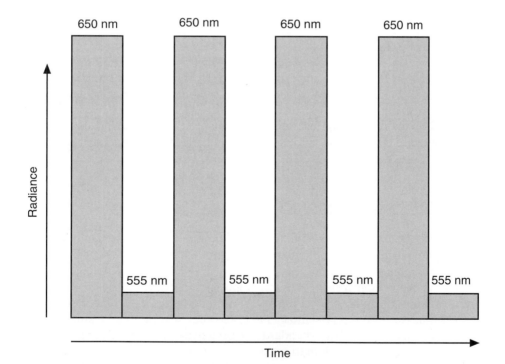

Figure 4–10. In heterochromatic flicker photometry, two monochromatic stimuli are temporally alternated. The observer's task is to adjust the radiance of one of these stimuli such that the perception of flicker is minimized.

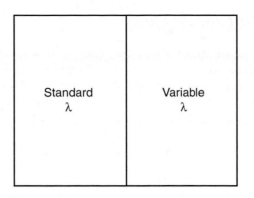

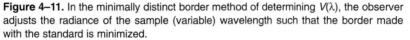

Figure 4–11. In the minimally distinct border method of determining $V(\lambda)$, the observer adjusts the radiance of the sample (variable) wavelength such that the border made with the standard is minimized.

cycles per second. This produces color fusion, whereby only one color is seen. In this case, the 555 nm (green) and 650 nm (red) fuse such that orange is perceived.

This orange color, however, is not seen as steady; rather, it is perceived as flickering. The flicker is due to a mismatch in the luminance of the two stimuli. The task in HFP is to adjust the radiance of the sample stimulus such that the flicker is minimized. When this is done, the standard and sample wavelengths are at equal luminance. This procedure, when repeated across the spectrum, yields a photopic luminosity function. HFP produces very reliable results.

Another approach to determining $V(\lambda)$ is the minimally distinct border (MDB) method devised by Boynton (1973) and illustrated in Fig. 4–11. Here, the standard wavelength and sample wavelength are placed side by side such that a border is formed where they meet. The observer's task is to adjust the radiance of the sample so that the visibility of the border is minimized. When repeated across the spectrum, a photopic luminosity function is obtained. As with HFP, MDB produces highly reliable results.

The HFP and MDB methods produce very similar results, and these results differ from those obtained using direct brightness matching (Wagner and Boynton, 1972). Importantly, the results of HFP and MDB follow Abney's law of additivity, whereas the results of direct brightness matching do not.

The $V(\lambda)$ curve represents the compilation and standardization of data from several laboratories, obtained largely with HFP, promulgated by the Commission Internationale de L'Eclairage (CIE). As such, the CIE $V(\lambda)$ curve does not represent luminosity for any one individual, but for an ideal standard observer. Without such a standard luminosity function, a workable photometric system would not be possible. It is important to keep in mind that $V(\lambda)$ is closely related to brightness, but for the reasons outlined earlier, it is not precisely the same as brightness.

SPECIFICATION OF LIGHT SOURCES

Modern light sources are divided into two categories: incandescent and luminescent. An **incandescent** source generates light through heat, whereas a **luminescent** source produces light through the excitation of individual atoms. A common light bulb, where a voltage differential across a filament causes the filament to become hot and generate light, is an incandescent source.

A frequently encountered **luminescent light source** is the fluorescent light tube, which is filled with gases whose atoms are energized into an excited state by a voltage differential applied across the tube. The unstable gas atoms release energy when they spontaneously revert to their unexcited state. This energy is in the form of short-wavelength ultraviolet radiation, which is absorbed by a phosphor that coats the inside of the bulb and then is re-emitted as longer-wavelength visible light. This phosphor can be varied to produce the desired spectral emission characteristics.

Figure 4–12 shows the spectral distributions of typical incandescent and fluorescent light sources. Note that the incandescent source shows a relative concentration of energy at long wavelengths. The fluorescent source, in contrast, does not show such a skewing of power toward the long-wavelength region of the spectrum. It does, however, show energy spikes across the spectrum. The spikes produced by certain fluorescent light bulbs may render them unsuitable for administering color vision tests (see Chap. 6).

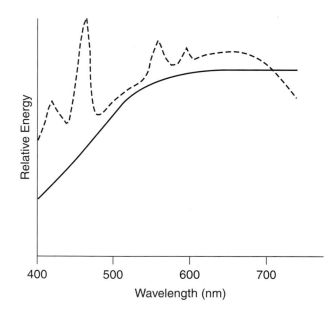

Figure 4–12. The solid curve represents the spectral distribution of a tungsten (incandescent) light bulb, and the dashed curve, the spectral distribution of a fluorescent light tube. Note the energy spikes in the fluorescent tube's spectral distribution.

Blackbody Radiators and Color Temperature

A blackbody radiator is a theoretical construct that has proven convenient for describing sources of electromagnetic radiation, including light sources. Its spectral output is determined by its temperature (T), as quantified by Wein's displacement law

$$\text{Peak wavelength} \propto 1/T$$

and the Stefan–Boltzman law

$$\text{Total power} \propto T^4$$

Figure 4–13A shows the spectral distribution of a blackbody radiator at three different temperatures. Note that as the temperature increases, the peak wavelength decreases, and the area under the spectral distribution curve, which represents power, increases.

When it comes to specifying light sources, the blackbody radiator's spectral output that is of most interest is in the visible spectrum, which is delineated by the dashed lines in Fig. 4–13A. This region is replotted in Fig. 4–13B with the three spectral distributions normalized to 555 nm. Note that a blackbody radiator with a temperature of 2000 Kelvin (K) has most of its power concentrated at longer wavelengths. In comparison, a blackbody radiator with a temperature of 10,000 K has its power concentrated at shorter wavelengths.

How can blackbody radiators be used to specify light sources? Suppose we wish to describe the spectral output of a tungsten–halogen light bulb, such as is found in an ophthalmoscope. One approach is to provide a graph of its spectral output. Alternatively, we could provide *the temperature of the blackbody radiator* whose spectral output matches that of the ophthalmoscope bulb, the so-called **color temperature (CT)** of the bulb.[8]

Commercially available light sources are frequently specified by their CT, which provides much information about the source. For example, although sources with CTs of 2000 K and 10,000 K both appear white, they do not match each other in appearance. From studying Fig. 4–13, it is seen that the 2000 K source will appear yellow-white because it has relatively more energy in the long-wavelength region of the spectrum, whereas the 10,000 K source will appear blue-white because there is relatively more energy in the short-wavelength region.

The term *color temperature* is only appropriate when specifying incandescent light sources. For the specification of nonincandescent sources, such as fluorescent bulbs, the proper term is **correlated color temperature.** The correlated color temperature of a fluorescent light tube depends on the nature of the phosphor that coats the bulb.

Merchandisers frequently illuminate products with bulbs whose CTs show their products to maximum advantage. For instance, a butcher may illuminate beef

---

8. Color temperature is often a source of confusion. Keep in mind that it refers to the temperature, in degrees Kelvin (K), of the blackbody radiator, not the light source.

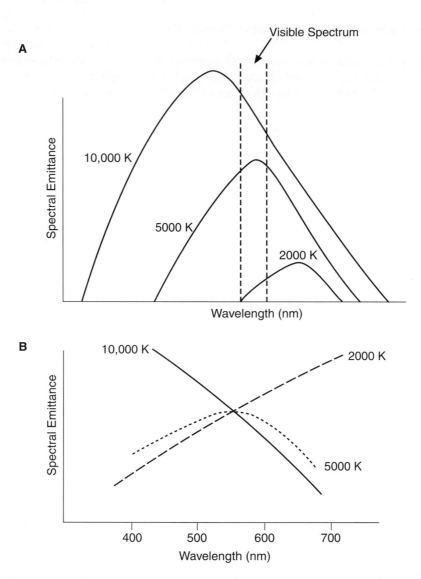

Figure 4–13. A. Approximate spectral distributions for blackbody radiators with temperatures of 2000 K, 5000 K, and 10,000 K. The dashed lines show the range of the visible spectrum. **B.** Approximate relative spectral distributions, for visible wavelengths, of the sources given in A. These distributions have been normalized to 555 nm.

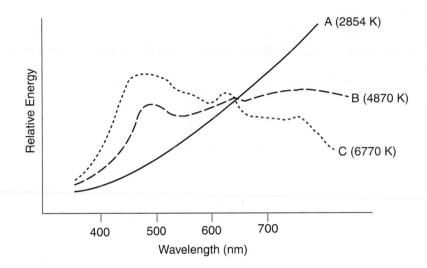

Figure 4–14. Approximate spectral distributions of standard illuminants A, B, and C, along with their color temperatures.

using a relatively low CT to accentuate the fresh, red color of the meat, while a jeweler may choose to illuminate his or her diamond display with a high CT to highlight the bluish nature of the diamonds.

Standard Illuminants

Several standard illuminants have been defined by international convention. Their spectral distributions are given in Fig. 4–14. Standard illuminant A, with a CT of 2854 K, represents an incandescent light bulb. Illuminants B and C represent sources with higher blue contents. Illuminant C is recommended for administering most color vision tests (see Chap. 6).

FILTERS

Colored Filters

A colored filter may absorb and/or reflect some wavelengths that are incident upon it, while transmitting others. As a result, the spectral distribution of the light emerging from the filter is not the same as that incident on it. In essence, the filter subtracts light to produce color.[9]

Figure 4–15A shows a filter that is illuminated by a tungsten bulb. The light incident on the filter appears white, but the light emerging from the filter is

---

9. The light is subtracted through absorption, reflection, and/or interference.

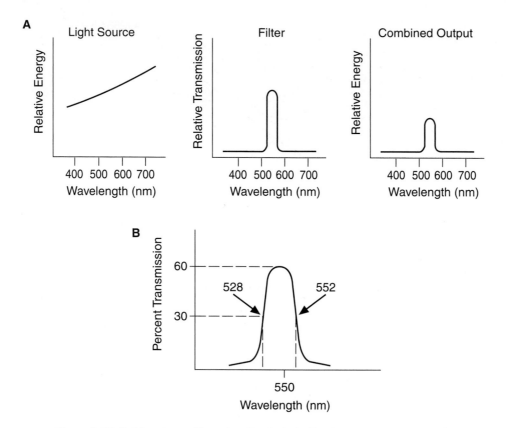

Figure 4–15. A. A band-pass filter, when illuminated with a tungsten source, transmits a band of light. The filter will appear green because the wavelengths it transmits are centered at 540 nm. **B.** The half-height bandwidth for this filter is 552 nm − 528 nm = 24 nm.

green. This is because the filter strongly absorbs most wavelengths, except those in the region of 540 nm. These wavelengths are transmitted, giving the filter its green appearance.

Figure 4–15A shows an example of a **narrow-band filter**—a filter that passes only a narrow spectral band of light. Filters of this type are typically specified by the location of their peak and their half-height bandwidth. As indicated in Fig. 4–15B, the half-height bandwidth is the spectral range over which the filter transmits 50 percent or more of its peak transmission percentage. The smaller the half-height bandwidth, the more selective is the filter. Like narrow-band filters, **broad-band filters** have a band-pass nature; however, the width of the band is greater for a broad-band filter (Fig. 4–16A).

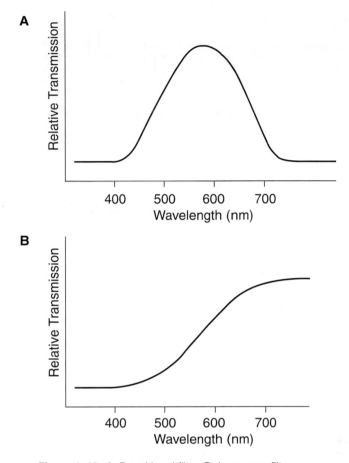

Figure 4–16. A. Broad-band filter. **B.** Long-pass filter.

Long-pass filters transmit long wavelengths, but not short wavelengths (see Fig. 4–16B). Filters of this sort are often used in sunglasses to block high-energy UV radiation. Because they transmit longer wavelengths, objects viewed through these filters may appear yellowish. Sunglasses that incorporate a long-pass filter are sometimes called blue-blockers.

Unlike those colored filters that absorb and/or reflect light, **interference filters** take advantage of the interference of light waves to produce a very narrow band of light. These filters may have a half-height bandwidth so narrow that, for practical purposes, they can be thought of as transmitting only a single wavelength of light. They are essentially monochromatic. Such filters have important applications in vision research.

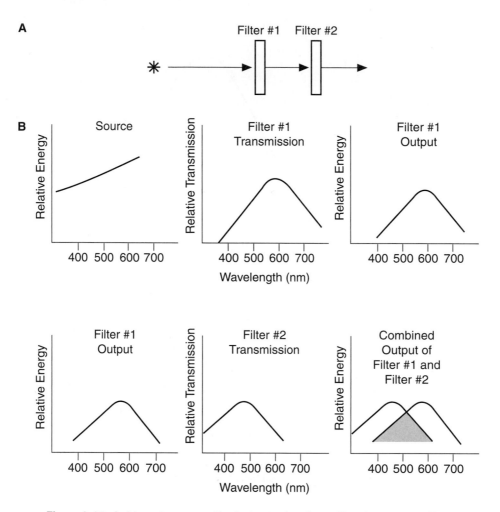

Figure 4–17. A. A tungsten source illuminates two band-pass filters in sequence. The first filter shows maximal transmission at 570 nm and the second at 470 nm. **B.** The top row shows the output of the first filter when illuminated with the tungsten source. Because the filter has a peak transmission of 570 nm, the peak output of this filter is at 570 nm. The bottom row shows the output of this same filter incident on the second filter. The second filter has its peak transmission at 470 nm. Only that light common to the two filters is transmitted. This is given by the shaded area of overlap of the two spectral distributions. This is an example of a subtractive color mixture.

Subtractive and Additive Color Mixtures

Consider two colored filters placed in sequence, as given in Fig. 4–17. The first filter transmits a broad band of light centered at about 570 nm, whereas the second filter's transmission is centered at 470 nm. When placed in sequence, the only light transmitted by the filter combination is that represented by the over-

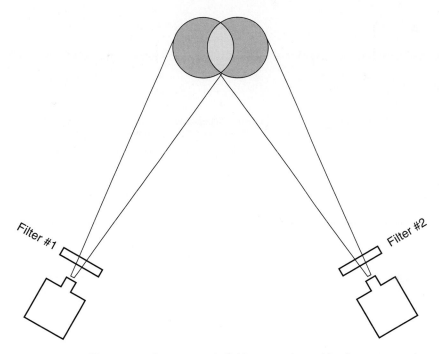

Figure 4–18. The output of two separate light sources is combined on a screen to produce an additive light mixture.

lap of the two transmission curves. In this case, the resultant spectral distribution peaks at about 520 nm.

Note that the filter combination transmits less light than either filter by itself. This is a natural result of the manner in which these filters work—they subtract light, resulting in what is called a subtractive color mixture. The pigments present in common paints, when mixed together, produce subtractive mixtures.

Subtractive mixtures should be distinguished from additive color mixtures in which light from two different sources is summed. For example, if we shine a light through each of the two filters in Fig. 4–17 and then combine the output on a screen, we have an additive mixture (Fig. 4–18). The additive mixture contains more light than that emitted by either of the filters. Most projection systems, such as found in televisions and movie theaters, use additive light mixtures.

Neutral Density Filters

A neutral density filter transmits all wavelengths equally, thereby minimizing color distortion (Fig. 4–19A). Whereas, objects viewed through, say, a broadband filter with a peak transmission at 570 nm may appear yellow, the same objects viewed through a neutral density filter would retain their natural colors.

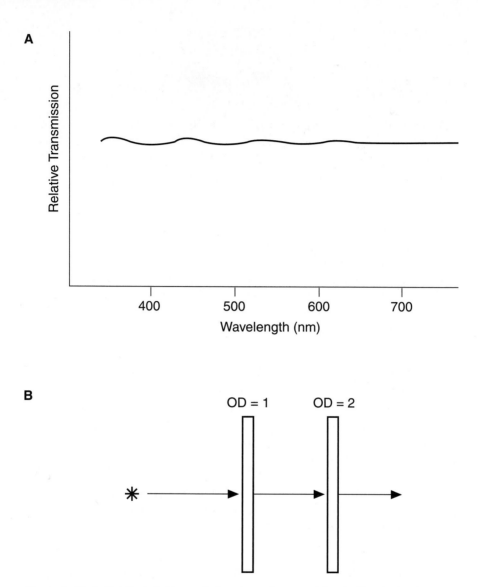

Figure 4–19. A. Relatively flat transmission curve of a neutral density filter. **B.** A combination of neutral density filters with optical densities of 1 and 2 produces an optical density of 3. This combination transmits 0.1 percent of the incident light.

Neutral density filters are specified by their optical density (OD), defined by the following relationship:

$$OD = \log(1/T)$$

where T is the fraction transmittance of the filter and OD is in log units.

Consider an example. A neutral density filter transmits 10 percent of the light incident on it. What is its OD?

$$OD = \log(1/0.10)$$
$$OD = 1.00$$

The advantage of specifying optical density in log units is that these values are additive. If we place a 1 log filter and a 2 log filter back to back, the combination is a 3 log filter (see Fig. 4–19B). Using the formula for OD, we can calculate the percent of light transmitted by this 3 log filter to be 0.1 percent.

CLINICAL CONSIDERATIONS

The crystalline lens absorbs a substantial amount of high-energy ultraviolet (UV) radiation, thereby contributing to the protection of the retina. This absorption of UV radiation, however, is thought to promote cataract formation (Weale, 1983). For this reason, it is common to prescribe spectacles that block UV radiation.

To produce a UV block, an ophthalmic lens is either coated or saturated with a substance that acts as a long-pass filter. For optimal protection, this substance should block both UV A and UV B. The resulting lens may be slightly yellow because the filter blocks some blue light. To provide patient comfort in the form of sunglasses, an additional filter, such as a neutral density filter, must be incorporated into the lens. Neutral density filters are especially suitable for this application because they block all wavelengths equally. Consequently, color distortion is minimized.[10]

SUMMARY

Radiometry refers to the power produced by an electromagnetic source. It does not take into account visibility. Photometry, in comparison, takes into account the visual efficiency (as given by the $V(\lambda)$ photopic luminosity function) of the various wavelengths that constitute a source.

The spectral distribution of a light source can be given by specifying its color temperature or correlated color temperature. Its spectral distribution can be altered by projecting it through filters that subtracts certain wavelengths of light, while transmitting others.

The discussion in this chapter represents a basic summary of photometry and radiometry. A more detailed treatment can be found in the work of Wyszecki and Stiles (1982).

---

10. When looking through sunglasses made of a high-pass filter combined with a neutral density filter, objects will tend to appear yellowish because the filter combination acts as a high-pass filter. If the sunglasses were made by combining a high-pass filter with a colored filter, rather than a neutral density filter, the color distortion may be worse.

Self-Assessment Questions

1. A light source and filter combination produces 1000 lumens. The filter is monochromatic with peak transmission at 600 nm. How many watts are transmitted by the filter?

2. A source produces 10 W at 500 nm, 5 W at 550 nm, and 20 W at 650 nm. How many lumens are produced?

3. For the data in question 2, give the number of scotopic lumens produced.

4. An illuminance probe is used to measure the lighting concitions in a class-room. The reading obtained is 70 foot-candles. The probe measures 3 × 3 cm. How many lumens are incident on the surface of the probe?

5. A device measures irradiance. You would like to convert this device into an illuminance probe. How do you do this?

6. A point source has an intensity of 100 cd. What illumination does it produce at a distance of 2 feet? Give your answer in both foot-candles and lux (lumens/m2). (Assume there are 10 lux per foot-candle.)

7. A point source of 50 cd is 1 foot from a sheet of paper. Another point source at 3 feet from this same piece of paper illuminates the paper equal to the first source. What is the intensity of this unknown point source?

8. An illuminance meter is tilted 60 degrees from the perpendicular position with respect to a point source of light. The meter reads 100 lux and is 2 feet from the source. What is the intensity of the point source?

9. A neutral density filter absorbs 75 percent of the light incident on it. What is the optical density of the filter?

10. A 0.5 neutral density filter is combined with a 1.0 neutral density filter. A. How much light (as a percentage) does the combination transmit? B. How much is absorbed?

Q ────────────────────

11. A matte surface with a reflectance factor of 0.7 has a luminance of 50 foot-lamberts. What is the illuminance falling on the surface?

12. By use of the inverse square law and an illuminance device, the intensity of a point source is determined to be 25 cd. Assume this uniform point source produces the same amount of light in all directions. How many total lumens does it produce?

13. A light source is located 3 feet from a matte surface. The illumination falling onto the surface is 100 lux. The luminance of this surface, at an angle of 30 degrees, is 5 foot-lamberts. What is the reflectance factor of this surface?

Color Vision

5

Sophisticated color vision presumably conferred an evolutionary advantage to our nonhuman primate ancestors.[1] Although not critical for survival in modern-day society, the ability to distinguish colors immeasurably enriches our visual world.

Color vision has been extensively studied for over two centuries. Much of what has been learned has important clinical implications.

TRICHROMATIC THEORY

Historical Considerations

From Chapter 2, we know that color is a wavelength-dependent perception. As we change the wavelength of a stimulus, its color also changes. What are the physiological mechanisms that underlie the relationship between wavelength and color?

Early investigators postulated that each color is coded by a cone that is uniquely responsive to that color. Because humans are capable of perceiving thousands of colors, thousands of different cone types would be required at all retinal locations. Given all the other stimulus characteristics that must be encoded and the finite processing capabilities of the retina, this is not plausible.

---

1. Some have suggested that highly developed color vision conferred an evolutionary advantage to monkeys in the detection and selection of tropical fruits and edible leaves (Osorio and Vorobyev, 1996).

Thomas Young, in 1802, proposed an alternative model of color vision. In Young's own words:

> As it is almost impossible to conceive each sensitive point of the retina to contain an infinite number of particles, each capable of vibrating in perfect unison with every possible undulation, it becomes necessary to suppose the number limited; for instance to the three principal colours . . . and that each of the particles is capable of being put in motion more or less forcibly by undulations differing less or more from perfect unison. Each sensitive filament of the nerve may consist of three portions, one for each principal colour (MacAdam, 1970, p. 51).

Although the terminology is dated, Young formulated a theory on which modern color vision science is based. He posited that color information is coded by a limited number of cone types, perhaps three, and that the relative activities of these different cone types encodes color. The theory that embodies this and related concepts is referred to as the **trichromatic theory.** Much of its support comes from psychophysical color matching experiments, our next topic.

Monochromacy

As a first step in understanding the trichromatic theory, let us learn why a person with only one photopigment has no color discrimination. Such a person is referred to as a **monochromat.** Figure 5–1 shows the absorption spectrum for the hypothetical photopigment of such an individual. This absorption spectrum displays the probability of a quantum being absorbed as a function of wavelength. For example, a quantum of λ_b has a 50 percent chance of being absorbed, whereas a quantum of λ_a has only a 25 percent chance of being absorbed.

When a photopigment molecule absorbs a quantum of light, it does not encode the wavelength of that quantum. All information regarding its wavelength is lost, the so-called **principle of univariance** (see Chap. 3).

Is an individual who has only one photopigment able to make wavelength-based discriminations? In other words, if we show this person two patches of light, one patch consisting of λ_a and the other of λ_b, can he or she distinguish between these two patches? This question can be answered by observing Fig. 5–2, which illustrates two patches of light, λ_a and λ_b, each of which emits 100 quanta of light. Because the probabilities of absorption of these two wavelengths are different, each patch results in a different number of quantal absorptions. For λ_a the probability of absorption is 0.25, resulting in 25 absorptions. Likewise, for the patch containing λ_b, the probability of 0.50 results in 50 quantal absorptions. Since the patch with λ_b produces twice as many quantal absorptions, it is brighter. The subject may interpret this difference in brightness as a difference in color.

Let us take this a step further. What happens if we were to double the intensity of the patch with λ_a such that it now emits 200 quanta, while keeping λ_b at the same intensity? As shown in Fig. 5–2, this results in 50 quantal absorptions for both wavelengths. Because both patches produce the same effect on the

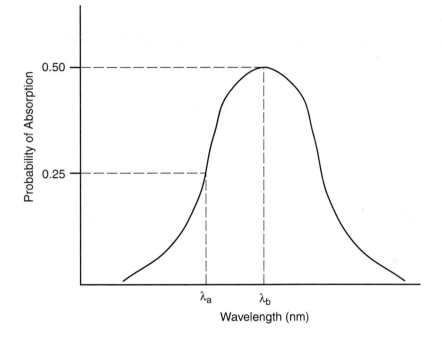

FIGURE 5–1. Absorption spectrum for the photopigment of a hypothetical mono-chromat.

visual system, they are indistinguishable. This example shows that a person with one photopigment cannot make wavelength-based discriminations because different wavelengths *can always be made to appear identical by adjusting their intensities.* This is the condition of monochromacy. The individual is totally colorblind—he or she is unable to distinguish objects on the basis of wavelength alone.

Although we know that people with monochromatic vision are unable to make distinctions based on wavelength, they may very well be able to correctly label colors. Consider the case of a **rod monochromat**, an individual who has only rods. As we learned in Chapter 3, the rhodopsin contained in rods peaks at 507 nm. Say that we show this person three patches of light, as indicated in Fig. 5–3, each of which emits 5000 quanta of light, and tell him or her that one patch is blue-green, one is yellow, and the other is red. To the rod monochromat, the 505-nm patch will appear bright, the 570-nm patch less bright, and the 600-nm dim. If we ask the subject to assign these color labels to the patches of light, he or she is likely to do so correctly.

What is happening here? The short answer is that the monochromat uses brightness to label colors. All of his or her life, this rod monochromat has noticed that other people label dim objects as red and bright objects as green. Therefore, he or she has learned to label colors on the basis of brightness.

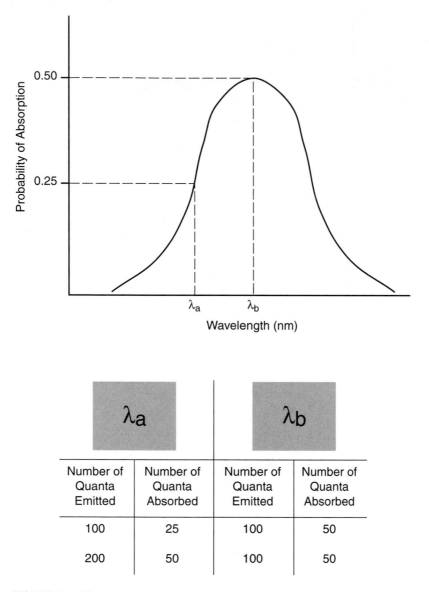

FIGURE 5–2. These two patches of light will be indistinguishable to this monochromat when each patch produces the same number of quantal absorptions.

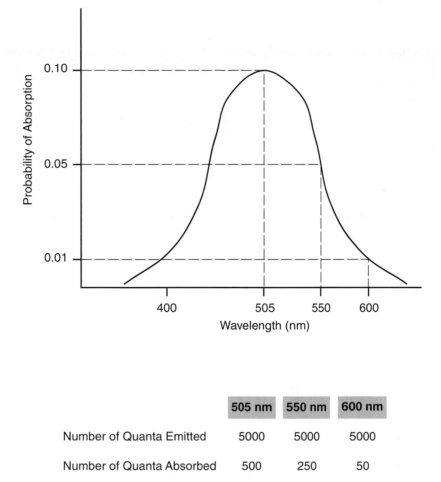

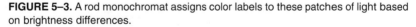

	505 nm	550 nm	600 nm
Number of Quanta Emitted	5000	5000	5000
Number of Quanta Absorbed	500	250	50

FIGURE 5–3. A rod monochromat assigns color labels to these patches of light based on brightness differences.

When confronted with natural objects, such as apples and bananas, the task of color labeling may be made easier by the presence of other cues, such as the shape of the fruit.

Does the monochromat perceive colors? We have no way of answering this question. After all, I cannot even be sure that you and I are perceiving the same color when we observe a red tomato. We do, however, know that monochromats can be fooled if we adjust the intensities of stimuli: they do not have the ability to distinguish stimuli on the basis of the wavelength alone.

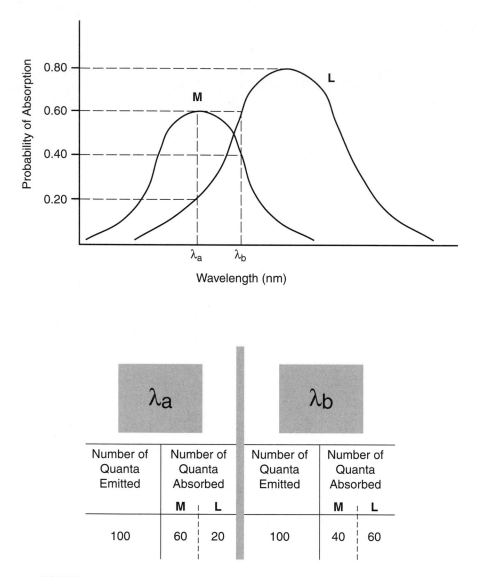

FIGURE 5–4. The two patches, λ_a and λ_b, can be distinguished by this dichromat based on differences in wavelength. The dichromat will not be able to adjust the intensities of the two patches so that they match.

Dichromacy

Consider the photopigment arrangement in Fig. 5–4. The individual has two photopigments, M and L, which peak at different wavelengths and have overlapping absorption spectra throughout much of the spectrum. In the following analysis, we will determine if this person is able to make wavelength-based discriminations.

Suppose the individual is given two patches of light, one consisting of λ_a and the other of λ_b. He or she is asked to adjust the intensity of λ_b so that the two patches appear identical. If the individual is capable of matching these two wavelengths, he or she does not have the ability to make wavelength-based discriminations. If, however, the person is unable to match these two patches of light, he or she possesses the ability to make discriminations based purely on wavelength.

From studying Fig. 5–4, it is clear that it is not possible to adjust the intensity of λ_b such that it will match λ_a. This is because there is no intensity at which the number of quanta absorbed by M and L for λ_b equals the number absorbed by these same photopigments for λ_a. No matter how the intensities of these two patches of light are adjusted, they never have identical effects on the visual system. They are distinguishable and, moreover, they are distinguishable solely because they are different wavelengths.

Now consider the situation in Fig. 5–5. In this case, we again have two patches of light; however, one patch consists of λ_b and the other consists of an additive mixture of λ_a and λ_c. The individual is able to control the intensity of each wavelength, independent of the other wavelengths. For example, he or she can adjust the intensity of λ_c without affecting the intensity of λ_a or λ_b. Given this situation, will the person be able to adjust the intensities of the various wavelengths such that the patch on the left is identical to that on the right? That is, can the intensity of the various wavelengths be adjusted such that each patch of light results in the same number of quantal absorptions by pigments M and L?

Careful examination of Fig. 5–5 shows that it is indeed possible for the subject to adjust the intensities such that *each patch has the same effect on the visual system*. (Each patch produces 200 quantal absorptions by photopigment M and 300 by L.) From the subject's perspective, these two patches of light, which are physically different, appear identical. Two stimuli that appear identical, but are physically different, are referred to as **metamers.**

The individual just described is a **dichromat.** These individuals have some degree of color discrimination, yet it is limited. A patch of λ_a always looks different than a patch of λ_b; however, a patch of λ_b may be matched by the proper combination of λ_a and λ_c. To state this more precisely, given at least three wavelengths, divided into two patches, a person with dichromatic vision (a dichromat) is able to adjust the relative intensities of these wavelengths such that the two patches appear identical.

Trichromacy

It is well established that most humans have trichromatic vision. The concepts underlying trichromacy are the same as those for dichromacy, the only difference being that there are three different photopigments with overlapping absorption spectra rather than two. A commonly accepted set of cone spectra for normal

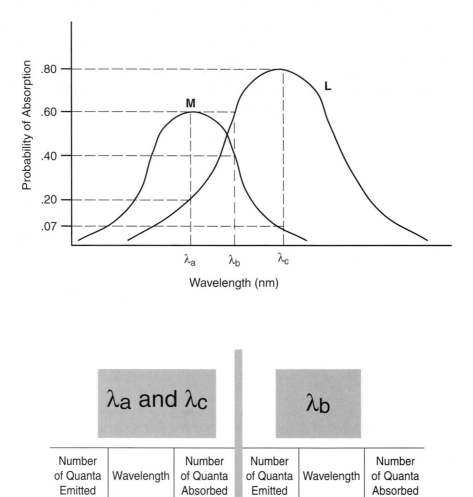

Number of Quanta Emitted	Wavelength	Number of Quanta Absorbed		Number of Quanta Emitted	Wavelength	Number of Quanta Absorbed	
		M	**L**			**M**	**L**
300	λ_a	180	60	500	λ_b	200	300
300	λ_c	20	240				
TOTAL		200	300	TOTAL		200	300

FIGURE 5–5. By proper adjustment of the intensities of λ_a, λ_b, and λ_c, the two patches will appear identical. This is because they will have the exact same effect on this dichromat's visual system. Each patch produces 200 quantal absorptions by photopigment M and 300 by photopigment L.

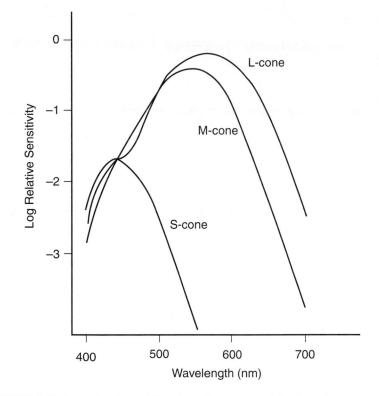

FIGURE 5–6. Approximations of the absorption spectra of the three human cones, based on the data of Smith and Pokorny (1975). (*From Boynton RM*. Human Color Vision. *New York: Holt, Rinehart, and Winston; 1979. Reprinted with permission of Dr. Boynton.*)

human trichromats is given in Fig. 5–6. These curves are based on data from a number of experimental approaches.

We will not perform a detailed analysis of a trichromat's wavelength discrimination abilities. It should, however, be apparent that we can extend those principles developed during our study of dichromacy to this situation. If we do so, we find that a trichromat shows wavelength discrimination that is superior to a dichromat, but still limited.

Let us formally define trichromacy. Given at least four wavelengths, divided into two patches, a person with trichromatic vision (a trichromat) is able to adjust the relative intensities of these wavelengths such that the two patches appear identical. An example is illustrated in Fig. 5–7. The two patches appear identical because they result in the same number of quantal absorptions by each of the three photopigments. They are metamers.

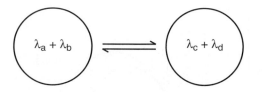

FIGURE 5–7. A trichromat is able to adjust the intensities of four wavelengths, divided into two patches, such that the two patches appear identical. These two patches, which are physically different but appear identical, are metamers.

Given three wavelengths, as illustrated in Fig. 5–5, a trichromat will not be able to create a match. Two patches that appear perfectly matched for a dichromat do not appear matched for a trichromat, demonstrating the trichromat's superior color discrimination. Given four wavelengths, however, a trichromat will be able to make a match, illustrating the limits of his or her ability to discriminate colors.

ABSORPTION SPECTRA OF THE CONE PHOTOPIGMENTS

The most direct measurements of the photopigment absorption spectra come from electrophysiological recordings of individual photoreceptors and molecular genetics. These data confirm and extend those obtained through other techniques such as color matching and retinal densitometry (see Chap. 3).

Electrophysiological Recordings

Membrane currents have been recorded from the outer segments of macaque monkey and human photoreceptors using an eyecup preparation in which the excised retina of an experimental animal or donated human eye is bathed in an enriched saline solution to maintain tissue viability (Schnapf and Baylor, 1987; Schnapf et al, 1987). A cone is isolated and exposed to monochromatic light, and the amount of energy required to elicit a criterion response is determined as a function of wavelength (Fig. 5–8). The reciprocal of this threshold function is the spectral sensitivity of the cone. The cone spectra obtained using this procedure are very similar to those derived through psychophysical matching experiments.

Molecular Genetics of Cone Photopigments

Each molecule of cone photopigment consists of the **chromophore** and an **opsin.** The chromophore, which is identical for all cone photopigments, is retinal, an aldehyde derivative of retinol (vitamin A). Light quanta are absorbed by the chromophore, initiating the series of events leading to vision (see Chap. 12). It is the opsin, a visually inert chain of amino acids that is

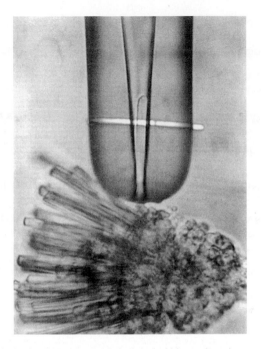

FIGURE 5–8. A single photoreceptor is isolated within a micropipette and exposed to monochromatic light (the white horizontal line). In this manner, the spectral sensitivity for a photoreceptor can be determined. This photograph shows the isolation of a rod, but the same principles apply to cones. (*From Schnapf JL, Baylor DA. How photoreceptors respond to light. Sci Am 1987;256:40–47. Reprinted with permission of authors.*)

interlaced into the disk membranes of the outer segment, that determines the absorption characteristics of the photopigment molecule. Each class of cones has a different opsin.

The genes that code for the opsins of the human photopigments have been identified and isolated with recombinant DNA techniques (Nathans et al, 1986b). For the M- and L-cones, the opsin genes were found on the X chromosome. This was not surprising because it has long been known that certain color vision deficiencies in which either the M- or L-cone photopigment is missing or altered (i.e., red-green color anomalies) are inherited in a sex-linked manner (see Chap. 6). The gene for the S-cone photopigment is located on chromosome 7, and the gene coding rhodopsin is found on chromosome 3.

The cone photopigment genes are homologous to the rhodopsin gene, suggesting that all four share the same ancestor (Fig. 5–9) (Nathans, 1986b). The M- and L-cone opsin genes are exceedingly similar to each other, showing a 98 percent homology (i.e., 98 percent of the DNA sequence is identical), suggesting that they evolved relatively recently. The homology of the S-cone opsin gene to the M- and L-cone opsin genes is 40 percent, indicating that it evolved earlier.

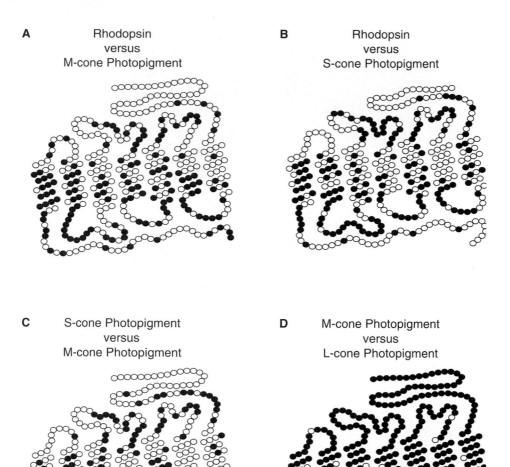

FIGURE 5–9. Comparison of amino acid sequences (deduced from nucleotide sequences) for **(A)** rhodopsin versus M-cone photopigment, **(B)** rhodopsin versus S-cone photopigment, **(C)** S-cone photopigment versus M-cone photopigment, and **(D)** M-cone photopigment versus L-cone photopigment. The closed circles represent amino acids that are the same in both photopigments, and the open circles represent amino acids that are different (Nathans et al, 1986b).

The X-chromosome typically has one copy of the L-cone opsin gene and one or more copies of the M-cone opsin gene. The presence of multiple copies of the M-cone opsin gene apparently does not affect color matching. The role of the extra copies is not understood at this time (Knau et al, 2002).

In a continuation of his pioneering work on the molecular genetics of color vision, Nathans determined the absorption spectra of human photopigments by transfecting tissue culture cells with the genes encoding the photopigments (Merbs and Nathans, 1992). The transfected cells produced the various human photopigments, and the absorption spectra of these pigments were then determined. The S- and M-cone photopigments peaked at 426 and 530 nm, respectively. Two variants of L-cone photopigments were found, with one peaking at 552 nm and the other at 557 nm. The finding of two L-cone photopigments was not surprising because it had been known for some time that people with normal color vision do not all show the same color matching data (Neitz and Jacobs, 1986).

GRASSMAN'S LAWS OF METAMERS

Grassman's laws of metamers describe the general characteristics of trichromatic vision (Fig. 5–10) (Grassman, 1854). These three laws follow from the previous discussion of the trichromatic theory. According to the **additive** property, when the same radiation is added in an identical manner to two metamers, they remain metamers. If they were perfectly matched before we added the new light, they are still matched following this addition.

Consider an example. Suppose that we have two patches of yellow light that appear identical to each other. One patch is monochromatic, say 570 nm, and the other patch is a mixture of 530, 560, and 600 nm. If we add an equal amount of 630 nm to each patch, they still appear identical to each other, but are now both orange. They remain metamers.

If the intensities of two metamers are increased (or decreased) by the same amount, they remain metamers—the so-called **scalar** property of metamers. Consider the two patches of yellow light just discussed. Each patch produces the same number of quantal absorptions in the three cones. If the intensities of the patches are increased by the same amount, each patch continues to result in the same numbers of absorptions as the other patch, thereby maintaining the metamerism. The patches will appear brighter, but still appear identical to one another.

Grassman's law regarding the **associative property** of metamers states that a match will be maintained if one metamer is substituted for another metamer. This makes sense when we consider that each metamer, by definition, has exactly the same effect on the visual system. Therefore, we are at liberty to substitute one metamer for another.

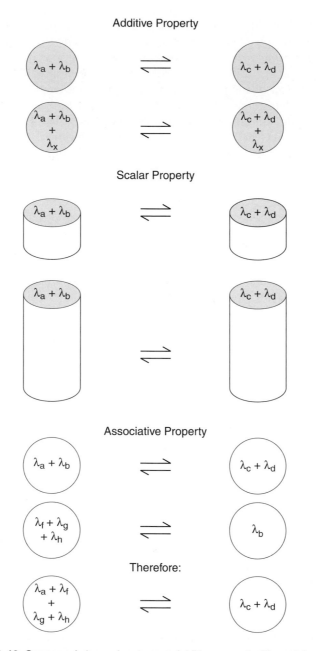

FIGURE 5–10. Grassman's laws of metamers. Additive property: The patches on the left and right side remain metamers after the addition of equal amounts of λ_x to each side. Scalar property: If the intensity of each side is increased by the same amount, the metamerism holds. Associative property: A metamer may be substituted for λ_b and the match still holds; the metamerism remains unchanged.

TABLE 5-1.   COLOR LABELS

	Hue	*Saturation*	*Brightness*
Definition	Layperson's term for color (i.e., blue, green, yellow, etc.)	Fullness or purity of color	Brightness
Physical stimulus	Wavelength (also intensity: Bezold-Brücke phenomenon)	Both wavelength and colorimetric purity (or excitation purity)	Radiance

COLOR LABELS

To say that a stimulus is, for example, blue is a rather incomplete description. Because there are many variants of blue, more detail is required. People who work in the field of color science often specify stimuli along three *perceptual* dimensions: hue, saturation, and brightness (Table 5–1). These perceptual attributes are not entirely independent of each other.

Hue

Hue is that perception most closely associated with wavelength. A stimulus of 540 nm has a hue of green, whereas a stimulus of 570 nm has a hue of yellow. Although it is common to use the terms color and hue interchangeably, color is a much broader term that includes hue, saturation, and brightness.

Desaturation and Saturation

A desaturated color *appears* as though it has been mixed with white; it does not look bold or full of color. Pastels are examples of desaturated colors. A saturated color, in comparison, appears to be full of color; it does not appear washed out like a desaturated color.

The perception of saturation is wavelength dependent, with a monochromatic stimulus of 570 nm appearing less saturated than a monochromatic stimulus of any other wavelength (Fig. 5–11) (Priest and Brickwedde, 1938; Kaiser et al, 1976).[2] Stated differently, unadulterated 570 nm appears to have white added to it, whereas other wavelengths appear more pure.

---

2. Stimuli consisting of a single wavelength are sometimes called monochromatic or spectral.

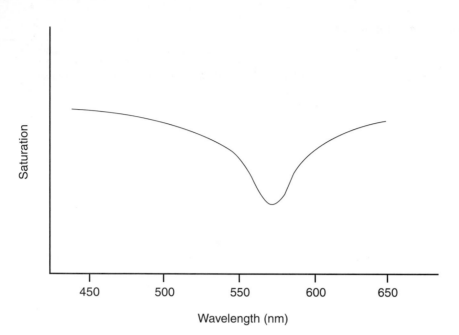

FIGURE 5–11. Saturation as a function of wavelength, showing that stimuli of 570 nm are less saturated than stimuli of other wavelengths (Wright, 1946).

Saturation is related to the physical property, **colorimetric purity** (*p*), by the following formula (Pokorny et al, 1979):

$$p = \frac{L_\lambda}{L_\lambda + L_w}$$

where

L_λ = luminance of the test wavelength

L_w = luminance of the white light that is combined
with the test wavelength

This relationship quantifies the amount of white that has been added to a wavelength and, therefore, gives us information regarding the saturation of the sample. If the sample is a pure spectral hue, with no white added, it has a colorimetric purity of 1. Keep in mind, however, that not all stimuli with a colorimetric purity of 1 appear equally saturated.

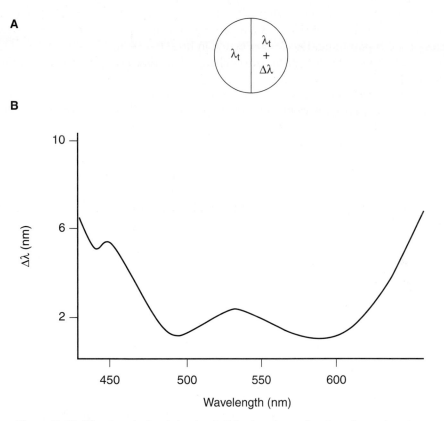

Figure 5–12. Wavelength discrimination (Δλ) is plotted as a function of wavelength. The upper figure **(A)** shows the stimulus conditions used to obtain the bottom graph. This graph **(B)** is an approximation (Pokorny and Smith, 1970).

Brightness

Brightness sensation closely follows the photopic luminance function (Wagner and Boynton, 1972). Under photopic conditions, a 555-nm stimulus is perceived as brighter than other equal energy monochromatic stimuli.[3]

WAVELENGTH DISCRIMINATION

The ability to distinguish one wavelength from another is better in some regions of the spectrum than in others (Wright, 1941; Pokorny and Smith, 1970). This can be demonstrated by using the stimulus configuration depicted in Fig. 5–12A. A

---

3. Although it is common to interchange the terms brightness and luminance, these terms have different definitions. As we learned in Chapter 4, the $V(\lambda)$ curve closely matches the sensation of brightness, but is not precisely the same function (Wagner and Boynton, 1972).

test wavelength, λ_t, is on the left side of a split field.[4] The right side is initially identical to the left, but then is changed by an amount, $\Delta\lambda$, such that the two sides of the bipartite field no longer match in hue. In essence, we determine how much a stimulus' wavelength must be changed so that it appears to be a different hue.[5]

The results of such an experiment are given in Fig. 5–12B. Because of its W-like shape, this curve is often referred to as the "W curve" of color discrimination. In the regions of best discrimination—at about 495 and 590 nm—two stimuli are different hues even if their wavelengths are just a few nanometers different. A stimulus of 490 nm, for example, may be distinguishable from 495 nm. However, a stimulus of 415 nm may be the same hue as 410 nm because hue discrimination is relatively poor in the short-wavelength region of the spectrum.

Why do wavelength discrimination thresholds vary across the spectrum? Although not settled, it may be that color discrimination is best where the slopes of the cone absorption spectra change most rapidly with respect to each other (see Fig. 5-6).

BEZOLD–BRÜCKE PHENOMENON

Most monochromatic stimuli show a slight change in hue as their intensity is adjusted. This is called the Bezold–Brücke phenomenon. To demonstrate it, an observer views a bipartite field with a variable wavelength, λ_v, on the left side and a control wavelength, λ_c, on the right (Fig. 5–13A). The right side, which remains constant throughout the experiment, is initially identical to λ_v. During the experiment, the intensity of λ_v is slowly increased. If its hue changes as the intensity increases, its wavelength is adjusted so that it continues to match the hue of λ_c.

Consider a greenish-yellow test wavelength of 550 nm. As the intensity of this wavelength is increased, it appears to be of a longer wavelength (i.e., it appears more yellowish). To maintain the initial hue appearance (greenish-yellow), it is necessary to reduce its wavelength. This is indicated in Fig. 5–13B by the line that starts at 550 nm and tilts toward shorter wavelengths as the intensity increases. All stimuli that fall on this line, referred to as a **hue contour line,** have the same hue (greenish-yellow).

Figure 5–13B displays hue contour lines for a number of different stimuli. Note that most of the lines are tilted. As the intensity of most monochromatic stimuli is increased (or decreased), the hue changes and, consequently, the wavelength must be changed to maintain a constant hue.

As indicated by the nontilted hue contour lines, three wavelengths do not change hue as their intensity is increased (see Fig. 5–13B) (Hurvich, 1981). These wavelengths—478, 503, and 578 nm—are referred to as **invariant wave-**

---

4. A split field is also called a bipartite field.

5. As the wavelength is changed, luminance is adjusted so that both sides of the bipartite field remain the same luminance. Therefore, only hue is varied as the wavelength is changed.

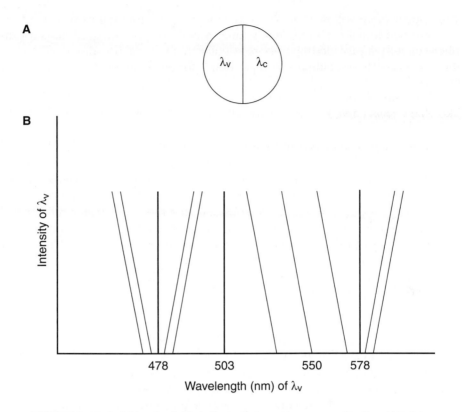

FIGURE 5–13. A. A bipartite field similar to that used to measure the Bezold-Brücke phenomenon. λ_v and λ_c initially have the same wavelength and equal intensity. As the intensity of λ_v is increased, its wavelength is adjusted to maintain a hue match with λ_c. **B.** Approximate results of such an experiment. Along each line, hue remains constant. These lines are referred to as hue contour lines. At the three invariant wavelengths (478, 503, and 578 nm), hue does not change as intensity is increased. This graph is an approximation (Hurvich and Jameson, 1955).

lengths, or **invariant points.** The hues associated with these wavelengths—blue at 478 nm, green at 503 nm, and yellow at 578 nm—are called **unique hues.** These hues look pure in that they do not appear to be mixed with another wavelength.

You may find the following simple rule useful: stimuli with a wavelength that is shorter than unique green (i.e., the violets, blues and greens below 503 nm) appear more blue as their intensity is increased, and stimuli longer than 503 nm appear more yellow as their intensity is increased. For example, a stimulus of 450 nm (initially violet) becomes bluish as its intensity is increased. To maintain the original violet hue, its wavelength must be decreased. Therefore, the hue contour line tilts to the left (see Fig. 5-13B). A stimulus of 585 nm (yellow-orange) will appear more yellow as its intensity is increased, requiring its wavelength to be increased to maintain the original hue. A possible physiological basis for this phenomenon is provided by opponent color theory, which is discussed later in this chapter. (Also, see discussion question 7 for this chapter.)

COLOR CONSTANCY

Consider a shirt with a colorful pattern. Whether viewed indoors under incandescent light or outdoors in natural sunlight, the shirt's colors appear almost the same. Even when viewed under a colored light, the shirt's appearance is surprisingly similar to its appearance under more natural conditions. This is an interesting phenomenon when one considers that the wavelengths reflected off the shirt are considerably different under the various lighting conditions. Color constancy refers to the approximately constant color appearance of objects as lighting conditions change (Land, 1964).

Color constancy assists us in identifying objects as lighting conditions vary. The world would be rather confusing if the color properties of objects changed dramatically as the lighting conditions varied. It is advantageous that an apricot appears approximately the same color both indoors and outdoors, and at various times of the day. The physiological basis for color constancy has not been fully elucidated (Zeki, 1993).

Color constancy is not absolute. As lighting conditions change, there are subtle, but important, changes in color appearance. When viewing a natural landscape, for instance, lighting conditions provide a cue that allows us to gauge the time of day (Zaidi, 1997).

PHYSIOLOGICAL BASIS OF COLOR VISION

Opponent Color Theory

Toward the end of the 19th century, a German physiologist, Ewald Hering, made a number of astute and important observations regarding the perception of colors (Hering, 1920/1964). He noted that red and green are not seen simultaneously, and the color label red–green is not used. Colors are either red or green, but not both. The same holds true for blue and yellow. These two hues are not seen in the same location and we do not use the color label blue–yellow. Hering also observed that a chromatic stimulus elicits an afterimage that is of a complementary color. For instance, a red stimulus elicits a green afterimage and a blue stimulus elicits a yellow afterimage.

These and similar observations led Hering to propose the opponent color vision theory, which posits that color is processed by bipolar hue channels referred to as the red–green and blue–yellow channels. By bipolar, it is meant that at any given instant the channel can signal only one of the two attributes it is capable of coding. For example, the red–green channel is capable of signaling only red or green but not both red and green simultaneously. The same is true of the blue–yellow channel—only blueness or yellowness is encoded, not both simultaneously. Hering also hypothesized that brightness is coded by a separate white–black channel.

For quite some time, Hering's theory was not considered seriously because he incorrectly suggested that a substance is present within the visual system that could signal either green or red, and another substance that could signal either blue or yellow. Even with the primitive understanding of physiology that existed in the 19th century, this was considered unrealistic. Moreover, the trichromatic theory, which was accepted by many of the great scientists of the time, explained much of what was known about color perception. It certainly was sufficient to explain color-matching data. Through the first half of the 20th century, many thought that the trichromatic and the opponent color theories were not compatible. As it turns out, both are true in their most fundamental aspects.

Quantitative data in support of color opponency comes from hue cancellation experiments (Hurvich, 1981). For a sample wavelength, the observer adjusts the amount of red or green *and* blue or yellow that is necessary to cancel the hue sensation produced by the sample wavelength. By cancel, we mean that hue (red or green *and* blue or yellow) is added to the sample until it turns white. This procedure, when repeated for many wavelengths across the visible spectrum, can be used to derive opponent color functions similar to those in Fig. 5–14, which shows the red–green and blue–yellow channels. Also plotted is the sensitivity of the proposed brightness channel, which has a shape very similar to the photopic luminosity function.

According to the opponent-color theory, the perception of color can be explained by the relative activity of the red–green, blue–yellow, and brightness channels. The model correctly predicts the locations of the unique hues, which are located at the crossover points of the red–green and blue–yellow channels (locate these in Fig. 5–14). At these points (e.g., 578 nm), only one of the two channels is active, resulting in the perception of a "pure" hue (e.g., yellow).

Electrophysiological Evidence for Color Opponency

Opponent color processing was placed on firm ground when Svaetichin (1956), using single-unit electrophysiological techniques, discovered horizontal cells in the fish retina that are activated by certain wavelengths of light and inhibited by others, a form of color opponency. Subsequently, color opponent cells were found in the primate retina and dorsal lateral geniculate nucleus (DeValois et al, 1966; Weisel and Hubel, 1966; Gouras, 1968).

In electrophysiological experiments, a visual neuron is isolated and its electrical activity recorded. When studying color vision, these experiments typically

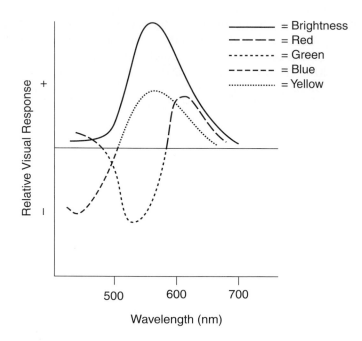

FIGURE 5–14. Approximations of the red–green, blue–yellow, and brightness channels proposed by Hurvich and Jameson (Hurvich and Jameson, 1955).

involve Old World monkeys (e.g., rhesus) because their color vision is exceedingly similar to humans. The fovea of the anesthetized animal is aligned with the fixation point "F" on a screen (see Fig. 5–15). A microelectrode capable of recording action potentials is inserted into the primate's dLGN (or retina), and a single cell is isolated.

To assess a neuron's color-coding capabilities, its receptive field[6] is exposed systematically to equal energy spectral stimuli. The neuron's response, as measured by its frequency of action potentials, is plotted as a function of wavelength. For the neuron in Fig. 5–16A, short-wavelength stimuli (below 570 nm) cause inhibition (a decreased firing rate of the cell), while long-wavelength stimuli (longer than 570 nm) produce excitation (an increased rate of neural firing). As this cell responds to one portion of the spectrum with excitation and another portion with inhibition, it is referred to as a **color opponent,** or spectrally opponent, neuron.

This cell has color-coding capabilities. If we are told that the neuron is excited by a stimulus, we know that the stimulus must be a long wavelength. Likewise, if the cell is inhibited by a stimulus, we can assume that the stimulus is a relatively short wavelength.

---

6. As discussed in Chapter 12, a neuron's receptive field is that area in visual space that influences the activity of the neuron.

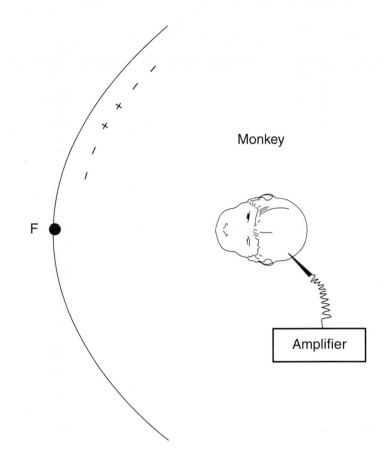

FIGURE 5–15. Basic setup for recording activity from an isolated neuron. The animal's fovea is aligned with the fixation point *F*. A microelectrode records the electrical activity of a single neuron, and this signal is amplified and recorded.

In addition to color opponent neurons, DeValois et al (1966) found another class of neurons that are **noncolor opponent.** An example of the spectral sensitivity of such a neuron is given in Fig. 5–16B. Note that it is not inhibited by any wavelength and responds to all spectral stimuli with excitation. This neuron does not have color-coding capabilities; it is monochromatic. Recall that a monochromat can adjust the intensities of any two wavelengths so that they appear identical. The same principle applies to this noncolor opponent neuron. By observing Fig. 5–16B, we see that a stimulus of 555 nm will produce more of an excitatory response than an equal-energy stimulus of 620 nm. If we were to increase the intensity of the 620-nm stimulus, however, we could increase the neuron's response such that it equals that produced by the 555-nm stimulus. Under these conditions, the neuron would not be able to distinguish between the two stimuli.

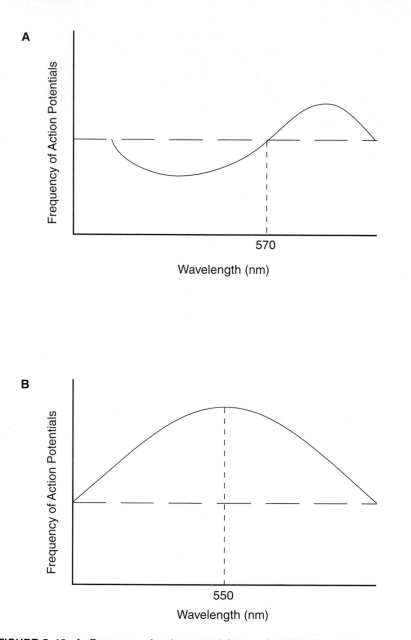

FIGURE 5–16. A. Frequency of action potentials as a function of wavelength for a color opponent neuron. Wavelengths below 570 nm cause a reduction in the frequency of action potentials, whereas longer wavelengths cause an increased rate of firing. **B.** Frequency of action potentials, as a function of wavelength for a noncolor opponent neuron. All wavelengths result in an increased frequency of action potentials. (These figures are schematics.)

The spectral sensitivity function for a typical noncolor opponent neuron has a broad peak in the midspectral region, at about 555 nm. This has led some scientists to conclude that it represents the addition of M- and L-cone inputs.

Modern Models of Color Vision

Thus far in our discussion of the physiology of color vision we established two facts: (1) color vision is normally trichromatic, and (2) opponent processing plays a critical role in coding color information. At first glance, it may appear that these two facts are incompatible, but this is not the case.

Trichromacy tells us that three classes of cones are sufficient to explain color-matching data. It does not, however, address the manner in which this information is encoded by the nervous system.

The presence of color opponent neurons in the retina and dLGN reveals that receptoral information (trichromacy) is encoded in an opponent fashion at postreceptoral levels. The three classes of cones are "wired" together to produce spectrally opponent neurons. This postreceptoral antagonism first occurs very early in the retina, at the level of the horizontal cells.

The recoding of trichromatic information in terms of color opponency is illustrated schematically in Fig. 5–17. L- and M-cones oppose each other to produce L-M opponent cells. These cells have spectral sensitivities similar to that illustrated in Fig. 5-16A. S-cones are opposed by an addition of L- and M-cones to produce S-(L+M) opponent cells.[7] The model in Fig. 5–17 also shows noncolor opponent cells, which sum the input of L- and M-cones, and are sometimes labeled L+M cells. Spectral sensitivity for a noncolor opponent cell is given in Fig. 5-16B.

Some investigators argue that the L-M and S-(L+M) cells are exclusively devoted to coding hue, and have no role in coding brightness information. In this view, the coding of brightness is performed by the noncolor opponent cells (Lee et al, 1988; Shapley, 1990). Saturation is coded by the ratio of activity of the opponent color to noncolor opponent cells.

Other researchers, however, believe that both hue and brightness are coded by the same cells (Ingling and Martinez-Uriegas, 1983; Kelly, 1983; Lennie, 1984; Derrington et al, 1984; Shapley, 1990). In this formulation, sometimes referred to as the "double-duty hypothesis," opponent color neurons do double-duty by coding both hue and brightness information.[8]

---

7. The L-M neurons are sometimes called red-green opponent cells, while the S-(L+M) neurons are called blue-yellow opponent cells.

8. The double-duty hypothesis does not rule out the possibility that luminance–not brightness—is coded by noncolor opponent neurons.

Cones

Bipolar Cells

Bipolar Cell
Receptive Fields

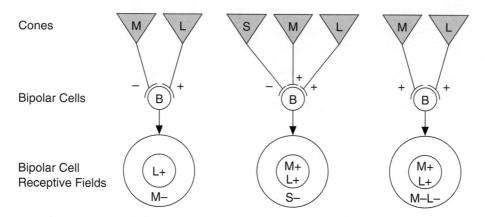

FIGURE 5–17. Simplified model of color processing. For clarity, contributions of horizontal cells are not shown. Inhibitory synapses are indicated by minus signs, and excitatory synapses by plus signs. The two columns on the left show the construction of color-opponent neurons, while the column on the right is for a noncolor-opponent neuron. For the noncolor-opponent cell, the inhibitory contributions to the receptive field surround are not illustrated. Receptive fields are discussed in Chapter 12. See text for further details.

As briefly discussed in Chapter 2, the retinocortical visual projection is organized along at least three major pathways: the parvo, magno, and konio pathways.[9] The neurons that constitute these three pathways manifest differences in the processing of color information, as well as detail and motion information. Of particular relevance to the current discussion is that parvo and konio cells tend to be color opponent, whereas magno cells are noncolor opponent (or weakly color opponent).

In summary, primate color vision is trichromatic, with the trichromatic signal encoded in an opponent fashion. This opponent processing may occur very early in the visual system, at the level of the horizontal cells. Although it is established that hue information is encoded by color opponent (parvo and konio) neurons, it is not clear whether brightness information is encoded by these neurons or by a separate class of noncolor opponent (magno) cells.

MUNSELL COLOR APPEARANCE SYSTEM

The ability to verbally describe color does not match our superior ability to perceive fine gradations in color. Suppose that a small area of your yellow living room wall needs to be repainted, and you would like the replacement paint to match the original color. Although this task may seem simple, anyone who has

---

9. The parvo and magno pathways are discussed in detail in Chapter 13.

attempted it will tell you otherwise. Because we are so good at discriminating colors, it is very difficult to find a perfect match. We could do our best to describe the color of the original paint to a salesperson, but without showing him or her an actual sample, it would be virtually impossible to find an acceptable match. There are hundreds of yellows that vary in hue, saturation, and brightness.

The Munsell color appearance system allows us to describe colors with a great deal of specificity along three physical dimensions: hue, chroma, and value (Boynton, 1979; Pokorny et al, 1979; Wyszecki and Stiles, 1982). **Hue** is related to the wavelength of the stimulus. **Chroma** can be thought of as being akin to colorimetric purity and is related to the saturation of the color sample. **Value** refers to the reflectance of the sample and is related to brightness.

The Munsell system can be conceptualized as a cylinder containing various color samples (Fig. 5–18). Hue varies continuously along the perimeter of the cylinder, with the primary hues being red, yellow, green, blue, and purple. These are further subdivided into intermediaries. Chroma is measured as a radius from the center of the cylinder and ranges from 1 to 14, with 14 denoting the highest purity. Value increases along the vertical dimension, with 0 indicating the least reflectance and 10 the most. In practical application, the Munsell system is laid out in a book, with each page containing a number of samples, all of the same hue. These samples are referred to as **Munsell chips.** In the case of the yellow paint we discussed earlier, the original paint color may specified by the hue, chroma, and value that correspond to a particular Munsell chip.

CIE COLOR SPECIFICATION SYSTEM

The CIE color specification system is based on the trichromacy of vision: a color is specified by the relative amounts of three primaries, which when mixed together, produce the color (Boynton, 1979; Pokorny et al, 1979; Hurvich, 1981; Wyszecki and Stiles, 1982). The CIE system can be challenging conceptually because the CIE primaries are not real, but are imaginary. They represent a mathematical transformation of real primaries. This conversion is performed to avoid specifying negative quantities of primaries.

R,G,B System

To understand the CIE system, first consider the **R,G,B** system of color specification. As illustrated in Fig. 5–19A, the wavelength to be matched (λ_v) is placed on one side of a bipartite field. On the other side are the red, green, and blue primaries: λ_r (645 nm), λ_g (526 nm), and λ_b (444 nm). The amounts of these three primaries are adjusted until a perfect match between the two sides of the field is obtained.

When this procedure is repeated for each wavelength, across the spectrum, we obtain **color matching functions,** which are illustrated in Fig. 5–19B. These color-matching functions show the amount of each primary required to match a

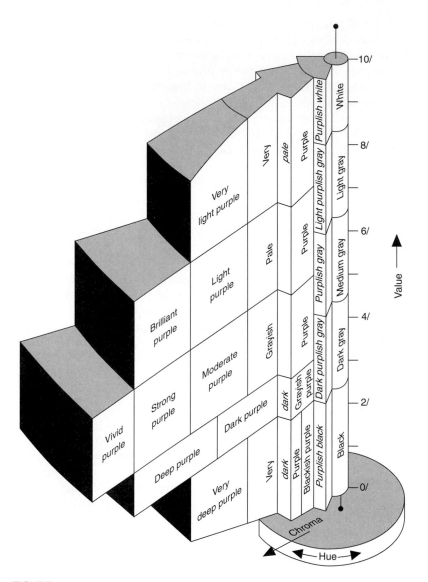

FIGURE 5–18. The Munsell color appearance system. Hue is specified along the perimeter of a cylinder, chroma as a radius from the center of the cylinder, and value as the vertical dimension of the cylinder. (From *Judd DB, Wyszecki G. Color in Business, Science, and Industry. Copyright © 1963. Reprinted by permission of John Wiley & Sons, Inc.*)

given wavelength. The quantity of each primary required for a match is referred to as the **tristimulus value.**

Note that for wavelengths in the region 450 to 550 nm, negative amounts of λ_r are required to obtain a match. This means that the required amount of λ_r must be added to λ_v, rather than to the mixture field, to obtain a match. No matter

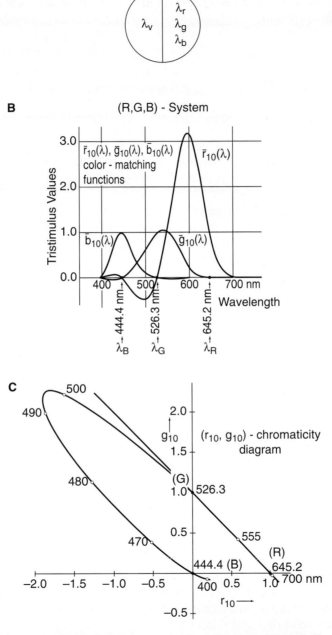

FIGURE 5–19. A. In the **R, G, B** system, a given wavelength, λ_v, is specified by the relative amounts of the three primaries (λ_r, λ_g, λ_b) required to match it. **B.** Color matching functions for the **R, G, B** system. Note that negative quantities of the primary **R** are required over much of the spectrum. **C.** Chromaticity diagram for the **R, G, B** system. (*From Wyszecki G, Stiles WS. Color Science: Concepts and Methods, Quantitative Data and Formulae. Copyright © 1982. Reprinted by permission of John Wiley & Sons, Inc.*)

which real primaries are chosen to generate matching functions, there will always be some regions of negative quantities. The CIE system was designed to overcome this problem.

Imaginary Primaries

Using matrix algebra, it is possible to transform one set of color matching functions into another. For the CIE system, the **R,G,B** matching functions are mathematically transformed into matching functions for three imaginary primaries called **X**, **Y**, and **Z**. These are given in Fig. 5–20A.[10] Note that all wavelengths can be matched with positive quantities of these primaries. It is not necessary to use negative quantities.

The **CIE chromaticity diagram** (see Fig. 5–20B) shows the relative amounts of the imaginary primaries required to match any real color. This chromaticity diagram is constructed by converting the tristimulus values to relative units, referred to as **chromaticity coordinates.**

The tristimulus values are given by uppercase letters, whereas the chromaticity coordinates are given in lowercase letters. The following equations show the relationship between the tristimulus values and the chromaticity coordinates:

$$x = \frac{X}{X + Y + Z}$$

$$y = \frac{Y}{X + Y + Z}$$

$$z = \frac{Z}{X + Y + Z}$$

where

$$x + y + z = 1$$

The sum of the chromaticity coordinates must equal 1. Therefore, if two of the coordinates are known, we can calculate the third. The chromaticity diagram shows only the x and y chromaticity coordinates. Coordinate z is calculated by subtracting the sum of x and y from 1.

---

10. The matching function for primary Y has the same form as the photopic luminance function.

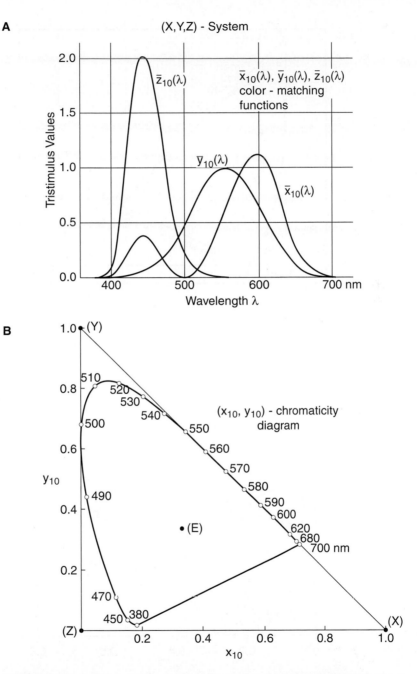

FIGURE 5–20. **A.** Color matching functions for the imaginary primaries **X, Y, Z**, which are mathematical transformations of the **R, G, B** primaries. **B.** Chromaticity diagram for this system. This diagram is commonly referred to as the CIE chromaticity diagram. (*From Wyszecki G, Stiles WS*. Color Science: Concepts and Methods, Quantitative Data and Formulae. *Copyright © 1982. Reprinted by permission of John Wiley & Sons, Inc.*)

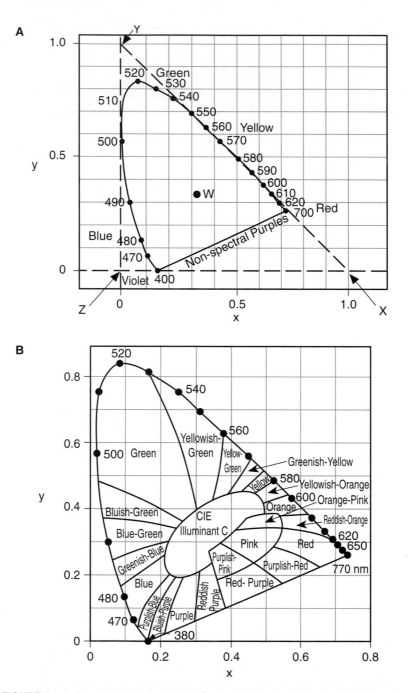

FIGURE 5–21. **A.** An approximation of the CIE chromaticity diagram. All physically realizable colors fall along the perimeter of this diagram, or within the diagram. The imaginary primaries (*X, Y, Z*) fall outside the diagram. **B.** Color labels applied to various regions of the CIE chromaticity diagram. (*From Judd DB.* Color in Business, Science, and Industry. *Copyright © 1952. Reprinted by permission of John Wiley and Sons, Inc.*)

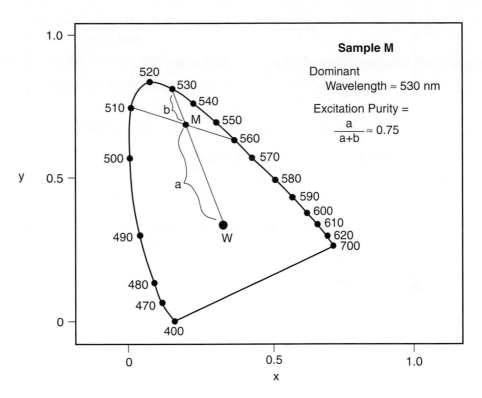

FIGURE 5–22. Equal amounts of 510 and 560 nm are combined to form a mixture, *M*. This mixture has a dominant wavelength of 530 nm and an excitation purity of 0.75.

Basic Attributes of the CIE Chromaticity Diagram

Contained within the CIE chromaticity diagram are all physically realizable colors (Fig. 5–21). Note that the imaginary primaries themselves (points *X, Y,* and *Z*) fall outside of the diagram because they are not physically realizable.

Spectral hues (monochromatic hues) are arranged along the arc of the perimeter of the diagram, which is referred to as the **spectral locus**. Nonspectral purples fall along the straight line connecting 400 and 700 nm. (Purples are not produced by a single wavelength but by mixtures of blue and red.) White falls in the center of the diagram and is indicated by *W*.[11]

Calculations

As we will learn in Chapter 6, the CIE diagram is invaluable for understanding defective color vision. It is also useful for calculating color mixtures. As indicated in Fig. 5-22, if we wish to mix equal amounts of 510 and 560 nm, we connect

---

11. Although white is designated as single point in Fig. 5-21, there are actually many variants of white, each with a different color temperature.

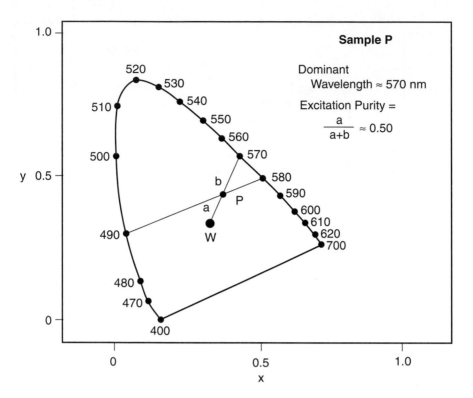

FIGURE 5–23. A mixture of three parts of 580 nm to one part of 490 nm produces a mixture, *P*. The dominant wavelength of this mixture is 570 nm, and the excitation purity is 0.50.

these two points with a line. The resultant mixture falls at the midpoint of this line, represented by the letter *M*. To specify this mixture, we connect point *M* with point *W*, which represents white, and extend the line to the perimeter of the diagram. In this case, it intersects 530 nm, which is referred to as the **dominant wavelength.**

The relative distance of the sample along the line that connects *W* to the perimeter of the CIE diagram is a measure of its colorimetric purity, and is referred to as the **excitation purity.** The excitation purity of sample *M* is given by $a/(a + b) = 0.75$.

Take another example. In this case, we mix 490 nm with 580 nm, such that there is three times more 580 nm than 490 nm. Figure 5–23 shows the determination of the dominant wavelength and excitation purity for this mixture. The first step is to connect 490 and 580 nm. The mixture point is three fourths of the way from 490 to 580 nm because of the relative amounts of these two wavelengths. Connecting this point with white gives us a dominant wavelength of 570 nm and an excitation purity of 0.50.

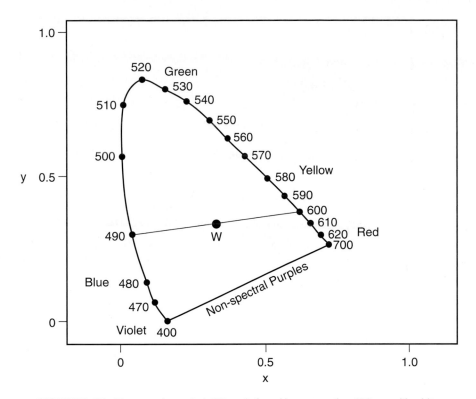

FIGURE 5–24. The complement of 490 nm is found by connecting 490 nm with white and extending this line to the opposite perimeter of the CIE diagram. This gives the complement of 490 nm as 600 nm.

The CIE diagram is useful for ascertaining a color's complement. **Complementary colors,** when mixed together, produce white. To determine the complement for a given wavelength, simply connect the wavelength, through white, to the opposite side of the CIE diagram (Fig. 5–24). In this case, we show that the complement of 490 is 600 nm. These two wavelengths, when mixed together, produce white.

Where Is White in the CIE Chromaticity Diagram?

Up to this point, we have assumed that white is a single point within the CIE diagram. From the discussion of color temperature in Chapter 4, however, it is clear that no single spectral distribution has exclusive claim to the label white. Indeed, the standard illuminants A, C, D_{65}, and so forth are all variants of white.

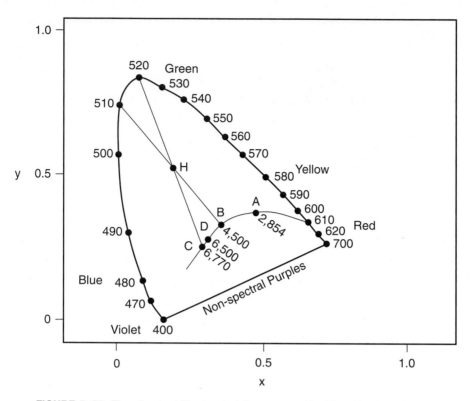

FIGURE 5–25. The standard illuminants fall on an arc (the Planckian locus) within the CIE diagram. The sample H can be made by combining 510 nm with illuminant B or by combining 520 nm with illuminant *C*.

Sources of various color temperatures form an arc within the CIE diagram, referred to as the **Planckian locus** (Fig. 5–25). The samples that fall on this locus, including the various standard illuminants, can be considered to be variants of white.[12]

Summary of the CIE Color Specification System

The CIE system can be one of the more challenging topics in vision science. If you are having difficulty understanding this material, do not feel alone. Countless others have struggled to comprehend this highly theoretical system.

---

12. An illuminant with a lower color temperature (e.g., illuminant A) appears reddish-white, while an illuminant with a higher color temperature (e.g., illuminant C) appears bluish-white.

Keep in mind the following:

1. The CIE diagram specifies the relative amounts of primaries necessary to match a color sample.
2. The CIE primaries do not really exist—they are imaginary.
3. The CIE system uses imaginary primaries to avoid the use of negative quantities.
4. Any set of color matching functions, real or imaginary, can be converted to another set of real or imaginary functions.

Now, go back to the beginning of this section on the CIE diagram and try it again. It is easier the second time through!

SUMMARY

It is firmly established that normal human vision is trichromatic. This trichromatic information is encoded in a color opponent fashion by postreceptoral visual neurons.

Color is perceived along the perceptual dimensions of hue, saturation, and brightness. Because of the ability to make fine color discriminations, sophisticated color appearance and color specification systems have been devised.

Knowledge of color vision physiology has facilitated the development of psychophysical tests to aid in the diagnosis and management of certain eye diseases. The role of color vision in the assessment of eye disease is discussed in the following chapter on defective color vision.

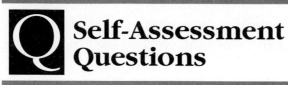

Self-Assessment Questions

1. A monochromat puts on a pair of red sunglasses. With these glasses on, will this individual behave as a monochromat or a dichromat? Explain.

2. A. What is the dominant wavelength of a mixture that consists of 60 percent of 490 nm and 40 percent of 540 nm? B. What is the excitation purity of this mixture? C. What is the complement to this mixture? (When making these calculations, do so with respect to illuminant C in Fig. 5–25.)

3. Answer all questions asked in question 2 for a mixture of one third of 490 nm and two thirds of 610 nm.

4. Note that illuminant D65 lies closer to the blue corner of the CIE diagram than illuminant A, which lies closer to the red corner of the diagram. Discuss this in terms of the color temperatures and chromatic appearances of these two illuminants.

5. A. How is it possible that a painter can match all hues with the use of only three primary colors? B. What is a limitation of using only three primaries for painting? Explain.

6. Hunters sometimes wear camouflaged clothing. Devise an instrument that would enable you to distinguish a camouflaged hunter from the natural background.

7. It has been mentioned that the Bezold–Brücke phenomenon could be explained by opponent color theory. Provide such an explanation. (Hint: Why do certain wavelengths change hue with increasing intensity, while others do not?)

6

Anomalies of Color Vision

Approximately 4.5 percent of the population manifest defective color vision (Pokorny et al, 1979). Most prevalent are **inherited defects,** which are nonprogressive and pose no threat to vision, but may have a profound effect on the performance of certain visually related activities, including those encountered at school and on the job.

Color vision anomalies that are not inherited are referred to as **acquired defects.** Less prevalent than hereditary defects, they are secondary to disease or drug toxicity, and can be an important diagnostic tool.

In this chapter, we discuss the classification and characteristics of the various anomalies of color vision. Clinical testing procedures are presented along with recommendations for the management of these frequently encountered conditions.

BASIC CLASSIFICATION

Table 6–1 provides a basic classification of color vision defects, showing a division into two general categories: **dichromacy** and **anomalous trichromacy.** Dichromats are missing one of the three retinal photopigments (Rushton, 1963a,b; 1965b). A **deuteranope** is missing chlorolabe, a **protanope** is missing erythrolabe, and a **tritanope** is missing cyanolabe. The missing photopigment is presumably replaced by a remaining photopigment. In the case of a deuteranope,

TABLE 6–1. BASIC CLASSIFICATION OF COLOR VISION DEFICIENCIES

| Photopigment Status | Red–Green Defects | | Blue–Yellow Defects |
	Protan Defect	Deutan Defect	Tritan Defect
Dichromat	Protanope (protanopia)	Deuteranope (deuteranopia)	Tritanope (tritanopia)
Anomalous trichromat	Protanomalous trichromat (protanomaly)	Deuteranomalous trichromat (deuteranomaly)	Tritanomalous trichromat (tritanomaly)

chlorolabe is replaced by erythrolabe. In a protanope, erythrolabe is replaced by chlorolabe. This is referred to as the **replacement model** of dichromacy.[1]

The replacement of the missing photopigment by a remaining photopigment is consistent with the normal resolution acuities of dichromats. If the M- or L-cones were simply missing, rather than replaced, dichromats would probably manifest clinically measurable reductions in visual acuity.

Anomalous trichromats have three photopigments, but the absorption spectrum of one of these photopigments is displaced to an abnormal position (Alpern and Torii, 1968a,b; Alpern and Moeller, 1977; Alpern and Wake, 1977). This is illustrated in Fig. 6–1. A **deuteranomalous trichromat** manifests a displacement of the chlorolabe spectrum toward longer wavelengths, whereas a **protanomalous trichromat** shows displacement of the erythrolabe spectrum toward shorter wavelengths.[2] These displacements of the cone photopigments from their optimal positions result in deficient color discrimination.

In the classification scheme in Table 6–1, the terms **protan, deutan,** and **tritan** refer to the affected photopigment. An individual who falls into one of these three categories is either a dichromat or an anomalous trichromat. For instance, a protan may be either a protanope or a protanomalous trichromat. If the erythrolabe is missing, the patient is a dichromat—a protanope. If the photopigment absorption spectrum is displaced, he or she is an anomalous trichomat—a protanomalous trichromat. Likewise, a deutan has a defect of chlorolabe such that she or he is either a deuteranope or a deuteranomalous trichromat.

Protans and deutans tend to confuse reds and greens, and are said to have a **red–green defect.** These defects are usually, but not always, inherited. Tritans, who confuse blues and yellows, are classified as having a **blue–yellow defect.** Such defects are almost always acquired.

---

1. The replacement hypothesis applies to protanopia and deuteranopia, not tritanopia.

2. Neitz and Neitz (2000) proposed that the abnormal photopigment found in an anomalous trichromat should be considered a variant of the remaining normal photopigment. In this view, a deuteranomalous trichromat has two forms of erythrolabe (rather than erythrolabe and a variant of chlorolabe). Likewise, they argue that a protanomalous trichromat has two types of chlorolabe (rather than chlorolabe and a variant of erythrolabe).

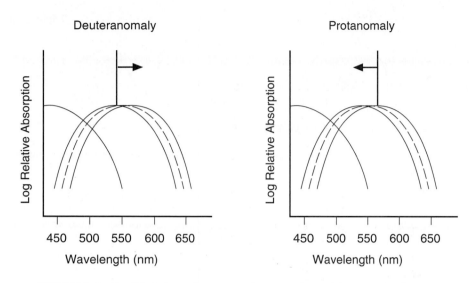

FIGURE 6–1. Simplified absorption spectra for anomalous trichromacy. In deutera-nomaly, the M-cone spectrum is displaced toward long wavelengths, and in protanomaly the L-cone spectrum is displaced toward short wavelengths. The solid curves show the normal positions of the cone absorption spectra, and the dashed curves show the locations of the displaced spectra.

BASIC DATA OF COLOR DEFICIENCY

People with anomalous color vision process chromatic information differently than individuals with normal color vision. Among the characteristics that distinquish anomalous color vision are spectral sensitivity, wavelength discrimination, color confusion lines, and the perception of saturation. The discussion that follows emphasizes data for inherited protan and deutan defects because these defects are common and well documented. Inherited tritan defects are extremely rare, making fewer data available.[3]

Spectral Sensitivity: Chromatic System

The color-opponent, or chromatic, system can be identified in human subjects by determining spectral sensitivity for large stimuli of long duration flashed on a photopic white background.[4] The stimulus configuration and results of such an experiment are given in Fig. 6–2.

---

3. Data are not provided for acquired defects because of the variable nature of these defects leads to inconsistent data.

4. To isolate the chromatic system, the monochromatic increments should be large (1 degree) and of long duration (200 msec), and the background moderately bright (1,000 trolands) (Sperling and Harwerth, 1971; King-Smith and Carden, 1976).

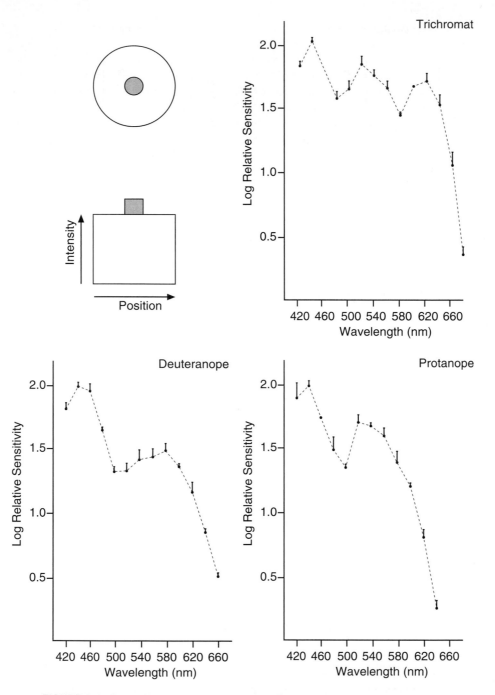

FIGURE 6–2. Chromatic increment spectral sensitivity functions for a normal trichromat, deuteranope, and protanope. Stimulus conditions are given in the upper left. (*Adapted from Schwartz SH. Spectral sensitivity of dichromats: role of postreceptoral processes.* Vision Res. *1994;34:2983–2990.*)

A normal trichromat shows a color-opponent spectral sensitivity function with three peaks (Sperling and Harwerth, 1971; King-Smith and Carden, 1976). The 440-nm peak corresponds to cyanolabe maximum absorption. The peaks at 520 and 620 nm presumably result from a subtractive, or opponent, interaction between the M- and L-cones, causing these peaks to be displaced from the absorption maxima of chlorolabe and erythrolabe (530 and 557 nm, respectively).

A strikingly different result is obtained when the experiment is repeated on dichromatic subjects (Verriest and Uvijls, 1977; Schwartz, 1994). A deuteranope shows only two peaks, corresponding to the remaining two photopigments, cyanolabe and erythrolabe. Likewise, a protanope manifests two peaks, one for cyanolabe and one for chlorolabe.

Spectral Sensitivity: Luminance Function

Figure 6–3 shows $V(\lambda)$ (photopic luminance) functions for normal trichromacy, deuteranopia, and protanopia. As we learned, the $V(\lambda)$ function of normal trichromats has a broad peak in the region of 555 nm. Dichromats, particularly

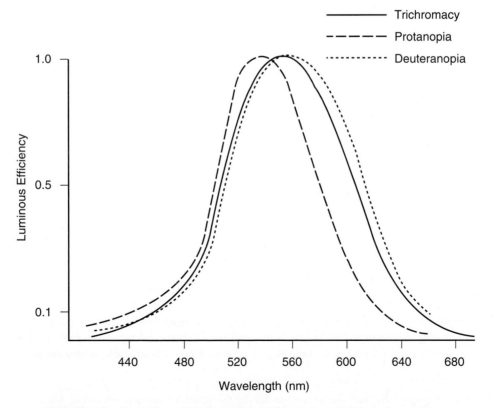

FIGURE 6–3. Photopic luminance functions, $V(\lambda)$, for normal trichromacy, deuteranopia, and protanopia (Hsia and Graham, 1957).

protanopes, manifest luminance functions that differ from this normal $V(\lambda)$ function (Hsia and Graham, 1957). The protanopic $V(\lambda)$ curve is substantially displaced toward shorter wavelengths, whereas the $V(\lambda)$ curve of deuteranopes shows a very slight displacement toward longer wavelengths. The displacement of the deuteranopic luminosity function is minimal, and for clinical purposes it may be considered normal.

The $V(\lambda)$ function of a normal trichromat presumably results from the addition of M- and L-cone inputs (see Chap. 3). Consequently, the absence of one of these cone types, as occurs in dichromacy, produces a displacement of the $V(\lambda)$ curve.[5] The absence of erythrolabe (protanopia) causes the luminance curve to be displaced toward shorter wavelengths, and the absence of chlorolabe (deuteranopia) causes the $V(\lambda)$ function to be displaced toward longer wavelengths. The greater dislocation of the luminance function in protanopia suggests that L-cones play more of a role in generating the normal $V(\lambda)$ function than do M-cones.

Because of the displacement of the protanopic $V(\lambda)$ function toward shorter wavelengths, these individuals may find it difficult to see certain red objects. This can be demonstrated in the laboratory by projecting a beam of 660-nm light (or a red laser) onto a screen. Whereas this stimulus is easily seen as a bright red spot by an observer with normal vision, it is invisible (or nearly invisible) to a protanope. Because erythrolabe is absent, the 660-nm quanta of light are simply not absorbed.

The luminosity functions of anomalous trichromats manifest the same general dislocation as dichromatic functions, but less pronounced. Protanomalous trichromats show displacement of the luminosity function toward shorter wavelengths, but less so than protanopes. Deuteranomalous trichromats manifest very minimal displacement of the luminosity function toward longer wavelengths; this displacement is even less than that found in deuteranopes.

Wavelength Discrimination

Figure 6–4A shows wavelength discrimination functions for normal, deuteranopic, and protanopic observers. Both protanopes and deuteranopes show relatively well-developed wavelength discrimination in the region of 490 nm, but at longer wavelengths—beyond about 545 nm—are not able to discriminate between stimuli on the basis of wavelength differences alone (Pitt, 1935; Wright, 1946).

As illustrated in Fig. 6–5, deuteranopes and protanopes have only one cone photopigment that absorbs beyond 545 nm, and thus behave as monochromats in this region of the spectrum. Nonetheless, red–green dichromats are able to discriminate

---

5. Since S-cones make little or no contribution to the photopic luminance function, tritans are
   expected to have a normal function.

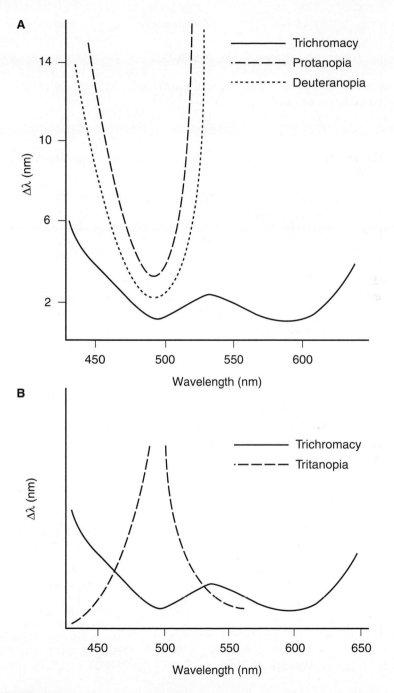

FIGURE 6–4. Wavelength discrimination functions for **(A)** deuteranopia and protanopia (Pitt, 1935) and **(B)** tritanopia (Wright, 1952). The solid curves represent wavelength discrimination for a normal trichromat.

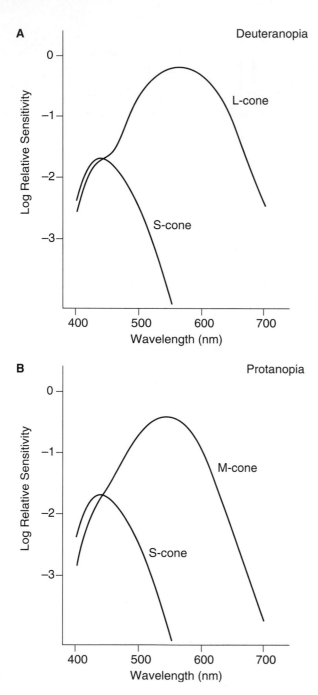

Figure 6–5. Approximations of the absorption spectra for the remaining photopigments in **(A)** deuteranopia and **(B)** protanopia. Note that beyond about 545 nm, red-green dichromats are essentially monochromatic. These absorption spectra are based on the data of Smith and Pokorny (1975).

between stimuli that are longer than 545 nm if these stimuli differ in luminance. A stimulus of 575 nm, for example, is brighter than an equal energy stimulus of 600 nm. When equated for luminance, however, these stimuli are indistinguishable.

Figure 6–4B shows a wavelength discrimination function for tritanopia. Unlike red–green dichromats, tritanopes show well-developed wavelength discrimination at longer wavelengths, but poor wavelength discrimination in the region of 495 nm (Wright, 1952).

Color Confusion Lines

The limited ability of dichromats to distinguish among colors can be illustrated by plotting their so-called color confusion lines on the CIE diagram. Figure 6-6 shows that the confusion lines for deuteranopia, protanopia, and tritanopia each originate from a different **copunctal point.** All colors falling along a confusion line are indistinguishable to the dichromat.

Figure 6-6 reveals that a deuteranope confuses greens with reddish purple, while a protanope confuses greens with red. This confusion of greens with red-

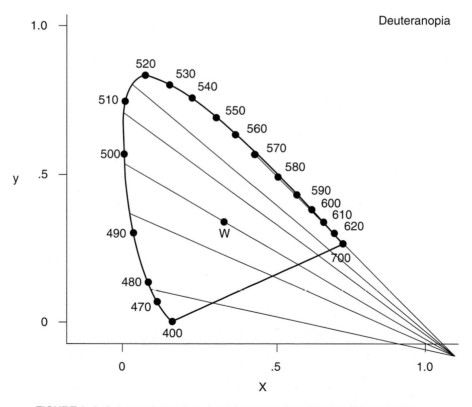

FIGURE 6–6. Color confusion lines for dichromats plotted on the CIE chromaticity diagram.

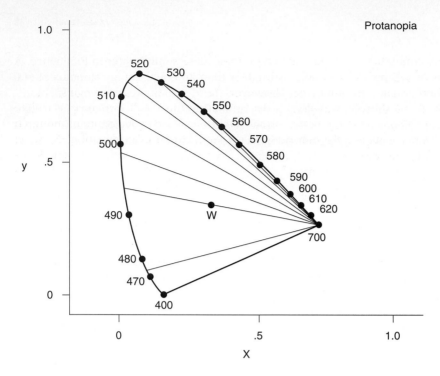

Protanopia

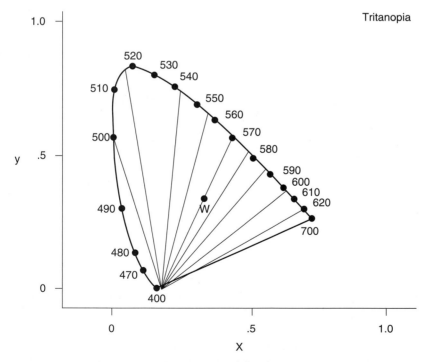

Tritanopia

FIGURE 6–6. Continued

136

dish colors is the reason that deuteranopes and protanopes are referred to as red–green dichromats. For a tritanope, blue-violet and yellow are confused with each other, hence the term blue–yellow defect.

Deuteranopes and protanopes share a confusion line that is tangential to the segment of the spectral locus that runs from about 545 to 700 nm, reinforcing an important point made in the discussion on wavelength discrimination. Namely, red–green dichromats are monochromatic from 545 nm upward, confusing stimuli ranging from 545 to 700 nm (see Fig. 6–15).[6] This confusion line is useful in the design of color vision tests utilized to diagnose red–green defects.

Saturation

Recall from the previous chapter that not all spectral stimuli appear equally saturated. For a normal trichromat, 570 nm appears less saturated (more whitish) than do other wavelengths. The saturation function for a normal trichromat, along with those for deuteranopes and protanopes, are given in Fig. 6–7A. Note that the deuteranopic function intersects the abscissa at about 498 nm, whereas the protanopic function intersects it at 492 nm. These particular wavelengths appear white, and are referred to as **neutral points.** (The neutral point for a tritanope is about 569 nm.)

Each class of dichromats has a confusion line that passes through white. All stimuli falling along one of these lines are confused with white. As can be seen in Fig. 6-6, these lines intersect the spectral locus at the neutral points.

Upon questioning, a dichromat may report that green traffic lights appear white (or whitish). These traffic lights are approximate metamers for the dichromatic neutral points.

Although anomalous trichromats do not manifest neutral points, they display abnormal saturation perception. As indicated in Fig. 6–7B, 498 nm is the least saturated wavelength for a deuteranomalous trichromat, whereas 492 nm is the least saturated for a protanomalous trichromat.

<u>COLOR LABELING</u>

Although red–green dichromats are essentially monochromatic for wavelengths beyond about 545 nm, they do remarkably well at labeling colors. This is especially true when other cues, such as context or brightness, are available. For example, a protanope (or deuteranope) has no difficulty labeling an apple as red and a banana as yellow. This is an easy task because these individuals have learned that others label apples as red and bananas as yellow.

---

6. While a red-green dichromat does not possess wavelength-based discrimination beyond 545 nm, he or she can still use luminance as a clue to distinguish among stimuli constituted of these wavelengths.

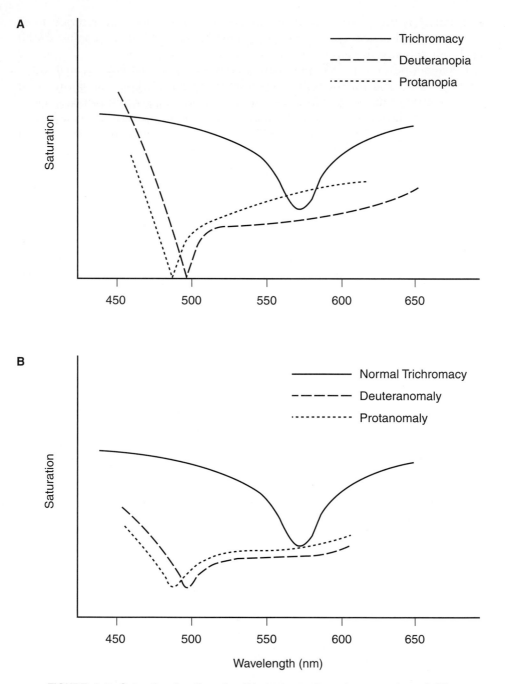

FIGURE 6–7. Saturation functions for **(A)** deuteranopia and protanopia and **(B)** deuteranomaly and protanomaly. The solid curves represent normal trichromacy. Note the intersections of the deuteranope's and protanope's functions with the abscissa at 498 and 492 nm, respectively. These wavelengths represent the dichromatic neutral points (Chapanis, 1944).

Dichromats have more difficulty assigning color labels to manufactured items, such as the pattern on a blouse or shirt, because they may not know how others would label the colors contained within the pattern. They know that others see an apple as red, but may not know how others see the stripes on a particular shirt. A dichromat may assign a color label to the stripes on the basis of brightness cues and, to some extent, the context in which the shirt is worn.

Consider the following example. Jose is known to be a conservative dresser and often wears gray patterns. Today he is wearing a shirt with pink vertical stripes. We ask his friend, who is a protanope, to tell us the color of the stripes. The pink stripes appear very dim to the protanope and could be labeled pink (red) or gray (black). Because conservative Jose is wearing the shirt, the protanope might assume that the stripes are gray. If, however, the context was different, the color label might well be different. If Richard, who is known as a less conservative dresser, wore the same shirt, the protanope might label the stripes pink.

Although a dichromat does not have wavelength-based discrimination for long-wavelength stimuli, we should be careful when drawing conclusions regarding his or her perceptions of these stimuli. A dichromat may label a tomato as red, as will a normal color observer. We could tell the dichromat that he or she is labeling the tomato as red based on brightness cues, but he or she may insist that it appears red. Just as we cannot be certain that any two normal trichromatic individuals are experiencing the same perception when viewing a red object, we cannot be certain of what a dichromat perceives when viewing this same object.

Figure 6–8 shows how the spectrum might appear to individuals with normal and abnormal color vision. The density of the vertical bars indicates wavelength discrimination: the more dense the bars, the better the wavelength discrimination. The color labels (V, B, G, Y, O, R) show the approximate regions of the spectrum that are assigned these color labels.

Consider the diagram for normal color vision. The bars are most dense at about 490 and 590 nm, indicating best wavelength discrimination in these regions of the spectrum (also see Fig. 6-4). In comparison, the diagrams for protanopia and deuteranopia show that the spectrum is divided into two parts: a blue region and a long-wavelength, "variable" region. These are separated by the neutral point wavelength, which is perceived as white. Wavelength discrimination is best in the region of the neutral point. The "variable" region represents that area of the spectrum over which these dichromats are monochromatic. As discussed, stimuli within this region are discriminated largely on the basis of context or brightness differences.

Because erythrolabe is absent, the protanopic visible spectrum is truncated at longer wavelengths, ending prior to the others. Consequently, protanopes (and certain protanomalous trichromats) may have difficulty seeing red tail, brake, and traffic lights.

Also given in Fig. 6–8 are the visible spectra for protanomalous and deuteranomalous observers. These individuals display wavelength discrimination

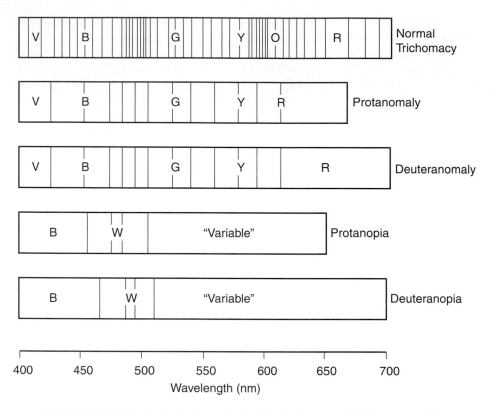

FIGURE 6–8. Color discrimination and color labeling by normal trichromats and the various classes of red–green color defectives (Heath, 1963). The density of the vertical lines is reflective of the individual's ability to discriminate wavelengths. Note that the spectrum for dichromats (protanopes and deuteranopes) is divided into a blue and "variable" region separated by the white neutral point. The term *variable* indicates that the subject labels these wavelengths on the basis of brightness and context cues. For both protanopia and protanomaly, the visible spectrum is truncated at longer wavelengths.

considerably superior to dichromats, but less well developed than normal trichromats.

INHERITED ANOMALIES OF COLOR VISION

The majority of red–green defects are inherited, transmitted in a X-linked recessive fashion (Nathans et al, 1986b; Nathans, 1989). Consequently, they are considerably more common in men than women, with prevalences of 8.0 and 0.4 percent, respectively.[7] Table 6–2 summarizes prevalence and inheritance of the

---

7. About 8 percent of Caucasian, 5 percent of Asian, and 5 percent of African males manifest red-green defects (Nathans, 1999).

TABLE 6–2. PREVALENCE AND INHERITANCE OF THE MOST COMMON
COLOR VISION DEFECTS

Classification	Prevalence in Males (%)	Inheritance
Deuteranopia	1	X-linked recessive
Protanopia	1	X-linked recessive
Deuteranomaly	5	X-linked recessive
Protanomaly	1	X-linked recessive
Tritanopia and tritanomaly	0.005	Autosomal dominant

Data from Verriest (1969).

various anomalies of color vision. Note that inherited tritan defects are extremely rare, and transmitted in an autosomal dominant fashion (Kalmus, 1955).

Figure 6–9 shows several examples of the transmission of red–green defects from parents to their offspring. When reviewing this figure, keep in mind that a heterozygous female ($\overline{X}X$) is a carrier, whereas a male with the defective gene has anomalous color vision ($\overline{X}Y$). Because the gene is recessive, a female must be homozygous ($\overline{X}\overline{X}$) to express the defect. Note that a boy always receives the defective gene from the mother. Patients often assume that color defects are transmitted from father to son.

MOLECULAR GENETICS OF RED–GREEN COLOR VISION ANOMALIES

Recent work on the molecular genetics of color vision may explain how color vision anomalies originated in our ancestors (Nathans et al, 1986a; Nathans, 1989; Neitz and Neitz, 1994). The highly homologous genes for the M- and L-cone photopigments are positioned on the X chromosome in a head-to-tail tandem array (Fig. 6–10A). This arrangement suggests that erroneous crossover of genetic information could occur when the pair of X chromosomes align and exchange genetic information during meiosis (i.e., unequal homologous recombination). For instance, the gene coding for the M-cone photopigment could erroneously align with the gene coding for the L-cone photopigment, leading to an unequal exchange of genetic information.

Figure 6–10B provides an example where the gene coding for the M-cone photopigment crosses over during meiosis (*intergenetic* crossover). As a result, one of the X chromosomes does not have the gene coding for the M-cone photopigment, and the offspring inheriting this chromosome will be deuteranopes. The other chromosome has multiple copies of the gene coding for the M-cone photopigment. Offspring inheriting this chromosome will have normal color vision.[8]

---

8. As discussed in Chapter 5, it is common for an individual to possess multiple copies of the M-cone opsin gene. Having multiple copies of this gene does not seem to impact color vision.

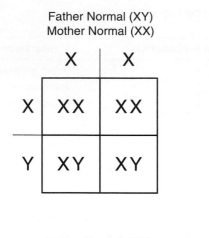

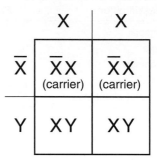

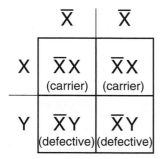

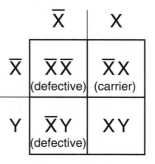

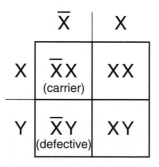

FIGURE 6–9. Examples of the transmission of X-linked, red–green defects from parents to offspring.

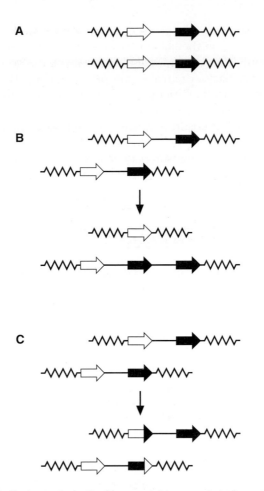

Figure 6–10. A. During meiosis, the M-cone and L-cone photopigment genes (black and white arrows, respectively) on one chromosome normally align the M-cone and L-cone photopigment genes on the paired chromosome **B.** Dichromacy could result when the M-cone photopigment gene erroneously aligns with the highly homologous L-cone photopigment gene, leading to the *intergenetic* crossover of the M-cone photopigment gene. As a result, one chromosome has no M-cone photopigment genes; the offspring who inherit this chromosome will be deuteranopes. The paired chromosome has two copies of the M-cone photopigment gene and one copy of the L-cone photopigment gene; the offspring who inherit this chromosome will have normal color vision. **C.** *Intragenetic* crossover results in hybrid genes (combination black–white arrows). Depending on the specific nature of the crossover, a hybrid gene may result in a normal photopigment, the loss of a photopigment (dichromacy), or a photopigment with an absorption spectra that is displaced from its normal location (anomalous trichromacy) (Nathans et al, 1986a; 1986b).

Hybrid genes[9] result from the *intragenetic* crossover of genetic material (see Fig. 6–10C). Depending on the specific nature of the intragenetic crossover, the resultant hybrid gene leads to a normal photopigment, the non-expression of the photopigment (dichromacy), or an aberrant photopigment. The latter may be the molecular basis of anomalous trichromacy. A hybrid gene that differs substantially from the normal gene may result in severe anomalous trichromacy, where the deviant photopigment absorption spectrum almost completely overlaps that of the other long wavelength photopigment.[10] When the hybrid gene is more similar to the normal gene, the result may be a milder form of anomalous trichromacy in which the location of the deviant absorption spectrum is almost normal (Neitz et al, 1996).[11]

ACQUIRED COLOR VISION ANOMALIES

Acquired defects of color vision are secondary to disease or toxicity. They may be either red–green or blue–yellow in nature. Because blue-yellow defects are so rarely inherited, it must be assumed that such a defect is acquired until proven otherwise.

Table 6–3 summarizes the major differences between inherited and acquired defects. Because inherited defects are secondary to stable physiological variations, they remain unchanged throughout life and result in clear-cut results on color vision tests. In comparison, the pathological processes that produce acquired defects are often variable in their course, resulting in color vision defects that may not be stable and may not produce clean test results.

Laterality

Whereas inherited defects are bilateral and symmetric in their presentation, acquired defects may be unilateral or asymmetric (Adams and Haegerstrom-Portnoy, 1987). Consequently, it must be assumed that any difference in the color vision of the two eyes, as demonstrated on a color vision test, is due to an acquired defect.

Because acquired defects may be asymmetric, it is important to perform color vision tests under monocular conditions. If a patient with a unilateral defect is tested binocularly, it may be missed because the results reflect the performance of

---

9. Hybrid genes are also called fusion or chimeric genes. See Neitz and Neitz (2000) for a more extensive discussion.

10. If there is *complete* overlap, the individual is a dichromat.

11. There is some interest in the development of genetic tests that are designed to diagnose red-green defects of color vision. The practicability and utility of such tests remains to be seen.

TABLE 6–3. DISTINCTION BETWEEN HEREDITARY AND ACQUIRED DEFECTS

Hereditary Defects	Acquired Defects
Almost always red–green	Red–green or blue–yellow
More prevalent in males	Equally prevalent in males and females
Symmetric: same in each eye	Asymmetric: often a difference in severity between the eyes
Color naming errors rare	Recent history of color naming errors
Defect is stable with time	Defect is unstable and changes over time
Easily classified with standard clinical color tests	Classification often not straightforward with standard clinical color tests; nonselective
Not associated with disease or toxicity	Associated with ocular or systemic disease or toxicity

the unaffected eye. The test should be first administered to the eye most likely to harbor disease (typically the eye with the worst corrected visual acuity) because it is more likely to manifest an acquired defect (Adams and Haegerstrom-Portnoy, 1987). When a color vision anomaly is found, the other eye should then be tested.

Köllner's Rule

According to Köllner's rule, outer retinal disease and media changes result in blue–yellow color vision defects, whereas disease of the inner retina, optic nerve, visual pathways, and visual cortex results in red–green defects (Köllner, 1912). This general guideline is not correct in every instance, and important exceptions have been reported (Schneck and Haegerstrom-Portnoy, 1997). Table 6–4 provides examples of the application of Köllner's rule.

It is not uncommon for a blue–yellow defect to be present in the early stages of an eye disease, and for it to change into a red–green defect as the disease progresses.[12] A patient may manifest both a blue–yellow and red–green defect simultaneously, a condition sometimes referred to as a **nonselective** loss. Although Köllner's rule predicts red–green deficiencies in optic neuritis, this malady may be associated with nonselective defects (Schneck and Haegerstrom-Portnoy, 1997).

ACHROMATOPSIAS

Achromatopsias are rare conditions where the patient behaves largely as a monochromat (Pokorny et al, 1979; Adams and Haegerstrom-Portnoy, 1987). The most common achromatopsia is **rod monochromacy (typical achromacy).** This

---

12. The reverse may also occur: an initially red-green defect may transform to a blue-yellow defect.

TABLE 6–4. COLOR VISION DEFECTS PREDICTED BY KÖLLNER'S RULE ALONG WITH EXAMPLES OF CONDITIONS EXPECTED TO PRODUCE THESE DEFECTS

Location	Defect	Condition
Media	Blue–yellow	Nuclear sclerosis
Outer retina	Blue–yellow	ARMD[a]
		Diabetic retinopathy
Inner retina	Red–green	Leber's optic atrophy
		Toxic amblyopia
Pathways	Red–green	Lesions

[a] Age-related macular degeneration.

label is a misnomer because these patients may have M- and L-cones, but in greatly reduced numbers (Haegerstrom-Portnoy, 1991). Rod monochromats manifest very poor color discrimination, nystagmus, photophobia, and visual acuity of about 20/200. This condition is inherited in an autosomal recessive fashion. Rod monochromacy is fully expressed at birth, differentiating it from rod–cone degenerations, such as retinitis pigmentosa, which typically develop later in life and are progressive.

Other achromatopsias include **blue-cone monochromacy** and **cone monochromacy.** In the former (also called incomplete congenital cone dysfunction or monocone monochromacy) only rods and S-cones are present. It is inherited in an X-linked recessive manner. Symptoms and signs are similar to those of rod monochromacy. This condition is very rare.

Cone monochromacy is an exceedingly rare disorder in which visual acuity is normal, yet the patient behaves as a monochromat. Although this condition is too rare to have been extensively studied, it appears to involve a defect in postreceptoral processing of color information.

CHROMATOPSIAS

Chromatopsias are not true color vision defects because they do not typically produce a decreased ability to discriminate colors. Rather, they represent a distortion of color vision, similar to looking through a colored filter. Patients report that objects have a colored tinge or halo.

Chromatopsia may follow cataract extraction. A nuclear cataract acts as a yellow filter, absorbing blue light. The patient has experienced this yellow filter, in all likelihood, for several years prior to extraction. Removal of the cataract exposes the retina to considerably more blue light than it has experienced in some time, resulting in the perception of blueness **(cyanopsia).** As the visual system adapts to the new distribution of radiant energy, the effect wanes.

Chromatopsias can occur secondary to various medications. For example, digitalis may produce **xanthopsia** (yellow vision). Fluorescein, used in fluorescein angiography, can also produce xanthopsia.

STANDARD COLOR VISION TESTS

Pseudoisochromatic Plate Tests

Pseudoisochromatic plate tests are the most commonly used color vision tests. They are relatively straightforward to administer and readily available.

The tests consist of a number of plates arranged into a booklet. Vanishing plates are the most common; they consist of a figure that must be distinguished from the background (Fig. 6–11). Patients with normal color vision can distinguish the figure from the background based on chromatic differences. Patients with anomalies of color vision, however, have difficulty seeing the figure. This is because the colors that make up the figure and those that constitute the background all fall on a common dichromatic confusion line (see Figs. 6–6 and 6–15). The colors are indistinguishable to patients with defective color vision; consequently, they do not see the embedded figure.[13]

Pseudoisochromatic plate tests do not distinguish between dichromats and anomalous trichromats. They may not be reliable for differentiating protan and deutan defects, although some tests have plates designed for this purpose.[14] For routine clinical practice, however, these limitations are of little importance.

Although certain pseudoisochromatic tests (e.g., the SPP2 and new HRR) include plates designed to detect blue-yellow defects, others do not. Because of the importance of detecting acquired defects, the lack of tritan plates is a serious limitation.

Farnsworth Dichotomous Test

The Farnsworth dichotomous test (Panel D-15) consists of 15 colored caps (or chips) that form a hue circle within the CIE diagram (Figs. 6–12 and 6–13). The patient arranges the colored caps such that they follow an orderly progression of color. To start, the examiner asks the patient to choose the colored cap that looks most like the affixed reference cap. The selected cap is placed next to the

---

13. Hidden digit and transformation plates are sometimes included in plate tests. The hidden digit is seen by a patient with anomalous color vision, but not by a patient with normal color vision. These plates work because under very specific circumstances, a patient with anomalous color vision can make color discriminations that cannot be made by a patient with normal color vision. For the transformation plate, patients with normal and abnormal color vision see different digits. For example, a patient with normal color vision may see an "8," whereas a patient with anomalous color vision labels the same digit as "3."

14. Consider a plate consisting of the number "85" where the digit "8" is red, the "5" is purple, and the background in which these two digits is embedded is gray. Since red falls along the protanopic confusion line that intersects white, a protan will not see the "8," but will see the "5." Likewise, since purple falls on the deuteranopic confusion line that intersects white, a deutan will not see the "5," but will see the "8." (Keep in mind that gray is a variant of white.) Refer to Fig. 6–6.

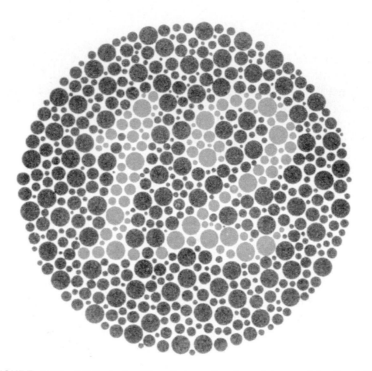

FIGURE 6–11. Black and white photograph of a plate used in the Ishihara pseudoisochromatic plate test.

reference, and the procedure is repeated using the selected cap as the new reference. The process continues until all caps are arranged in an orderly sequence of color. Like the desaturated D-15 test and the 100-hue test, which are described later, the Farnsworth D-15 test is referred to as an **arrangement test.**

The test is scored by connecting the cap numbers in the sequence arranged by the patient (see Fig. 6–13). When a patient with defective color vision arranges the caps, there may be crossovers on the hue circle that correspond to color confusion lines. The axis of these crossovers can be used to determine if the defect is protan, deutan, or tritan in nature. In nonselective defects, there may not be a clearly definable axis.

Although the Farnsworth D-15 test does allow the differentiation of protan, deutan, and tritan defects, it does not allow the differentiation of dichromats from anomalous trichromats. The anomaloscope, which is discussed later in this chapter, is the only clinical instrument that allows this diagnosis. Because the Farnsworth D-15 test does not detect minor defects, certain anomalous trichromats pass the test. This may not be a serious disadvantage because these minor defects are unlikely to have practical consequences for the patient. A distinct advantage of the Farnsworth D-15 test is its capacity to detect tritan defects.

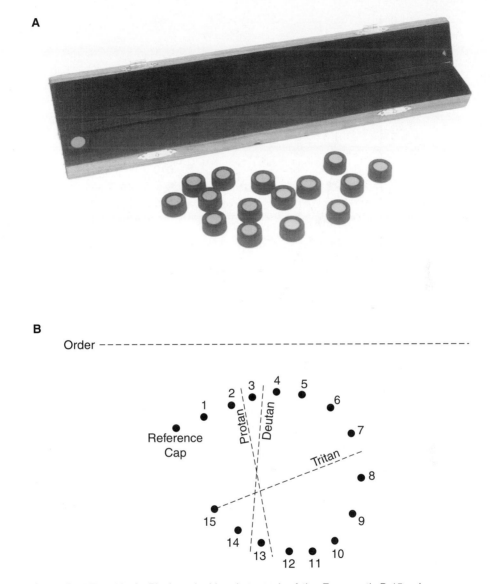

FIGURE 6–12. A. Black and white photograph of the Farnsworth D-15 color vision test. Note the reference cap that is affixed to the tray. **B.** Score sheet used to grade the Farnsworth D-15 test. Points are connected in a sequence corresponding to the arrangement of caps by the patient. Diagnosis of a defect as protan, deutan, or tritan is given by the axis of the crossovers.

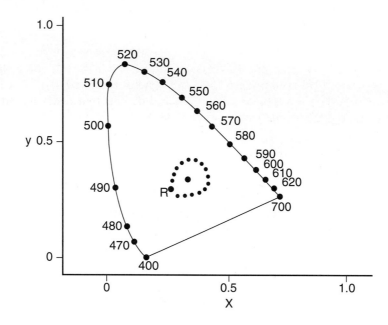

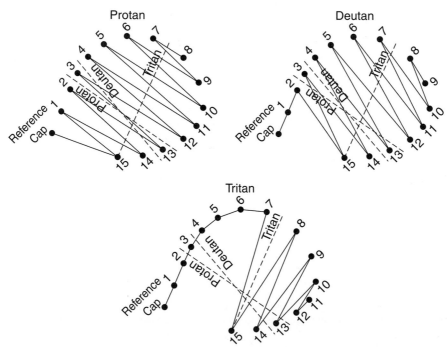

FIGURE 6–13. The top diagram shows the locations of the chips used for the D-15 test plotted on the CIE chromaticity diagram. These chips form a hue circle. "R" is the reference cap. The bottom three diagrams show the arrangement of caps for protan, deutan, and tritan anomalies. Diagnosis of the defect is made by noting the axis of the crossovers. In a selective color vision loss, the axis corresponds to the protan, deutan, or tritan color confusion lines (see Fig. 6–6).

Desaturated D-15 Test

In the desaturated D-15 test, the chips are less saturated than those in the standard D-15 test.[15] Because the task is more difficult, it detects anomalies that would be missed by the standard D-15 test. The desaturated D-15 test is especially useful in the detection of subtle acquired defects that occur in certain eye diseases, such as glaucoma (Adams et al, 1982).

Farnsworth–Munsell 100-Hue Test

Despite its name, the 100-hue test consists of only 85 color chips. These chips, which form a hue circle in the CIE diagram, are divided among four separate trays. The patient arranges, according to color, the chips contained within each tray. The test is graded by plotting the data on a scoring sheet and calculating a total error score. When the total error score is greater than the norms provided by the manufacturer, a diagnosis of a color anomaly is made. The axis indicates whether it is a protan, deutan, or tritan defect. Although the error score indicates the severity of the anomaly, this test does not distinguish dichromacy from anomalous trichromacy.

Administration of the 100-hue test is time consuming, and for most routine clinical applications, provides little advantage over the tests discussed thus far. Although rarely used in clinical practice, on occasion it is utilized in certain industries for screening employees.

NAGEL ANOMALOSCOPE

The Nagel anomaloscope is the only clinical instrument that can provide a complete diagnosis of red-green color vision anomalies, including the differential diagnosis of dichromacy from anomalous trichromacy. It is a superb teaching tool because it requires the integration of many different concepts regarding color vision.

Through the eyepiece, the patient views a bipartite field that is composed of an upper mixture field and a lower test field (Fig. 6–14) (Pokorny et al, 1979). The patient's task is to match the two fields so that they appear identical to each other.

The mixture field consists of variable amounts of 546 nm (green) and 670 nm (red). Turning a knob controls the relative amounts of 546 and 670 nm. If the mixture knob scale is set at zero, the mixture field consists of only 546 nm, and when set at 73, the mixture field consists exclusively of 670 nm. Mixture scale settings between 0 and 73 represent various combinations of 546 and 670 nm. An important feature of the mixture field is that its luminance, as measured for a normal trichromat, does not change. Whether the mixture field consists of pure 546 nm, pure 670 nm, or any combination thereof, the luminance is the same.

---

15. The radius of the hue circle formed by the desaturated chips is less than that formed by the chips that constitute the standard D-15 test (see Fig. 6–13).

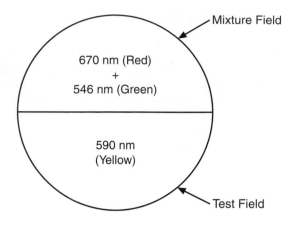

FIGURE 6–14. Bipartite field of the Nagel anomaloscope. The top field (mixture field) consists of 670 nm, 546 nm, or any combination of these two wavelengths. The luminance of this field, measured for a normal trichromat, does not change as the wavelength mixture is varied. The bottom field (test field) consists of 590 nm. This test field's radiance can be adjusted from a very low (dim) to a very high (bright) setting.

The lower test field consists of 590 nm (yellow) of variable radiance. Turning a knob controls the radiance. A test knob scale setting of 0 represents very dim yellow, whereas a scale reading of 87 represents bright yellow.

None of the Nagel anomaloscope's three primaries are absorbed by the S-cones (see Fig. 5–6). Therefore, for the region of the spectrum covered by these three primaries, normal trichromats behave as dichromatics. The primaries fall along a shared deutan and protan confusion line (Fig. 6–15) and constitute what is referred to as the **Rayleigh equation** (Rayleigh, 1881).

Normal Trichromats

When asked to match the mixture and test fields so that they appear identical, a normal trichromat adjusts the mixture field such that it appears yellow. He or she then adjusts the radiance of the test field to match this mixture field. Normal trichromats generally set the mixture scale to a value of about 45 and the test scale to about 17. Although there is some variability between individuals with normal color vision, the variability is not very large.

This is a simple color matching procedure, similar to those discussed in the previous chapter. Because a normal trichromat is dichromatic from about 545 to 700 nm, he or she is able to match any single wavelength (in this case 590 nm) by combining two other wavelengths (546 and 670 nm).[16]

---

16. Another way of understanding this match is to note that 590 nm falls on the uncurved portion of the spectral locus that connects 546 and 670 nm (see Fig. 5–21A). Therefore, a proper combination of 546 and 670 nm matches 590 nm.

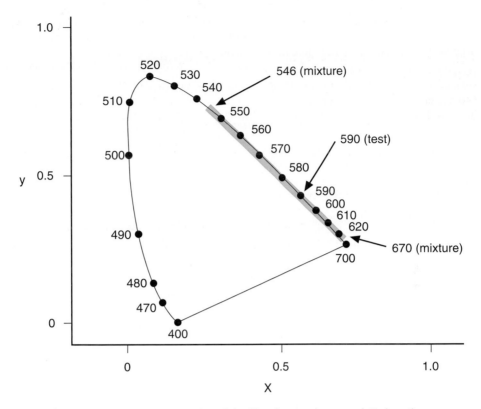

FIGURE 6–15. The three primaries of the Nagel anomaloscope plotted on the CIE chromaticity diagram. The line formed by connecting these three primaries corresponds to a color confusion line shared by deuteranopes and protanopes (Pokorny et al, 1979).

Dichromats

General Principles. If the mixture field is set to pure 546 nm, can a red-green dichromat adjust the test field radiance so this field matches exactly the mixture field? The answer is yes. When viewed by a person with normal color vision, the top appears green and the bottom, yellow. Yet, to a dichromat the two fields appear identical.

If the mixture field is set subsequently at pure 670 nm, can the dichromat now adjust the radiance of the test field so that the two fields appear identical? Again, the answer is yes. To an observer with normal color vision, the top field appears red and the bottom field yellow, but to the dichromat, they appear perfectly matched. In fact, no matter what combination of 546 and 670 nm is present in the mixture field, the dichromat is able to adjust the radiance of the 590-nm test field such that it matches the mixture field.

Because all three anomaloscope primaries fall on a common color confusion line, they appear identical to each other when their radiances are properly adjusted (see Fig. 6–15).[17] Recall that from about 545 to 700 nm, red-green dichromats have only one photopigment and behave as monochromats (Fig. 6–5). In this region of the spectrum, one wavelength can be matched to any other wavelength (or combination of wavelengths) if the relative radiances are adjusted appropriately. Therefore, a stimulus of 546 nm, 670 nm, or any combination thereof, will match 590 nm of the proper radiance.

Deuteranopes versus Protanopes. For a deuteranope, who has essentially the same luminance function as a person with normal color vision, the brightness of the mixture field is the same regardless of its setting (i.e., pure 546 nm, pure 670 nm, or any combination thereof is the same brightness to a deuteranope).[18] Therefore, once the deuteranope adjusts the test field radiance to match a particular mixture field (e.g., pure 546 nm), he or she does not need to change the test field setting to match any other mixture field setting. What test field setting does the deuteranope choose? Because his or her luminance function is similar to that of a person with normal color vision (see Fig. 6–3), he or she uses the same value, about 17.

Because a protanope has a luminance function that is very different than that of a person with normal color vision, the 546- and 670-nm mixture field stimuli do not have the same brightness (see Fig. 6–3).[19] The 546-nm stimulus appears bright, whereas the 670-nm stimulus appears very dim. Therefore, a protanope adjusts the 590-nm test field to a relatively high radiance when matching 546 nm and to a very low radiance when matching 670 nm.

In summary, both deuteranopes and protanopes are able to adjust the radiance of the test field such that this field matches any mixture field (546 nm, 670 nm, or any combination of these two wavelengths). For a deuteranope, brightness is approximately constant for all mixture field settings; therefore, he or she uses the same test field setting to match any mixture field. A protanope, however, finds it necessary to reduce the radiance of the test field when matching 670 nm, and to increase it when matching 546 nm, because his or her luminance function is displaced toward shorter wavelengths relative to a normal observer's luminance function.

Anomalous Trichromats

General Principles. If asked to adjust the mixture field so that it has the same color as the test field, anomalous trichromats generally select a mixture scale setting

---

17. Since protans and deutans share this color confusion line, the Nagel anomaloscope is useful for diagnosing both protan and deutan defects.

18. As already discussed, the luminance of the mixture field is designed to remain constant for a person with normal color vision as the field is adjusted from 546 to 670 nm.

19. For a protanope, the luminance function is displaced toward shorter wavelengths.

different than that selected by normal trichromats. Due to his or her displaced M-cone photopigment absorption spectrum, a deuteranomalous trichromat may require more 546 nm in the mixture field, setting the mixture scale, say, at 20, rather than the normal 45. In comparison, a protanomalous trichromat, because of his or her displaced L-cone spectrum, may set the mixture scale at, for example, 60.

A normal trichromat is very particular when making a match, setting the mixture scale at about 45. If we were to adjust the mixture field to 50 and ask a normal trichromat to adjust the yellow test field so that it matches the mixture field, he or she would not be able to do so. The top would appear reddish and the bottom yellow; adjusting the radiance of the test field would not cause the fields to match each other.

Anomalous trichromats are less specific in their matches than normal trichromats, but more specific than dichromats. Consider a deuteranomalous trichromat who matches the 590-nm test field by adjusting the mixture scale to 35. If we were to reset the mixture scale to 20, this patient might still be able to adjust the test field so that it matches the mixture field. He or she would, however, manifest more specificity than a deuteranope. For instance, if the mixture field was set to 73 (pure 670 nm), the deuteranomalous individual would not be able to match the test field to the mixture field, whereas a deuteranope would be able to do so.

Deuteranomaly versus Protanomaly. As we have discussed, the mixture scale setting is very helpful in distinguishing deuteranomaly from protanomaly. Deuteranomalous trichromats add extra amounts of 546 nm to the mixture field, typically adjusting the mixture scale between 0 and 40. Protanomalous trichromats, in comparison, add more 670 nm to the mixture field, resulting in mixture scale readings that typically range from about 50 to 73.

The test field setting also distinguishes deuteranomaly from protanomaly. Because a deuteranomalous person manifests essentially the same luminosity function as an individual with normal color vision, he or she adjusts the test scale to a normal setting, about 17. A protanomalous observer, however, has a luminance function similar to that of a protanope—it is displaced toward shorter wavelengths. When he or she matches the test field by adding "extra" 670 nm to the mixture field, the mixture field appears dim. To match this dim mixture field, the protanomalous trichromat sets the test field radiance to a low value, less than 15.

The expected anomaloscope results for various classes of color deficiencies are summarized in Table 6–5 and Fig. 6–16. These results are predictable based on basic principles of color matching.

ADDITIONAL CLINICAL CONSIDERATIONS

Inherited Defects

Although inherited deficiencies of color vision remain stable throughout life and pose no threat to vision, they can interfere with the performance of many visu-

TABLE 6–5. SUMMARY OF EXPECTED RESULTS USING THE NAGEL ANOMALOSCOPE TO DIAGNOSE RED–GREEN COLOR DEFECTS[a]

Condition	Mixture Field		Test Field	
	Setting	Appearance to a Normal Trichromat	Setting	Appearance to a Normal Trichromat
Normal trichromat	45	Yellow	17	Yellow
Deuteranope	Any setting from 0 to 73 will be matched	Green (0) to yellow (45) to red (73)	17	Yellow
Protanope	Any setting from 0 to 73 will be matched	Green (0) to yellow (45) to red (73)	35–5	Bright to dim yellow
Deuteranomaly	0–45	Greenish	17	Yellow
Protanomaly	45–73	Reddish	10	Dim yellow

[a]The appearances given are those reported by a normal observer, not a color defective. Values given are approximations.

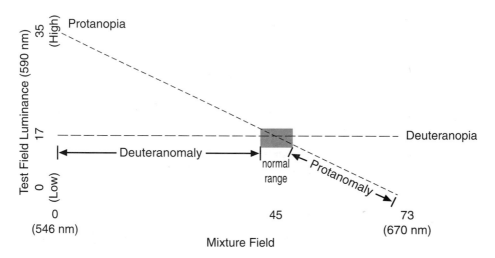

FIGURE 6–16. Anomaloscope results presented graphically. As indicated by the dashed line, a deuteranope matches all mixture fields with a constant test field luminance. The protanope is also able to match all mixture fields; however, he or she must adjust the luminance of the test field, increasing it when matching 546 nm, and decreasing it when matching 670 nm. Anomalous trichromats may reject the normal match and add either 546 nm (deuteranomaly) or 670 nm (protanomaly). The protanomalous observer needs to reduce the luminance of the test field as he or she adds 670 nm. The deuteranomalous observer does not need to adjust the luminance of the test field as he or she adds 546 nm.

ally related activities. School lessons are sometimes taught through the use of color-coded visual aids, potentially placing a color-deficient child at a serious disadvantage. Children with color vision anomalies are sometimes labeled as slow learners, possibly resulting in psychological trauma.

A pseudoisochromatic plate test should be administered at a child's preschool eye examination. Because inherited defects remain stable, it is not usually necessary to repeat the test on subsequent visits.[20] Parents should be reassured that inherited color vision anomalies are common, stable, and pose no threat to vision. They should be encouraged to have their other children tested. With the parent's permission, the child's teacher and the school administration should be notified and informed that color-coded learning tasks may pose an undue burden for the child.

Parents often ask if defective color vision will limit their child's occupational options. Certain occupations related to public safety (e.g., airline pilot, firefighter) may have color vision standards that exclude individuals with anomalous color vision. For other professions, including electrical engineering, pharmacy, optometry, ophthalmology, dentistry, and surgery, normal color discrimination can be an advantage.

Individuals with red–green defects may have difficulty distinguishing between colors that are dark (e.g., socks) or desaturated (pastels) if these colors fall along the red–green confusion lines (Table 6–6). The ability of protans and deutans to discriminate and name colors is improved by increasing the level of illumination (Adams and Haegerstom-Portnoy, 1987).

Protan defects have been associated with an increased frequency of rear-end automobile accidents due to the diminished ability to see red tail and brake lights (Birch, 1993). Protans may also have difficulty seeing red traffic lights.

Acquired Defects

It is best to screen adults with a test that detects acquired defects, which are often blue–yellow in nature. The Standard Pseudoisochromatic Plate test (SPP), the new HRR plate test, and the D-15 test are designed for this purpose.[21]

To establish baseline data for future reference, all patients should be screened on their first visit to an office. As was discussed previously, testing should be performed monocularly, first testing the eye with the worst corrected visual acuity or the eye suspected of manifesting a disease process. When a defect is found, the other eye should be tested to determine if the defect is asymmetric.

---

20. It is important to keep in mind that a child may manifest an acquired defect (either red-green or blue-yellow).

21. The SPP consists of two parts: the SPP1, which tests for red-green defects and the SPP2, designed to detect blue-yellow defects.

TABLE 6–6. COLORS FREQUENTLY CONFUSED BY DEUTANS AND PROTANS

Light grayish purple (mauve)–gray
Pink–gray
Green–white
Green–gray
Light yellowish brown (beige)–green
Dark purplish red (maroon)–brown
Olive–brown
Light green–light yellow
Light green–light orange
Light yellow–light orange
Light yellowish green (chartreuse)–pink
Light purple–light blue
Light orange–light red

Lighting Conditions for Color Vision Testing

Commonly used color vision tests are designed for administration under standard illuminant C lighting conditions. The **MacBeth lamp** provides illumination very similar to that provided by illuminant C and serves as an excellent light source for administering color vision tests. Unfortunately, this lamp is not readily available.

If an unfiltered incandescent source is used, it is likely that the patient will perform better than if the proper illumination were utilized. Because of its uneven wavelength profile, standard fluorescent lighting is generally not advisable (Adams and Haegerstrom-Portnoy, 1987).

Several practical lighting options are available for routine clinical practice. A nonstandard fluorescent tube, the Varilux F15T8/VLX, appears to provide appropriate illumination for color vision testing (Rodenstock and Swick, 1974). If an incandescent source is used, the patient should view the test through an appropriately colored filter that renders the lighting conditions suitable (Higgins et al, 1978). Such filters, mounted in plastic spectacle frames, are commercially produced for this purpose. Alternatively, color vision testing can be performed using (indirect) sunlight (Adams and Haegerstrom-Portnoy, 1987).

X-chrom Lens and Colored Filters

The X-chrom lens is a red contact lens, worn on one eye, that is designed to improve color discrimination. Although this contact lens is prescribed for dichromats or anomalous trichromats, it is most easily understood by considering its effect on a monochromat. Figure 6–17 shows the absorption spectrum for a hypothetical monochromat (left) and the spectral transmission curve for a red contact lens (center). The lens is a long-pass filter, blocking short wavelengths and transmitting longer wavelengths. The curve on the right is absorption spectrum of the eye while it is wearing the contact lens. It is the product of the photopigment absorption spectrum and the red lens transmission curve. Note that the contact lens has caused the original absorption curve to become displaced toward longer wavelengths.

How does this lens aid in color discrimination? Consider the two patches of light in Fig. 6–17, each of which emits 1000 quanta of light. These two patches are indistinguishable when viewed with the eye that is not wearing the contact lens because they each bleach the same amount of photopigment. When viewed by the eye wearing the red lens, however, the 590-nm patch bleaches more photopigment than the 490-nm patch, making the patches distinguishable. If we were to increase the intensity of 490 nm, such that when viewed through the contact lens it matches 590 nm, the match would no longer hold for the other eye. From this analysis, we can conclude that when wearing the red contact lens on one eye, the monochromat is able to distinguish the two patches if he or she compares the two eyes.

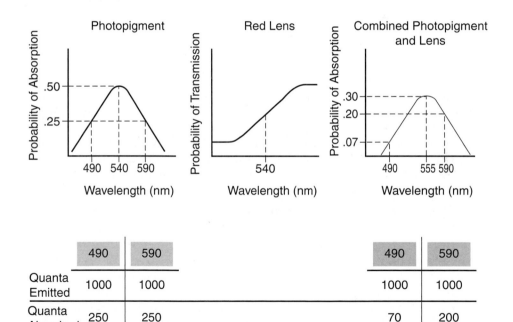

	490	590		490	590
Quanta Emitted	1000	1000		1000	1000
Quanta Absorbed	250	250		70	200

FIGURE 6–17. Use of a colored contact lens to improve color discrimination. The left curve shows the absorption spectrum of a hypothetical monochromat. The middle curve is the transmission curve for a red lens. This is followed by the absorption spectrum of an eye of this monochromat when wearing the lens. The lens displaces the absorption spectrum, effectively making the individual a dichromat if he or she compares the two eyes.

When comparing the two eyes—one eye with the red lens and the other without—a monochromat behaves like a dichromat. Each eye has a different absorption spectrum, resulting effectively in two photopigments (one in each eye). Likewise, if a dichromat wears a red contact lens on one eye and alternates viewing between the two eyes, he or she behaves like a tetrachromat (i.e., as if there were four photopigments). It is sometimes assumed that when one eye wears a red contact lens there is involuntary alternating viewing between the two eyes (somewhat akin to binocular rivalry; see Chap. 17). Although this may seem reasonable, there are limitations. Some patients may suppress the eye that is wearing the red contact lens. Others tend to fuse the images of the two eyes rather than alternate between them, behaving as if one large red filter has been placed in front of both eyes (i.e., as if viewing binocularly through a large colored filter).

Based on improved performance on pseudoisochromatic plate tests, it has been claimed that the X-chrom lens improves color vision. The same claim has also been made for binocular viewing through a large colored filter. It is true that viewing binocularly through a large colored filter may improve a dichromat's performance on a plate test; however, this does not indicate improved color discrimination. It does show that the filter has shifted the dichromatic confusion lines to a new location. The patient is still a dichromat, but the standard plate test is not designed for this "new" type of dichromat. An appropriately redesigned plate test would detect the patient's dichromacy.

Whereas a red contact lens is of questionable usefulness, a hand-held red filter may be helpful to certain patients. When properly used, the red filter may allow the patient distinguish objects that he or she cannot normally distinguish. For example, an electrical technician may have difficulty distinguishing two color-coded wires. When viewed through the red filter, however, these wires are more easily differentiated. It is critical that the patient understand that the filter will be useful only if objects are alternatively viewed with and without the filter.

Short Wavelength Automated Perimetry

The S-cone system is apparently more vulnerable to certain pathological processes than the M- and L-cone systems (Adams et al, 1990). This may be due to vulnerabilities in the S-cones themselves or the blue–yellow opponent pathway. The paucity of S-cones may be a factor.

Short wavelength automated perimetry (SWAP) has been developed to assess S-system function in certain eye diseases, particularly glaucoma (Johnson et al, 1992; Johnson, 1995). The commonly used Humphrey visual field apparatus can be adapted for this function by replacing the standard white stimulus with a short-wavelength stimulus to maximize S-system sensitivity. To suppress the M- and L-cones, the background is yellow rather than the standard white.[22]

---

22. Yellow preferentially bleaches the M- and L-cone photopigments, thereby reducing M- and L-cone sensitivities.

In glaucoma, elevated (or normal) intraocular pressure may damage the optic nerve, causing loss of vision. The diagnosis is often based on visual field loss as measured with a white stimulus on a white background. A substantial number of the optic nerve fibers are, however, apparently damaged by the time visual field defects are first noted (Quigley et al, 1982).

Current research suggests that SWAP is a more sensitive measure of glaucomatous nerve damage than standard, white-on-white visual fields, with patients in the early stages of glaucoma more likely to manifest S-cone field loss than standard field loss (Johnson et al, 1995). It seems likely that SWAP or similar procedures may, in the near future, play a larger role in the diagnosis and management of glaucoma.

Increment Spectral Sensitivity

As discussed earlier in this chapter, the color-opponent system may be isolated by determining threshold as a function of wavelength for monochromatic increments flashed on a white background (see Fig. 6–2). Spectral sensitivity for the color-opponent system in diabetics is illustrated in Fig. 6–18 (Adams et al, 1990). Note that as in glaucoma, the S-cone system is most vulnerable. The reason for this vulnerability is not fully understood.

SUMMARY

Inherited and acquired color vision defects are frequently encountered in clinical practice. They are detectable with readily available clinical tests.

Patients with inherited defects should receive counseling that includes reassurance and practical suggestions that may be of use at work or in school. In certain instances, it may be appropriate to discuss the potential impact of a color defect on career options.

Acquired defects are secondary to eye disease or drug toxicity, making screening for such defects a useful clinical tool in at-risk populations. In those instances where disease is suspected, but the diagnosis is uncertain, the finding of an acquired defect may be confirmatory.

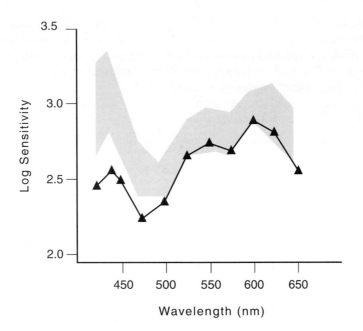

FIGURE 6–18. The shaded area shows the normal ranges of spectral sensitivity for the chromatic system, and the solid triangles show spectral sensitivity for the chromatic system of diabetic patients. Note the reduction in sensitivity at short wavelengths. (*Adapted from Adams AJ, Bodis-Wollner I, Enoch JM, et al. Normal and abnormal mechanisms of vision: Visual disorders and visual deprivation. In: Spillman L, Werner JS, eds.* Visual Perception: The Neurophysiological Foundations. *1990. Reprinted with permission of Academic Press and Dr. Anthony Adams.*)

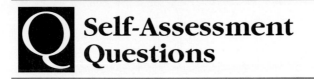

Self-Assessment Questions

1. A color-defective patient is unable to read the numbers given in a pseudoisochromatic plate test. **A.** Will he or she be able to read these numbers when viewing them through a red filter? **B.** Explain your answer.

2. A normal trichromat matches the mixture and test fields in the Nagel anomaloscope. **A.** Will the two fields appear matched when they are viewed through a red filter? **B.** Describe the appearance of the mixture and test fields when viewed through this red filter. **C.** Explain these results.

3. A normal trichromat matches the mixture and test fields in the Nagel anomaloscope. He or she then observes a large, bright red, adapting light for several minutes. Following this red adaptation, he or she observes the original match. **A.** Does the match between the mixture and test field still hold? **B.** Describe the appearance of the mixture and test fields. **C.** Provide an explanation.

4. A rod monochromat is tested on a Nagel anomaloscope. **A.** Describe the test field settings that are expected to match 546 and 670 nm. **B.** Explain your answer.

Spatial Vision

Spatial vision refers to the detection and analysis of variations in brightness across space. Examples include the resolution of detail (visual acuity) and the perception of borders, patterns, forms, and textures.

The clinical measurement of spatial vision is of fundamental importance in routine eye care. Virtually all patient visits include the determination of visual acuity, a highly sensitive measure of visual function.

SINE WAVE GRATINGS

How do we study the exceedingly complex processes of spatial vision? The key is to choose simple stimuli that can serve as building blocks to construct more complex stimuli. Sine wave gratings serve this purpose.

A sine wave grating is given in Fig. 7–1 along with its luminance profile. The grating consists of alternating bright and dark bars. Note that the peak of the luminance profile corresponds to a bright bar of the grating, whereas the trough of the profile corresponds to a dark bar. The transition from bright to dark bars is a gradual (sinusoidal) transition, not an abrupt transition. To fully describe a sine wave grating, it is necessary to specify its frequency, contrast, phase, and orientation.

Frequency

Compare the two gratings in Fig. 7–2. In the space taken up by the photograph, there are more alterations, or cycles, in the bottom grating. This bottom grating is

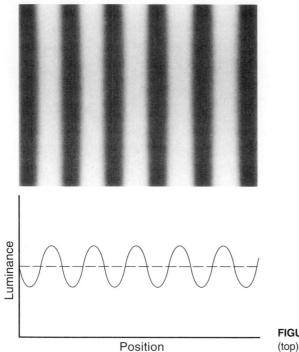

Luminance

Position

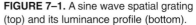

FIGURE 7–1. A sine wave spatial grating (top) and its luminance profile (bottom).

said to have a high spatial frequency, while the top grating has a comparatively low spatial frequency.

The spatial frequency of a grating can be specified by giving the number of cycles per degree of visual angle (e.g., 30 cycles per degree) or the number of cycles per unit of space (e.g., 4 cycles per centimeter). As we shall see, the specification of spatial frequency in terms of cycles per degree offers many practical advantages.

Contrast

The top of Fig. 7–3 shows a grating of low contrast along with its luminance profile. The bottom of this figure shows a grating of the same spatial frequency, but of a higher contrast. The dashed lines across the luminance profiles represent the average luminances of the gratings (the average of the peaks and troughs). While the average luminance (l_{ave}) is the same for both gratings, the bottom one has a larger difference between its peak and the average luminance value, indicative of higher contrast.

Contrast can be defined by following formula:

$$\text{contrast} = \frac{\Delta l}{l_{ave}} \qquad (7\text{–}1)$$

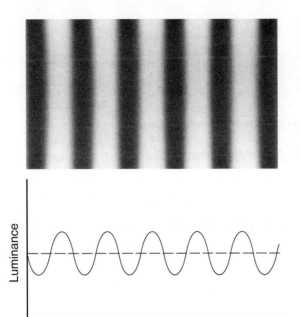

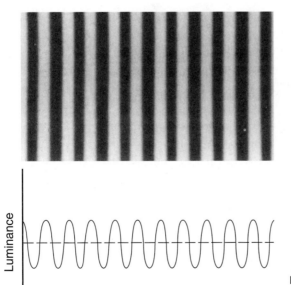

FIGURE 7–2. A low-frequency spatial grating (top) and a higher-frequency grating (bottom). Both gratings have the same contrast.

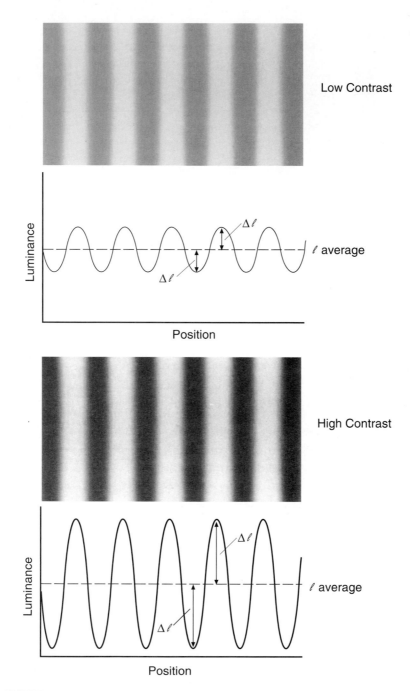

FIGURE 7–3. A low-contrast spatial grating (top) and a higher-contrast grating (bottom). Both gratings are of the same spatial frequency.

where

Δl = the difference between the peak and average luminance
l_{ave} = the average luminance of the grating (the average of the light peaks and dark troughs)

Although this formula is useful for defining and understanding contrast, it is not very practical for the measurement of contrast. Rather, it is more practicable to measure the maximum luminance (l_{max}) and the minimum luminance (l_{min}) and, from these values, calculate the contrast. The formula used is

$$\text{contrast} = \frac{l_{max} - l_{min}}{l_{max} + l_{min}} \qquad (7\text{--}2)$$

where

$$l_{max} = l_{ave} + \Delta l$$

$$l_{min} = l_{ave} - \Delta l$$

It can be demonstrated that Formula 7–2 provides the same result as Formula 7–1. Substituting for l_{max} and l_{min}, we have

$$\frac{(l_{ave} + \Delta l) - (l_{ave} - \Delta l)}{(l_{ave} + \Delta l) + (l_{ave} - \Delta l)} = \frac{\Delta l}{l_{ave}}$$

Contrast ranges between 0 and 100 percent. It cannot be greater than 100 percent because of the physical impossibility of making Δl greater than l_{ave}. (The trough of the luminance profile is at zero luminance when $\Delta l = l_{ave}$. It is not possible to have less than zero luminance.)

Phase and Orientation

Phase refers to the position of a sine wave grating with respect to another sine wave grating. For instance, if two gratings are in phase, the peaks and troughs of their luminance profiles will be in alignment. If two gratings are 180 degrees out of phase, the peak of one luminance profile will be aligned with the trough of the other profile.

Orientation describes the angle made by a grating with respect to a reference, such as the horizontal. In this chapter, only examples where all gratings are of the same orientation are presented.

FOURIER ANALYSIS: BASIC INTRODUCTION

Through a mathematical process referred to as **Fourier** (or **linear system**) **analysis**, sine waves of the proper frequency, contrast, phase, and orientation

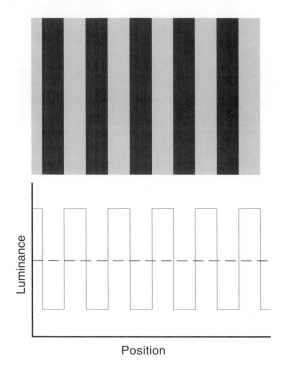
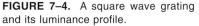

FIGURE 7–4. A square wave grating and its luminance profile.

can be used to construct other more complex spatial stimuli. Although it is not intuitively obvious, any achromatic scene—a black and white photograph of a house, forest, or face—can be thought of as consisting of sine waves of the appropriate frequency, contrast, phase, and orientation.

Consider the square wave grating in Fig. 7–4. Its luminance profile shows abrupt changes between bright and dark bars, sometimes referred to as "step" changes in luminance. Like any other complex spatial stimuli, a square wave can be constructed by adding together appropriate sine waves. Figure 7–5 shows how this is done. The sine wave that is of the same frequency as the square wave is referred to as the fundamental. The higher frequency sine waves are referred to as harmonics. (The third harmonic has three times the frequency of the fundamental and one third of its contrast, the fifth harmonic has five times the fundamental frequency and one fifth of its contrast, and so on.) The addition of the fundamental sine wave, and just a couple of odd numbered harmonics (third and fifth), produces a wave that is almost indistinguishable from a square wave. (Adding up the fundamental and all odd numbered harmonics out to infinity would produce an exact square wave.) Constructing a square wave is a far cry from constructing a face. The same principles, however, apply in both cases.

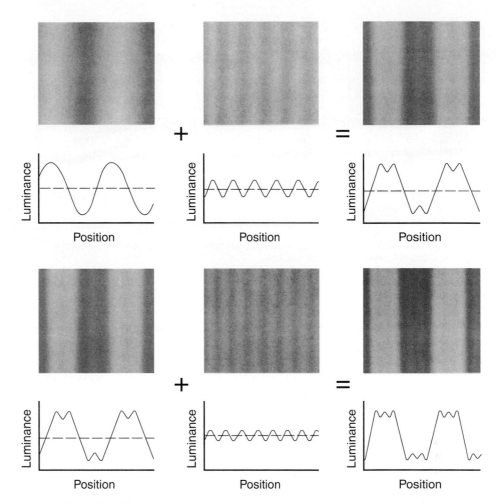

FIGURE 7–5. Construction of a square wave grating from the appropriate combination of sine wave gratings. (Levine and Shefner, 1991.)

SPATIAL MODULATION TRANSFER FUNCTION OF A LENS

A spatial modulation transfer function (SMTF) tells us how well an optical lens (or system) transfers information. How would we go about determining an SMTF? A grating of a specified spatial frequency and contrast serves as the object for the lens (Fig. 7-6). The image contrast is measured and then divided by the object contrast.[1] This ratio tells us how well the lens transfers the infor-

---

1. The image is in perfect focus.

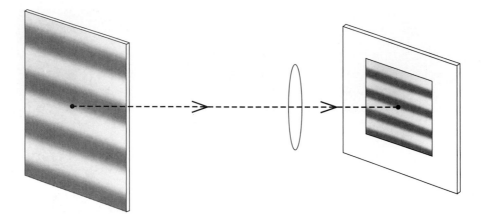

FIGURE 7–6. A spatial grating is focused by an optical lens to determine the spatial modulation transfer function for the lens.

mation (i.e., contrast) contained in the object. If the lens were perfect (and no lens is perfect), the image contrast would equal the object contrast. In reality there is some image degradation, resulting in a reduction in contrast.

This procedure is repeated for a spectrum of spatial frequencies, ranging from low to high frequencies. The result is a SMTF such as represented by the solid line in Fig. 7–7. You may think of this curve as representing the quality of image reproduction as a function of spatial frequency.

The SMTF given in Fig. 7–7 is characteristic of an optical lens. For low and moderate spatial frequencies, the image is transferred with good fidelity (little image degradation). Due to the aberrations inherent in any optical system, the image becomes more degraded at higher frequencies. These same aberrations have comparatively little effect on optical image quality at low and moderate spatial frequencies.

What is the effect of optical defocus on the SMTF? The solid line in Fig. 7–7 shows the SMTF for a lens in perfect focus, and the dashed curve shows the SMTF for the same lens when the image is out of focus. (For example, the image screen is moved away from the plane of focus.) Note that defocus results in a reduction in image quality primarily at high spatial frequencies, with low and moderate frequencies less affected. As we shall learn, this has important clinical implications.

Suppose we paint a spectacle lens with clear nail polish so that it is translucent, as is occasionally done when treating amblyopia. The image formed by this lens is much degraded. Its SMTF reveals an overall reduction in image contrast at all spatial frequencies (dash-dotted curve in Fig. 7–7). This effect, which could also be obtained by roughening the surface of the lens with sandpaper, is due largely to the scattering of light at the lens surface.

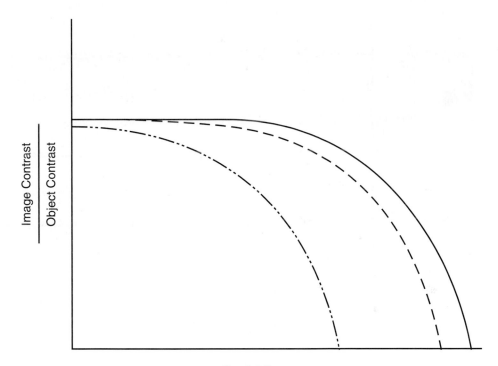

FIGURE 7–7. The solid line represents the spatial modulation transfer function (SMTF) for an optical lens in focus. The dashed line is for the same lens when out of focus. The dash-dotted line represents the SMTF for a translucent lens.

THE HUMAN CONTRAST SENSITIVITY FUNCTION

The human SMTF is often referred to as a contrast sensitivity function (CSF) because sensitivity, not image contrast, is measured. A subject is asked to view a monitor that initially displays a spatial grating that is below threshold—it has such low contrast that it is not visible. Instead, a screen with even luminance across its surface is seen. The examiner slowly increases the contrast until a point is reached where the grating is seen (it appears to emerge out of the background). The reciprocal of this threshold contrast is the contrast sensitivity for the grating. Thresholds are determined for a large number of different spatial frequencies, resulting in a graph that shows contrast sensitivity as a function of spatial frequency, a CSF.

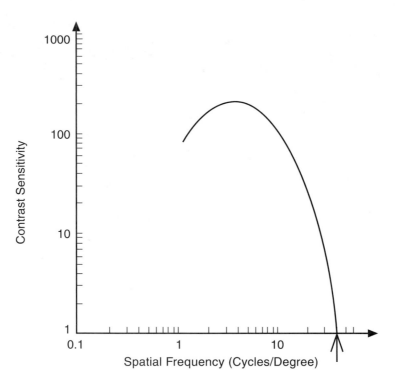

FIGURE 7–8. Typical human contrast sensitivity function. The arrow points to the high-frequency cutoff. Note that the coordinates are plotted in log units. The abscissa represents 100 percent contrast. (Contrast sensitivity is the reciprocal of threshold percent contrast.)

A typical adult human CSF is shown in Fig. 7–8. It is a band-pass function, showing peak sensitivity at about 4 cycles/degree and decreasing sensitivity on either side of this peak (Campbell and Robson, 1968). Humans detect a grating of 4 cycles/degree at a contrast lower than that required for the detection of other frequencies. This is further illustrated in Fig. 7–9, which shows, from left to right, gratings of increasing spatial frequency. From bottom to top, the contrast decreases. Note that gratings of moderate frequencies are seen at lower contrast levels (higher on the diagram) than are other frequencies.

CSF High-Frequency Cutoff

The high-frequency cutoff in sensitivity reflects the visual system's limited ability to resolve detail, even if the detail is at 100 percent contrast. As the spatial frequency of a 100 percent contrast grating is increased, a point is reached where the grating can no longer be resolved. For a young, healthy adult, the high-frequency cutoff can be about 60 cycles/degree, indicated by the arrow in Fig. 7–8.

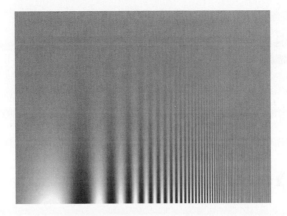

FIGURE 7–9. A plate that demonstrates the contrast sensitivity function. Contrast increases going from top to bottom, and spatial frequency increases going from left to right. Note that when held at arm's length, moderate spatial frequencies are seen at lower contrasts than low or high spatial frequencies (Campbell and Robson, 1964). Also see Dr. Izumi Ohzawa's Web site: http://www.bpe.es.osaka-u.ac. jp/ohzawa-lab/izumi/ CSF/A_ JG_RobsonCSFchart.html

Let us compare this to visual acuity,[2] which is determined by requiring a patient to resolve the details of visual characters, called **optotypes**,[3] designed for this purpose. The optotypes are typically of very high contrast. As the patient reads down an eye chart, the optotypes become smaller and their details become finer (i.e., the high spatial frequency content increases). Even at 100 percent contrast, a point is reached where the details of the optotypes can no longer be resolved (Fig. 7-10). In essence, visual acuity is the high-frequency cutoff determined using optotypes rather than gratings. As we learn later in this chapter, it is straightforward to convert from visual acuity to the high-spatial frequency cut-off.

Figure 7–11 illustrates the relationship between visual acuity and the CSF. The gratings are at 100 percent contrast. Directly above these gratings is a horizontal row of optotypes also at 100 percent contrast. The optotypes diminish in contrast as they approach the envelope of the CSF. In a typical acuity measurement, all optotypes would be at 100 percent contrast (or close to it), and the patient would be instructed to read the smallest letter that he or she can resolve.

An important limitation of a typical acuity measurement is that only a small portion of the patient's CSF is examined. It does not assess the ability to detect

---

2. As we learn later in this chapter, there are several forms of visual acuity. The form of acuity measured with a standard eye chart is referred to as recognition acuity.

3. Optoytpes often take the form of stylized letters, such as those on a standard Snellen visual acuity chart.

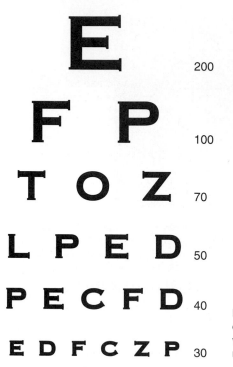

200

100

70

50

40

30

FIGURE 7–10. Snellen acuity chart. Each line is designated by its foot-size, which is the distance at which each of its optotypes subtends an angle of 5 min arc.

moderate spatial frequencies (e.g., 4 cycles/degree) even though we are the most sensitive to these frequencies. We return to this later in the chapter.

Why does the visual system show a reduction in sensitivity for high frequencies? We have already discussed one reason—optical limitations. Any optical system, including the eye, will show a high-frequency limitation due to optical aberrations. This is the case even when the eye is in perfect focus.[4]

Another factor that plays a role in the high spatial frequency cutoff is the packing density of retinal photoreceptors. Consider the schematic illustrations of photoreceptors packed at low and high densities in Fig. 7–12. A grating is superimposed on each of these matrices. If it is assumed that each photoreceptor sums up all the light that falls on it, it is hard to imagine how the coarse matrix on the left could resolve this grating. The finer matrix could, however, resolve this grating because the photoreceptors are packed sufficiently densely to allow bright bars to fall on alternate rows of photoreceptors. When stated more formally, this is referred to as the Nyquist theorem (Williams, 1986).

---

4. The correction of the eye's optical aberrations can lead to visual acuity beyond the typical 20/20 or 20/15, a condition referred to as supernormal vision (Schwartz, 2002). Although it is possible to create supernormal vision in the laboratory, its clinical attainment with custom contact lenses or laser refractive procedures (e.g., LASIK) has not been fully explored.

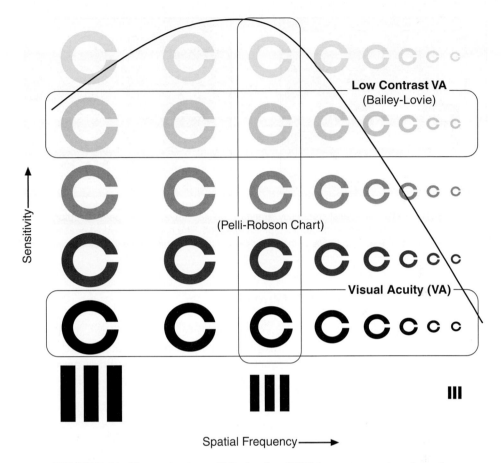

FIGURE 7–11. The contrast sensitivity function (CSF) forms an envelope for opto-types (letters) of various contrast and size. The bottom row of optotypes and the spatial gratings are both at 100 percent contrast. Contrast decreases as the envelope of the CSF is approached. Note that a horizontal array of low-contrast optotypes, of diminishing size, serve as the stimuli for the Bailey–Lovie chart. For the Pelli–Robson chart, all stimuli are the same size, but of diminishing contrast. This is represented by a vertical column of optotypes. (*Reproduced with permission from Adams AJ, Impact of emerging instrumentation on optometry. Optom Vis Sci. 1993;70:272–278.*)

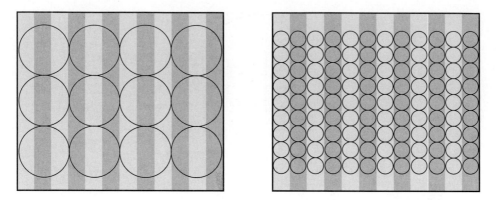

FIGURE 7–12. A spatial frequency grating projected on a coarse photoreceptor matrix (left) and on a finer photoreceptor matrix (right). The finer matrix would enable resolution of the grating because the bright bars of the grating fall on every other row of photoreceptors.

CSF in Uncorrected Refractive Errors

What happens to the high-frequency cutoff if the eye is out of focus, such as an uncorrected myopic eye? As with an ophthalmic lens that is out-of-focus, there is a reduction in the high-frequency cut-off (see Fig. 7-7). The solid curve in Fig. 7–13 shows the CSF for a myope who is fully corrected, and the dashed curve

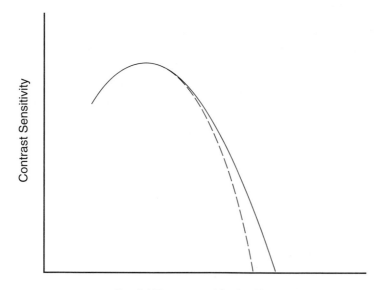

FIGURE 7–13. Contrast sensitivity functions for an eye in focus (solid line) and an eye out of focus (dashed line).

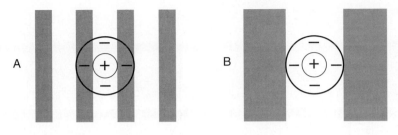

FIGURE 7–14. The spatial frequency grating on the left is a more optimal stimulus for this ganglion cell than the lower spatial frequency grating on the right. This is because the large bright bar of the low-frequency grating falls both on the receptive field's center and surround. This results in lateral inhibition, which reduces the neuron's response.

shows the CSF for the same myope without spectacles. Note the reduction in the high-frequency cut-off, which is consistent with our common-sense understanding that an uncorrected myope has reduced visual acuity.

CSF LOW-FREQUENCY DROP-OFF

Consider the response of a ganglion cell to light that falls on its receptive field, the area in space that influences its activity.[5] A typical ganglion cell receptive field consists of a center region that responds to illumination with either excitation or inhibition and a surround region that responds with the opposite sign. The result is spatial antagonism, which is also called lateral inhibition. For the receptive field in Fig. 7-14, light falling on the center causes excitation, while light falling on the surround causes inhibition.[6] This cell will be optimally activated when a bright bar falls on the center of its receptive field and a dark bar on its surround, as depicted in Fig. 7–14A. A lower spatial frequency—where the bright bar falls on both the receptive field's center and surround, thereby causing lateral inhibition—results in a smaller response, accounting for the CSF's low-frequency drop-off (see Fig. 7-14B).[7]

---

5. See Chapter 12 for a more complete description of receptive fields.

6. For a ganglion cell, excitation is defined as an increase in the frequency of action potentials (indicated by plus signs) and inhibition as a decrease in the frequency (indicated by minus signs).

7. As discussed in more detail in Chapter 12, when light falls on both the center and surround, the excitatory center response is offset by the inhibitory surround response. When dark bars fall on the surround, they block light that would otherwise fall on it, causing the inhibitory response of the surround to be minimized.

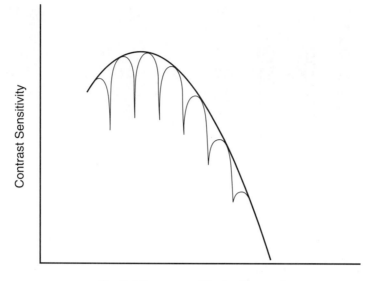

FIGURE 7–15. The contrast sensitivity function can be thought of as an envelope for a number of independent narrow spatial frequency channels.

THE VISUAL SYSTEM AS A FOURIER ANALYZER

In one view of visual information processing, the visual system is considered to be a Fourier analyzer. That is, the visual system is thought to deconstruct the retinal image into its spatial frequency components.[8]

This view is supported by the existence of independent spatial frequency channels within the visual system, as illustrated in Fig. 7–15. Rather than consisting of a single channel that is maximally sensitive to 4 cycles/degree, we can think of the CSF as forming an envelope that encompasses several narrow channels. Each of these channels is presumably independent.

The effect of prior adaptation to a spatial frequency grating supports this model (Blakemore and Campbell, 1969). Suppose a subject's CSF is determined and he or she then views an adapting grating (which is sinusoidal) for about a minute prior to the redetermination of the CSF.[9] The results of this experiment are given in Fig. 7–16A. Note that there is a discrete reduction in sensitivity at the specific frequency to which the observer was adapted. This is the result predicted by the multiple-channel hypothesis.

---

8. This is also referred to as linear system analysis.

9. The adapting grating drifts across the computer screen to prevent the formation of a retinal afterimage.

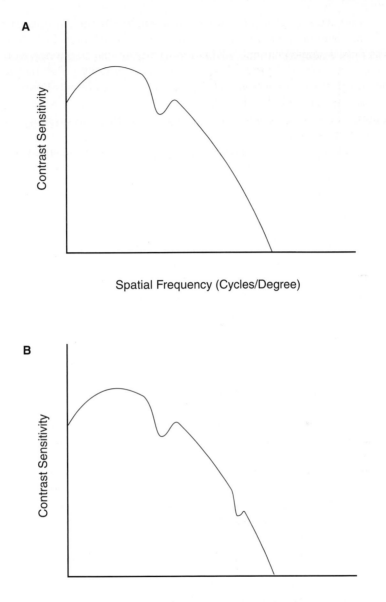

FIGURE 7–16. A. Prior adaptation to a sine wave grating of 6 cycles/degree results in reduced sensitivity at this frequency. **B.** Prior adaptation to a square wave grating of 6 cycles/degree produces a reduction in sensitivity at both the fundamental frequency (6 cycles/degree) and the third harmonic (18 cycles/degree).

What would we expect if there was only a single channel? In this case, there would be an overall reduction in the CSF across all frequencies. Moreover, if there was only a single channel, adaptation to any spatial frequency would have the same effect—it would produce a reduction in sensitivity for all frequencies.[10]

Further support for the notion that the visual system performs Fourier analysis comes from an ingenious experiment in which the observer adapts to a square wave grating rather than a sine wave grating (Blakemore and Campbell, 1969). Figure 7–16B shows the results when an observer adapts to a square wave grating of 6 cycles/degree. As expected, there is a reduction in sensitivity at the fundamental frequency of the square wave, 6 cycles/degree; however, note that there is a secondary reduction in sensitivity at 18 cycles/degree. We can account for this reduction by recalling that a square wave is composed of a fundamental sine wave of the same frequency and harmonic sine waves of odd multiples of this fundamental frequency. The secondary reduction in sensitivity represents adaptation to the third harmonic, which has a frequency of 18 cycles/degree.[11] It appears that a complex stimulus, the square wave, is broken down by the visual system into its components (a fundamental and its harmonics). This has been interpreted to indicate a form of Fourier analysis.

Mach bands demonstrate the usefulness of considering the visual system as a Fourier analyzer. As indicated by the luminance profile, the transition between the bright and dark regions in Fig. 7–17A is gradual. It is not, however, perceived as such. Instead, observers typically report bright and dark bands at the junctions of the bright and dark regions. These perceived bands, which do not actually exist, are referred to as Mach bands.

This illusion can be explained by assuming that the visual system performs a Fourier analysis of the stimulus. The gradual transition between the bright and dark regions consists of low spatial frequencies. Since the CSF manifests reduced sensitivity to these frequencies,[12] there is a relative enhancement of high spatial frequencies, resulting in the perception of enhanced boundaries (Mach bands).

Single-unit electrophysiological data from the primate visual cortex are consistent with the notion that the visual system could act as a Fourier analyzer.[13] Neurons in striate cortex appear to be finely tuned to specific spatial frequencies (DeValois et al, 1982). A collection of such neurons could form the physiological basis for the spatial frequency channels we discussed.

---

10. The same principle holds true for a photopigment. Bleaching rhodopsin with 507 nm does not cause a discrete reduction in sensitivity at 507 nm, but a reduction in sensitivity for all wavelengths. Furthermore, any wavelength that is absorbed by rhodopsin could cause this same overall reduction.

11. Reductions in sensitivity to the fifth, seventh, and other odd harmonics are not noted because of the low contrast of these harmonics.

12. Recall that this reduced sensitivity to low frequencies is due to lateral inhibition within the retina.

13. See Chapter 14 for a discussion of the receptive fields of cortical neurons.

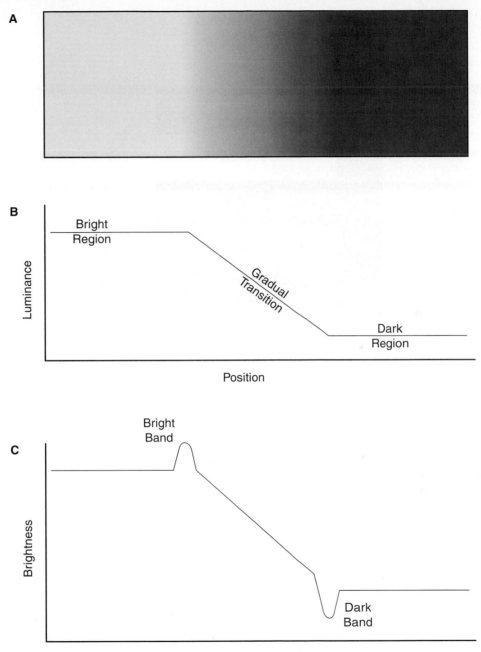

FIGURE 7–17. A. Although the decrease in luminance from left to right is gradual, bright and dark bands are observed. (The bright band is seen about one third of the distance from the left edge of the diagram and the dark band at about one third of the distance from the right edge of the diagram.) These bands, which are not physically present, are referred to as Mach bands. They represent a perceptual enhancement of borders. **B.** Luminance profile for the pattern in A. Note the gradual transition between the bright and dark regions of the pattern. **C.** Brightness of the pattern as perceived by a typical observer. The bright and dark bands, which are not physically present, are Mach bands.

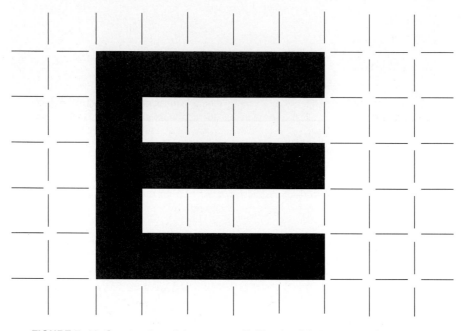

FIGURE 7–18. Construction of the optotype **E.** The detail (a bar or a gap) is one fifth of the overall size of the optotype.

Does the visual system actually act as a Fourier analyzer? The jury is still out on this question. Although the preceding experimental evidence is consistent with this model, it does not prove that it is correct. Nonetheless, the CSF is a useful and important tool for understanding how the visual system processes spatial information.

RELATIONSHIP OF THE CSF TO SNELLEN ACUITY

As we learned, visual acuity, as determined with optotypes, is equivalent to the CSF high-frequency cutoff. A typical optotype is designed such that its overall size is five times that of its detail (Fig. 7–18). The legs of the optotype **E** can be thought of as bars of a spatial grating (Fig. 17-19). To read the **E,** the patient must resolve its detail (e.g., bars and gaps). The angle that *just resolvable* bars (or gaps) make with the eye is called the **minimum angle of resolution (MAR).**

Visual acuity is often recorded in the form of the **Snellen fraction.** The numerator is the distance at which the measurement is taken, for example, 20 ft. The denominator is the **foot-size** of the smallest optotype that the patient can resolve. Foot-size is defined as the distance at which an optotype subtends 5 min

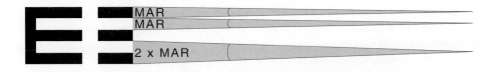

FIGURE 7–19. The optotype **E** may be thought of as consisting of the bright and dark bars of a grating. The smallest resolvable bar (or gap) subtends the minimum angle of resolution (MAR) at the eye. The combination of the bar and a gap, which is equivalent to one complete cycle of a grating, is twice the MAR.

arc. At this same distance, the optotype detail subtends one fifth of this value (1 min arc).[14]

An important advantage of the Snellen fraction is that it allows easy calculation of the patient's MAR, which is simply the reciprocal of the Snellen fraction. What information does a Snellen fraction of 20/40 provide? It tells us that the measurement was taken at 20 ft; the smallest letter the patient can read subtends 5 min arc, overall, at 40 ft (i.e., it has a foot-size of 40 ft); and the patient's MAR is 2 min arc.

What is the expected high-frequency cutoff of a patient with 20/40 acuity? Referring back to Fig. 7–19, note that the combination of a bar and a gap corresponds to a cycle of a spatial grating. A patient with 20/40 acuity can just barely resolve a grating whose bars (or gaps) subtend 2 min arc; therefore, a just resolvable grating subtends 4 min arc.[15] Since spatial frequency is typically given in cycles per degree, we must make the following conversion:

$$\left(\frac{1 \text{ cycle}}{4' \text{ arc}} \right) \left(\frac{60' \text{ arc}}{1 \text{ degree}} \right) = 15 \text{ cycles/degree}$$

This tells us that Snellen acuity of 20/40 is equivalent to a high-frequency CSF cutoff of 15 cycles/degree.

CLINICAL IMPLICATIONS OF THE CSF

We have spent a considerable amount of time developing the concepts associated with the human CSF. What is the clinical value of this knowledge? Of pri-

---

14. Each line on a Snellen chart is designated by its foot-size. In Fig. 7–10, the big **E** has a foot-size of 200, meaning that at a distance of 200 ft it subtends 5 min arc overall, while its detail subtends 1 min arc. If this is the smallest optotype a patient can read at a distance of 20 ft, his or her visual acuity is 20/200. The second line from the top consists of optotypes with foot-sizes of 100 ft. If this same patient was tested at 10 ft, the expected visual acuity is 10/100. In both cases, the MAR is 10 min arc.

15. Since the MAR is 2 min arc, each bar (or gap) of the threshold optotype **E** subtends 2 min arc at the patient's eye.

mary interest is that the optical correction of refractive errors improves only a limited aspect of a patient's spatial vision. Visual acuity is improved, but there is little effect at low frequencies.

In a highly visual society such as ours, high-frequency resolution is critical. Reading road signs, blackboards, computer screens, and books and watching movies and television are all dependent on a high level of visual resolution. Consequently, the demand for the correction of refractive errors is great. It is, however, important to realize that a reduction in acuity, secondary to a refractive error, is often well-tolerated by patients whose acuity demands are not high. Eye care practitioners are occasionally frustrated by the patient whose acuity can be substantially improved, yet prefers his or her old correction that produces worse visual acuity. These patients illustrate the critical fact that there is more to spatial vision than high-frequency resolution.

Consider the world about you. Certainly many objects are highly detailed and require good acuity to resolve. Yet many objects can be recognized by their moderate frequency content. Consider the tree across the street, the dog in the driveway, or the outline of your spouse's body. These objects may be recognized without high-frequency acuity.

The novice clinician is sometimes surprised by how well a patient with central (macular) vision loss (say, 20/200 acuity) performs certain visual tasks. The patient's high-frequency spatial resolution is severely impaired, but he or she retains vision at low frequencies. This patient will have difficulty reading, driving, and inserting a key into a keyhole, but may be capable of performing certain of the essential tasks of life, such as ambulation.

Studies of visual disability suggest that reductions in visual acuity and contrast sensitivity contribute independently to the performance of visually guided activities (West et al, 2002). Consider a patient who has a deficit at moderate frequencies with only minimal reduction in sensitivity at high frequencies. He or she may present with symptoms of substantially reduced vision. Yet when we perform a standard acuity test, we may find normal or near-normal visual acuity.

A reduction in sensitivity to moderate frequencies is typically accompanied by a reduction in acuity or other symptoms and signs. Patients with early cataract formation may complain of a profound reduction in their ability to see; however, visual acuity may be only slightly reduced (Fig. 7–20) (Hess and Woo, 1978). The discrepancy between the severe complaint and the slight reduction in acuity occurs because the cataract acts as a diffuser, reducing image contrast across all frequencies.[16] The patient is handicapped not only at high frequencies, but at moderate and low frequencies as well. Consequently, the patient's complaints are disproportionate to the reduction in acuity.

---

16. This is similar to the example discussed earlier in this chapter, where an optical lens is coated with clear nail polish.

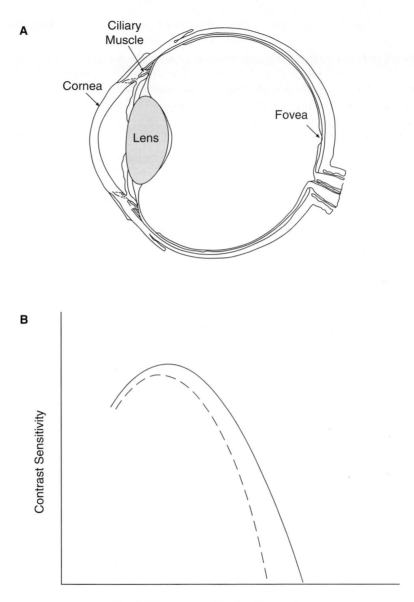

FIGURE 7–20 A. A cataract is an opacity of the crystalline lens. **B.** This opacity reduces the overall retinal contrast such that the resultant CSF has the form of the dashed curve.

Shining a light into the eye causes light scatter—a so-called **veiling glare**—that can reduce the contrast of the retinal image. This is the basis of the brightness acuity tester (BAT), a clinical instrument that shines diffuse light into the eye as the patient views an eye chart. While the diffuse light has minimal effects on visual acuity in the healthy eye, there can be a marked reduction in acuity if there is a cataract, even an early cataract.[17] A substantial reduction in the patient's visual acuity during BAT testing suggests that extraction of the cataract may be warranted. Along these lines, it should be noted that patients who have undergone cataract surgery are involved in significantly fewer motor vehicle accidents than cataract patients who have not undergone surgery (Owsley et al, 2002).

Contact lenses may produce corneal edema, with swelling of the corneal stromal layers (or epithelial cells) resulting in increased light scatter similar to that produced by a cataract (Hess and Carney, 1979; Woo and Hess, 1979). There is a resultant reduction in contrast sensitivity across all frequencies. Not surprisingly, these patients often have normal or near-normal acuity, but complain of poor vision. For example, the patient may have 20/20 vision yet complain of blur.

Scarring of the stromal layers secondary to trauma or refractive laser procedures (e.g., incisions from refractive keratometry) can cause clinically significant light scatter, with a resultant reduction in contrast sensitivity at moderate frequencies. Swelling of the stroma, as occurs in Fuchs endothelial dystrophy, can also lead to loss in sensitivity at moderate frequencies. Again, it is important to keep in mind that patients with reductions in contrast sensitivity at moderate frequencies may have only a slight reduction in acuity (e.g., 20/25), yet complain of severe visual impairment.

In summary, we must be aware that Snellen acuity samples only a small portion of the patient's spatial vision. Cataracts, corneal edema, and other conditions commonly produce reductions in contrast sensitivity at spatial frequencies other than those measured in an acuity task (Bodis-Wollner and Camisa, 1980). Consequently, complaints of reduced vision that are not proportionate to the reduction in Snellen acuity warrant careful investigation.

CLINICAL DETERMINATION OF THE CSF

Determination of a CSF is not a common clinical procedure. It is time consuming and often provides information that could be determined more efficiently through other related procedures.

The most accurate clinical methods display gratings on a video monitor that is

---

17. A similar effect can be found by comparing the patient's visual acuity as determined in a dark room with the acuity determined when the lights are turned on. A patient with a cataract is expected to show a more profound reduction in visual acuity with the lights on than a patient who does not have a cataract.

driven by a microprocessor. Such instruments are typically available only in large eye clinics. More accessible methods employ gratings displayed on a chart (VIS-TECH) or a series of cards (Arden plates). The reliability and validity of the latter tests have been called into question (Reeves et al, 1991).

Alternatively, visual acuity may be determined with low-contrast optotypes rather than the high-contrast optotypes typically used. The Bailey–Lovie low-contrast acuity chart may be used for this purpose (Bailey and Lovie, 1976). The concepts associated with this test are illustrated in Fig. 7–11. A variation on this theme is the Pelli–Robson approach, which measures threshold contrast using optotypes, not gratings (Pelli et al, 1988). Rather than the optotypes becoming smaller as the patient reads down the chart, they remain the same size and their contrast decreases. The concepts associated with this task are also illustrated in Fig. 7–11. Either the Bailey–Lovie low-contrast chart or the Pelli–Robson test would be appropriate for the typical eye-care office. They are efficient and alert the clinician to reductions in contrast sensitivity at moderate frequencies.

OTHER FORMS OF VISUAL ACUITY

The discussion of visual acuity has centered on resolution and recognition acuity. **Resolution acuity** involves distinguishing a pattern (e.g., a grating) from a uniform patch of light of equal luminance (see Fig. 17–9). When gratings are used, the acuity is sometimes referred to as **grating acuity.** The CSF high-frequency cutoff is an example of grating acuity. For a young, healthy adult, the high-frequency cutoff is from 40 to 60 cycles/degree, which is equivalent to a MAR of 0.75 to 0.50 minutes of arc.

Recognition acuity is a form of resolution that requires a patient to be familiar with an optotype and to recognize it. Snellen acuity is an example of recognition acuity because the patient must be familiar with the alphabet to read the optotypes on the chart. Young, healthy adults typically manifest Snellen acuities of 20/15 to 20/10.

Grating and recognition acuity are by far the most commonly utilized clinical measures of acuity. This is primarily because of their utility in the diagnosis and amelioration of refractive errors.

Other forms of visual acuity also provide useful information regarding the limitations of spatial vision. **Minimum detectable acuity** refers to the smallest object that can be seen. Imagine a thin wire against a blue sky. How thin could this wire be and still be visible? (In this task, the subject does not need to recognize the object, only to detect it.) Figure 7–21 illustrates how we can approach this question. Minimum detectable acuity can be considered to be equivalent to an increment threshold task.[18] Due to optical imperfections of the eye, the wire

---

18. See Chapters 3 and 11.

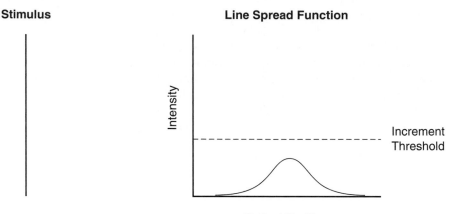

Stimulus   **Line Spread Function**

Increment
Threshold

Retinal Position

FIGURE 7–21. Minimum detectable acuity is determined by making a line progressively thinner, until it is no longer visible. A line spread function (LSF), with a maximum height that diminishes as the line becomes thinner, is formed on the retina. Viewed in this manner, minimum detectable acuity can be considered to be an increment threshold task. In the example illustrated, the line would not be detectable because the LSF's peak retinal intensity falls below the increment threshold.

is not in perfect focus on the retina; its image takes the form of a **line spread function.** In order for the line to be detected, the height of the line spread function must be of a critical value. It turns out that this critical value is the same as ΔI in an increment threshold experiment.

Minimum detectable acuity is limited by how thin a line (or small a dot) can be made and still emit sufficient light so that the increment threshold is reached. This has been determined to be about 1 second of arc (Westheimer, 1979). Note that this value is considerably smaller than that for resolution acuity.

Optical defocus, such as caused by an uncorrected refractive error, will result in a reduction in the height of the line spread function, with a resultant reduction in minimum detectable acuity. This reduction, however, is not as marked as with resolution acuity.

The final type of acuity that we discuss is **hyperacuity,** so named because of the exquisite sensitivity manifested in this form of acuity. Several different hyperacuity tasks are given in Fig. 7–22. Because of humans' excellent abilities at detecting tilt, a form of hyperacuity, it can be very difficult to align a picture on a wall so that it does not appear tilted.

Hyperacuity apparently depends on the visual system's ability to sense direction. Consider the **vernier acuity** task in Fig. 7–22A. Each bar represents a different direction. When these two bars represent sufficiently different directions, a threshold for this hyperacuity task is reached.

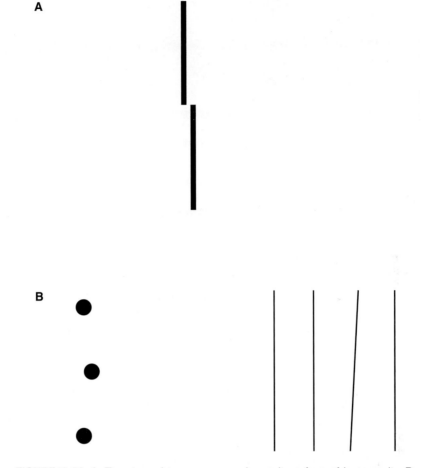

FIGURE 7–22. A. Target used to measure vernier acuity, a form of hyperacuity. **B.** Other targets that measure hyperacuity. For the target on the left, the task is to determine which circle is out of alignment. For the target on the right, the task is to determine which line is tilted.

Thresholds for hyperacuity are very low, on the order of 3 seconds of arc (Westheimer, 1979). These low thresholds are presumably related to the visual system's ability to average luminance information across space to arrive at a sense of direction. This process occurs at postreceptoral levels, including the retina and, perhaps, the visual cortex (Levi et al, 1985).

Hyperacuity is very resilient to optical defocus. Whereas refractive errors greatly reduce resolution acuity, they have minimal effects on hyperacuity. Figure 7–23 provides a possible explanation for this observation. For the resolution task, optical defocus causes the blur circles to overlap, thereby interfering with the resolution of the two lines. In comparison, optical defocus does not interfere with

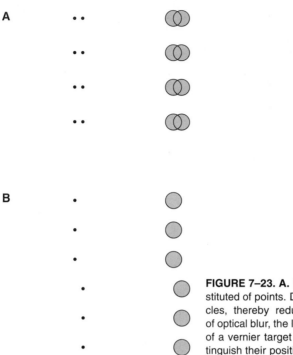

FIGURE 7–23. A. Each line can be considered as constituted of points. Defocus leads to overlapping blur circles, thereby reducing resolution acuity. **B.** In spite of optical blur, the luminance profiles of the blurred lines of a vernier target provide sufficient information to distinguish their positions.

the averaging of information across the retina that enables the positions of the two lines to be determined. The peaks of the luminance profiles are in different positions, and this leads to the perception of a different location for each line.

There is evidence that performance on vernier acuity tasks is adversely affected in glaucoma (McKendrick et al, 2002). The disease apparently results in damage to retinal circuits involved with the processing of position information.

SUMMARY

Contrast sensitivity functions provide a powerful tool for characterizing spatial vision capabilities. The common clinical measurement of visual acuity assesses only a limited aspect of a patient's spatial vision. Reductions at high spatial frequencies, however, prompt the most visual complaints, and if optical in nature, are amenable to correction. Nonetheless, it should be kept in mind that reductions at frequencies other than the highest frequencies do occur and are of clinical importance.

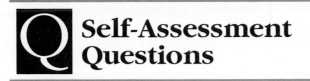

Q Self-Assessment Questions

1. Determine the predicted high-frequency contrast sensitivity function cutoff, in cycles/degree, for the following visual acuities: **A.** 20/15. **B.** 20/80. **C.** 20/150.

2. Visual acuity is to be measured at 20 ft with a Snellen chart. Calculate the expected Snellen fractions for patients with the following high spatial frequency cutoffs: **A.** 5 cycles/degree. **B.** 20 cycles/degree. **C.** 60 cycles/degree.

3. A patient's visual acuity is 20/100. **A.** What is the overall physical size, in mm, of the smallest letter the patient can read on a Snellen chart at a distance of 20 ft? **B.** What is the size of the detail, in mm, of this letter?

4. A patient has a Snellen fraction of 20/80. What would you predict the Snellen fraction to be when acuity is measured at 10 ft?

5. A patient shows a high-frequency contrast sensitivity function (CSF) cutoff of 30 cycles/degree when tested at 20 ft. **A.** What is the expected high-frequency CSF cutoff, in cycles/degree, when the procedure is repeated at 10 ft? **B.** What is the width of a single bar of the threshold grating, in mm, when the test is performed at 20 ft? **C.** What is the width of a single bar of the threshold grating when the test is performed at 10 ft?

6. You measure a patient's visual acuity with a projected Snellen chart. In a dark room, the acuity is 20/20. **A.** What happens to the measured visual acuity when you turn on the overhead room lights? **B.** Why?

8

Temporal Aspects of Vision

Whereas spatial vision is concerned with changes in luminance across space, temporal vision—time-related vision—is concerned with changes in luminance over time. Temporal vision is closely related to the ability to perceive motion.

Recent studies suggest that temporal and motion vision are analyzed by the magno retinocortical visual pathway, which feeds into motion analysis areas within the cerebral cortex. This knowledge has been used to develop clinical tests that may aid in the diagnosis of certain diseases of the visual system.

STIMULUS CONSIDERATIONS

Temporal vision is often studied with stimuli whose luminance varies sinusoidally over time (sometimes called temporal sinusoids) (Fig. 8–1). These stimuli are the temporal equivalent of spatial sine wave gratings. Whereas a spatial grating manifests a sinusoidal change in luminance across space, a temporal sinusoid manifests a sinusoidal change in luminance over time.[1] Sinusoidal stimuli permit the use of linear system analysis.

---

1. Quickly turning a light source, such as an incandescent lamp, on and off creates a temporal square wave. If the light source, however, turns on and off with a sinusoidal time course, the resultant stimulus is a temporal sinusoid.

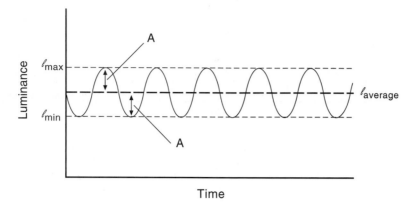

FIGURE 8–1. Luminance profile for a stimulus whose luminance is temporally modulated sinusoidally over time. A computer screen that turns on and off with a sinusoidal time course would produce a luminance profile similar to that given in this figure. "A" refers to amplitude of modulation.

Depth of Modulation

The visibility of a temporally modulated stimulus is related to its depth of modulation. The stimulus in Fig. 8–2A has a relatively small depth of modulation. A light source that is modulated at this small depth may appear steady, with no flicker noted.[2] In comparison, the stimulus in Fig. 8–2B manifests a relatively large depth of modulation. A light source modulated at this greater modulation depth is not perceived as steady. It is seen as flickering.

The preceding example is analogous to the detection of spatial gratings. A spatial grating of very low contrast appears as a uniform gray surface. Only when the contrast is sufficiently high is the grating resolved. Likewise, a temporally modulated stimulus of low modulation depth is not resolved; it appears steady. As the modulation depth is increased, it is resolved and seen as flickering.

The **percentage depth of modulation** of a temporally modulated stimulus is given by the following relationship:

$$\text{percentage modulation} = \frac{A}{l_{\text{ave}}}(100)$$

where

$$A = \text{amplitude of modulation}$$
$$l_{\text{ave}} = \text{time-averaged luminance}$$

Note that this formula is essentially the same as that for spatial contrast, except that the stimulus is temporally, rather than spatially, modulated.

---

2. Flicker is a perception that can be elicited by the temporal modulation of a stimulus.

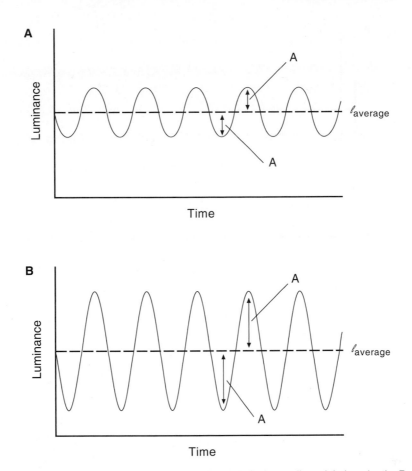

FIGURE 8–2. **A.** Temporal sinusoid with a relatively small modulation depth. **B.** Temporal sinusoid with a relatively large modulation depth.

Temporal Frequency

Just as it is possible to vary the frequency of a spatial grating, it is also possible to vary the frequency of a temporal sinusoid (Fig. 8–3). A low temporal frequency stimulus is seen as flickering at a low rate, whereas a higher temporal frequency stimulus flickers at a higher rate.

As the temporal frequency is increased, a frequency is reached at which flicker can no longer be resolved, the **critical flicker fusion frequency (CFF).** The CFF is analogous to spatial resolution acuity. As the frequency of a spatial grating is increased, it appears to consist of increasingly thin bars. At the high spatial frequency cutoff, the bars are not resolvable, and the stimulus appears as a uniform gray surface. Likewise, as the frequency of a temporally modulated stimulus is increased, the flicker appears more rapid. A frequency is eventually reached that cannot be resolved, and the stimulus appears steady. This temporal

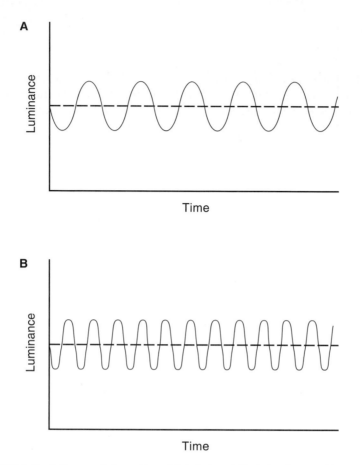

A

Luminance

Time

B

Luminance

Time

FIGURE 8–3. A. Temporal sinusoid modulated at a relatively low temporal frequency. **B.** Temporal sinusoid modulated at a relatively high temporal frequency.

frequency, the CFF, represents the high temporal resolution limit of the visual system for a given depth of modulation. Temporal frequency is typically given in hertz (Hz). One hertz is equal to one cycle per second.

TEMPORAL MODULATION TRANSFER FUNCTIONS

The advantage of sinusoidal stimuli is that they allow the application of linear system (Fourier) analysis (de Lange, 1958). In Chapter 7, we learned that any spatial stimulus can be constructed by the proper combination of spatial sine wave gratings. Similarly, a temporal stimulus can be constructed by the appropriate combination of temporal sinusoids.

Whereas spatial vision is characterized by the contrast sensitivity function (CSF), temporal vision is characterized by the temporal modulation transfer function (TMTF). To determine a TMTF, an individual views a light source (e.g., a computer screen) that is modulated sinusoidally at a given temporal rate. Initially, the modulation depth is very small, and the screen appears steady. The depth of modulation is slowly increased until the subject reports that the screen is flickering. The percentage modulation at which the person first sees flicker is the threshold. Its reciprocal represents the relative sensitivity (relative to the background illumination) for flicker resolution. This procedure is repeated for a large number of temporal frequencies, from low to high, to obtain a TMTF.

A typical human TMTF is given in Fig. 8–4. This graph shows relative sensitivity as a function of temporal frequency. Stimuli that fall outside of the TMTF are seen as fused or steady; they are not resolved temporally. Those stimuli that fall under the graph are resolved temporally and perceived as flickering.

Like the CSF, the TMTF has a band-pass shape; sensitivity for the detection of flicker falls off at both low and high temporal frequencies. Stimuli of moderate frequencies are detected at a smaller percentage modulation than are other stimuli.

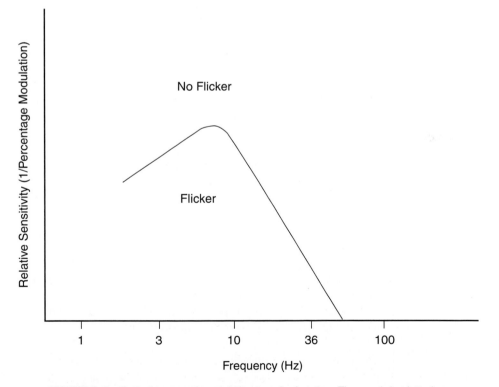

FIGURE 8–4. Typical temporal modulation transfer function. The graph is plotted on log coordinates.

Reduction in Sensitivity for Low Temporal Frequencies

Can we point to visual experiences that are consistent with the shape of the TMTF? Consider the low-frequency reduction in sensitivity, which reveals that very gradual or slow changes in illumination are not seen. Now, contemplate the change in illumination that occurs as the sun sets. Although we are aware of the changing illumination, we do not actually perceive the change itself. Observe the minute hand on a watch. Although we know that the minute hand moves, we do not actually see it move.

Another manifestation of the visual system's reduced sensitivity to low temporal frequencies is the inability to perceive stabilized retinal images (Riggs et al, 1953). Consider the retinal blood vessels that lie on top of the photoreceptors. Relative to the retina, these vessels are stabilized—they move as the eye moves and manifest a temporal frequency of zero. Only when a moving light is shined into the eye, which casts moving shadows on the photoreceptors, is it possible to visualize our own retinal vessels.[3] The retinal vasculature, when visualized in this manner, is referred to as the **Purkinje tree,** a manifestation of the **Troxler phenomenon,** the disappearance of low temporal frequency stimuli (Troxler, 1804).

Figure 8–5 demonstrates our reduced sensitivity to low temporal frequencies. Steady fixation of the top fixation point causes the blurred border to disappear; however, fixation of the bottom fixation point does not cause the sharply focused border to disappear. These phenomena are due to the interaction of eye movements with the stimulus border.

Even when fixating a target, small involuntary eye movements occur continuously (Ratliff and Riggs, 1950). When these eye movements occur across a blurred border (see Fig. 8–5A), the changes in retinal illumination at the border are of a very low temporal frequency, approaching 0 Hz. Because we are not sensitive to low temporal frequencies, the border disappears. Eye movements across the sharply focused border, as shown in Fig. 8–5B, result in the introduction of moderate temporal frequencies. Because we are very sensitive to these frequencies, the border does not disappear.

Reduction in Sensitivity for High Temporal Frequencies

An example of the high-frequency drop-off of the TMTF is the inability to perceive the temporal modulation displayed by household incandescent light bulbs. These bulbs are modulated at 60 Hz, yet appear steady due, in part, to our relative insensitivity to this high-frequency temporal modulation.[4]

[3.] To observe your retinal vasculature, place a penlight against your closed eyelid and jiggle it.

[4.] The modulation depth for an incandescent light bulb is small because the filament does not have time to cool down when the current is reversed. Its intensity diminishes, but not to zero.

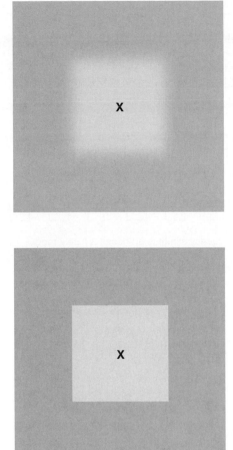

A

B

FIGURE 8–5. A. Steadily fixate the "X." Note that the blurred border disappears. **B.** The sharply focused border usually does not disappear when the "X" is fixated (Cornsweet, 1970).

It bears repeating that the TMTF is analogous to the CSF. For both, sensitivity is plotted as a function of frequency. In the case of the CSF, sensitivity, expressed in terms of spatial contrast, is plotted as a function of spatial frequency. For the TMTF, sensitivity, expressed in terms of percentage modulation, is plotted as a function of temporal frequency.

Both the CSF and TMTF show a band-pass shape, with maximal sensitivity to moderate frequencies. For spatial vision, this means that a sinusoidal grating of about 4 cycles/degree is seen at a lower spatial contrast than are gratings of lower or higher spatial frequencies. Likewise, a stimulus modulated temporally at moderate rates is seen as flickering at a lower percentage modulation than are stimuli of lower or higher temporal frequencies.

Both the CSF and the TMTF manifest a high-frequency cutoff. For the CSF, this high-frequency cutoff represents the highest spatial frequency that can be

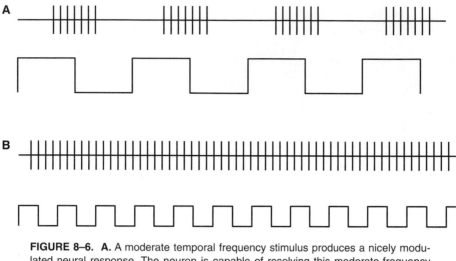

FIGURE 8–6. A. A moderate temporal frequency stimulus produces a nicely modulated neural response. The neuron is capable of resolving this moderate-frequency stimulus. **B.** The neuron's response is neither sufficiently fast nor transient to allow temporal resolution of this high-frequency stimulus.

resolved at 100 percent spatial contrast. For the TMTF, this high-frequency cutoff represents the highest temporal frequency that can be resolved at 100 percent modulation.

Origins of the Low- and High-frequency Drop-offs

The high-frequency cutoff of the TMTF is due to neural constraints in coding high temporal frequency information (Fig. 8–6). The faster a neural system responds and the more transient its response, the greater is its temporal resolution.

The reduction in sensitivity to low frequencies is due to lateral inhibitory interactions (lateral inhibition) within the retina (see Chap. 12). Low temporal frequency stimuli can maximize these inhibitory interactions with a resultant reduction in sensitivity (Ratliff et al, 1963).

CRITICAL FLICKER FUSION FREQUENCY

The critical flicker fusion frequency is the highest or lowest temporal frequency, at a given percentage modulation, that cannot be resolved. The example in Fig. 8–7 shows the CFF for 4.0 percent modulation, which corresponds to a relative sensitivity of 1/4.0, or 0.25. A line extended from this point intersects the TMTF at two points: 4 and 10 Hz. These frequencies represent the low and high-frequency CFFs for 4.0 percent modulation. At this percentage modulation, stimuli of 4 Hz or less, or 10 Hz or greater, are seen as fused. Other frequencies are

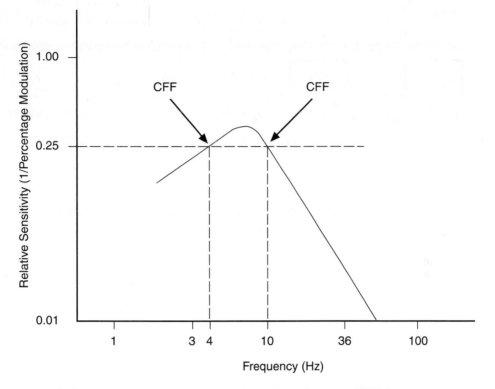

FIGURE 8–7. The low-frequency critical flicker fusion frequency (CFF) for 4 percent modulation is 4 Hz; the high-frequency CFF is 10 Hz. Stimuli of 4 percent modulation that are 4 Hz or less, or 10 Hz or greater, are not resolved; they appear steady.

resolved and perceived as flickering. When not specified, the CFF almost always refers to the high-frequency CFF.

Effect of Illumination on the Critical Flicker Fusion Frequency

Figure 8–8A displays TMTFs obtained under various levels of retinal illumination. Note that increasing the background illumination has different effects on relative sensitivity for low and high temporal frequencies (Kelly, 1961). For low temporal frequencies, increasing the illumination has no effect on relative sensitivity. This is demonstrated by the overlap of the low-frequency aspects of the TMTFs.

In comparison, high-frequency relative sensitivity increases as the background illumination increases, with the CFF increasing approximately linearly with the log of the retinal illumination (see Fig. 8–8B) (Ferry, 1892; Porter, 1902).[5] This is

---

5. This is referred to as the Ferry–Porter law.

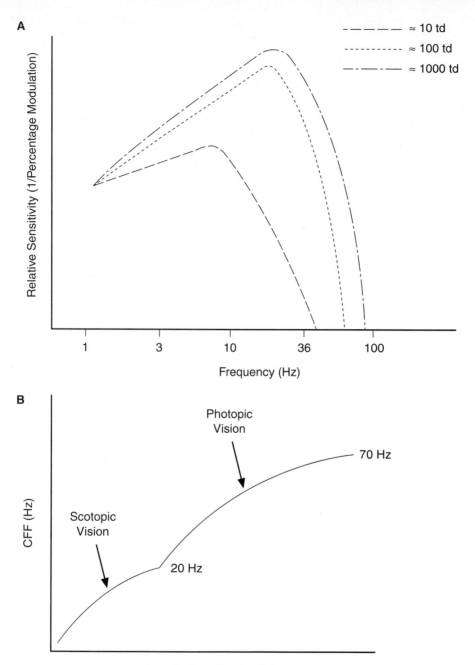

FIGURE 8–8. **A.** Temporal modulation transfer functions for background retinal illuminations of 10, 100, and 1000 td. Note that increasing illumination has no effect on low-frequency sensitivity and enhances high-frequency sensitivity (Kelly, 1961). **B.** Graphical representation of the Ferry–Porter law showing that the critical flicker fusion frequency (CFF) increases with the log of the retinal illumination. The CFF for scotopic vision is about 20 Hz; for photopic vision it is 70 Hz.

probably related to a general speeding up of retinal processes that occurs at increasing levels of light adaptation.

Effect of Stimulus Size on the Critical Flicker Fusion Frequency

The CFF increases with the log of the stimulus area (Granit and Harper, 1930).[6] Consequently, for a given percentage modulation, flicker is more likely to be perceived if the stimulus is large.

The extrafoveal retina is apparently better suited to detect flicker and movement than the foveal retina, contributing to the so-called **"where" system,** which alerts us to the presence of visual stimuli that require our immediate attention (Livingstone and Hubel, 1987, 1988).

Retinal parasol (magno) ganglion cells display high sensitivity to high temporal frequencies, and may thereby contribute to the peripheral retina's superior sensitivity to these stimuli.[7] Parasol cells synapse in the magno layers of the dorsal lateral geniculate nucleus (dLGN), which project to specific locations in striate cortex that, in turn, project to specific areas in higher visual cortex, forming the cortical where pathway.

Once a stimulus is detected by the where system, it is examined with foveal vision, which displays highly developed visual acuity. Contributing to the high visual acuity are the midget (parvo) ganglion cells, which are most concentrated in the fovea. The midget cells synapse in the parvo layers of the dLGN, which project to specific locations in striate cortex. This area projects to specific higher cortical areas, forming the cortical **"what" system** that enables us to examine a visual stimulus in detail such that it can be identified (Livingstone and Hubel, 1987, 1988). The where and what pathways are discussed in considerably more detail in Chapters 13, 14, and 15.[8]

OTHER TEMPORAL VISUAL EFFECTS

In this section, we introduce several assorted temporal phenomena that are frequently referred to in the vision science and perception literature.

Broca–Sulzer Effect

Suprathreshold flashes of light with a duration on the order of 50 to 100 milliseconds appear brighter than stimuli of either shorter or longer durations, a

---

6. This is referred to as the Granit–Harper law.

7. Parasol neurons respond in a transient manner, providing a mechanism for encoding high temporal frequencies (Fig. 13-6).

8. The where and what systems can be thought of as cortical processing streams. Note that they are not independent from each other—there is commingling of information

phenomena referred to as the Broca-Sulzer effect (Broca and Sulzer, 1902, 1904). It can be demonstrated by asking an observer to compare the brightness of two flashes (pulses) of light, a test flash and a comparison flash. The test flash is of variable duration and constant intensity. The comparison flash is of constant duration and variable intensity. The observer's task is to adjust the intensity of the comparison flash so that it matches the brightness of the test flash. Over the course of an experiment, the test flash is presented at a large number of durations, and for each, the observer adjusts the intensity of the comparison flash to match it. The result is a plot of brightness as a function of pulse duration that reveals durations of about 50 to 100 milliseconds to be the brightest (Fig. 8–9A).

Can the Broca–Sulzer effect be explained by the temporal response profiles of ganglion cells? Figure 8–9B shows the response of a ganglion cell when exposed to a flash of light. These data are replotted in Fig. 8–9C to show the frequency of action potentials as a function of time. This function has a form very similar to the Broca–Sulzer effect, leading some to conclude that the Broca–Sulzer effect can be explained by the frequency of action potentials generated in visual neurons (LeGrand, 1968). This correlation is, however, a false correlation (Wasserman and Kong, 1974; Schwartz, 1992). Note that the independent variables for the two experiments are not the same. For the psychophysical Broca–Sulzer effect, the independent variable is duration, whereas for the neural discharge, the independent variable is time. Because the independent variables are different, the psychophysical and physiological results should not be directly compared to each other.

To determine if the frequency of action potentials accounts for the Broca–Sulzer effect, it would be necessary to repeat the physiologic experiment using duration as the independent variable. If this were done, one would find that there is no aspect of the neural response that increases to a peak and then decreases as the duration is further increased. Consequently, the action potential profile of a ganglion cell does not provide a straightforward explanation for the Broca–Sulzer effect.

Action potential profiles may, however, explain reaction time distributions (RTDs) to long duration, near-threshold flashes of light (Schwartz and Loop, 1982; Schwartz, 1992). Reaction times are determined by asking an observer to view a barely visible flash that lasts for 1 second, and to press a button when the flash is first seen. If presented with a large number of trials (say, 250), a RTD is obtained (Fig. 8–10) that has a form similar to the action potential profile in Fig. 8–9c. Note that the independent variable is time (not duration). Thus it appears that RTDs are more closely correlated to the temporal profile of ganglion cells than is the Broca–Sulzer effect.

As this discussion illustrates, it is challenging to establish reliable linkage between psychophysical phenomena and the underlying physiology. Models of visual function that propose such linkage must be examined critically.

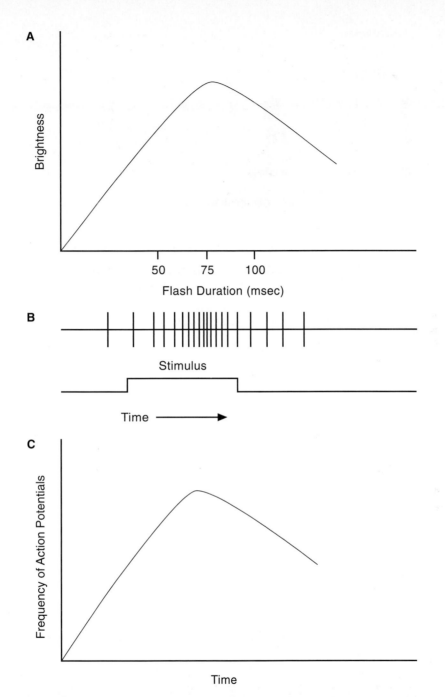

FIGURE 8–9. A. Graphical representation of the Broca–Sulzer effect. Stimuli with a duration of 50 to 100 milliseconds are perceived as brighter than stimuli with a duration of less than or greater than this value. **B.** A flash elicits action potentials in a ganglion cell. The frequency of these action potentials gradually increases and then decreases. **C.** The neural response in B is replotted as frequency of action potentials as a function of time. Note the similarity of this function to the form of the Broca–Sulzer effect; however, also note that the independent variables for these two phenomena are different. For the Broca–Sulzer effect, the independent variable is duration; for the neural response, it is time.

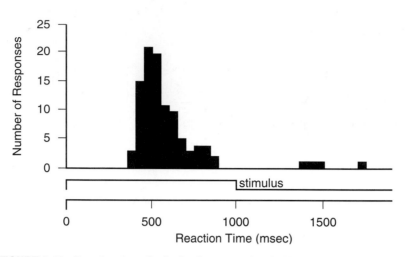

FIGURE 8-10. Reaction time distribution for a near-threshold, 1000-msec increment flashed on a spatially coincident background (Schwartz and Loop, 1982; Schwartz, 1996).

Brücke–Bartley Effect

A flickering light of approximately 10 Hz appears brighter than a steady light of the same average luminance. This so-called Brücke–Bartley effect is a manifestation of the Broca–Sulzer effect (Bartley, 1938).[9] The relationship between the two is illustrated in Fig. 8–11, which shows a temporal square wave stimulus with a frequency of 10 Hz. Each cycle is one tenth of a second, or 100 milliseconds. Therefore, the duration of each increment of light is 50 milliseconds, approximately the same duration associated with the Broca–Sulzer effect. For both effects, stimuli of about 50-millisecond duration appear brighter than stimuli of other durations.

Talbot–Plateau Law

A temporally modulated stimulus that is fused (i.e., not resolved) has the same brightness as a steady light of equal time-averaged luminance (Fig. 8–12). For this law, the Talbot–Plateau law, to apply, the temporally modulated light must be presented at a rate beyond the CFF.

MASKING

Masking involves the use of one stimulus, the **mask,** to reduce the visibility of another stimulus, the **target** (Breitmeyer, 1984). Masking phenomena provide

---

9. The Brücke-Bartley effect is sometimes referred to as brightness enhancement.

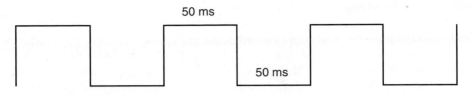

FIGURE 8–11. A square wave stimulus of 10 Hz can be thought of as consisting of half-cycles of 50-millisecond duration.

information regarding both spatial and temporal processing of visual information. Although we briefly touch upon physiological explanations for certain phenomena, detailed explanations are beyond the scope of this textbook. The various types of masking are briefly summarized here.

Simultaneous Masking

In simultaneous masking, both the mask and the target are present at the same time. An example is the use of spatial gratings (the mask) to interfere with the detection of a stimulus composed of similar frequencies (the target). Since both frequencies share the same spatial frequency channels, there is a reduction in the visibility of the target gratings.

Simultaneous masking is more pronounced in patients with amblyopia than in patients whose vision developed normally (see Chap. 17). Consequently, the acuity of an amblyopic eye is better when measured with isolated optotypes than when determined with a row of optotypes, such as found on a typical eye chart. This reduction in acuity caused by surrounding spatial patterns is referred to as the **crowding phenomenon** (Flom et al, 1963).

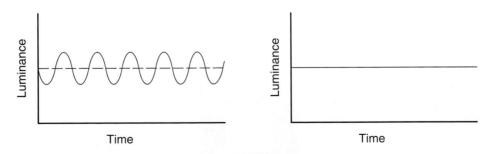

FIGURE 8-12. The Talbot–Plateau law states that the brightness of a fused temporally modulated stimulus is equal to the brightness of a steady light of the same average luminance.

Backward Masking

In backward masking, the target precedes the mask. Even so, the mask reduces the visibility of the (previously presented) target. This may occur when the mask is substantially brighter than the target, enabling the mask's neural response to reach central visual areas first, thereby interfering with detection of the target.

Forward Masking

In the case of forward masking, the mask precedes the target. The mask reduces the visibility of the subsequently presented target.

Metacontrast

Metacontrast is a form of backward masking where the mask and target are spatially adjacent. The visibility of a briefly presented target is reduced by the subsequent presentation of a spatially adjacent mask (Fig. 8–13). Lateral processing (inhibition) within the retina is thought to contribute to metacontrast. In addition, stimulation of the faster magno pathway appears to be critical for producing this effect (Breitmeyer, 1992).

Paracontrast

Paracontrast is a form of forward masking where the target and mask are spatially adjacent. A mask reduces the visibility of a subsequently presented, spatially adjacent target.

Target   Mask

     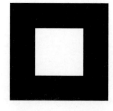

FIGURE 8–13. In metacontrast, the visibility of the target is reduced by the subsequent presentation of a spatially adjacent mask.

CLINICAL CONSIDERATIONS

The diagnosis of primary open angle glaucoma (POAG) is often problematic. Increased intraocular pressure (IOP) is correlated with visual field loss, but it is not a reliable predictor of whether an individual will develop such loss. Whereas not all patients with elevated IOPs develop visual field defects, other patients with normal IOPs do develop these defects. Moreover, visual field testing is not as sensitive an indicator of ganglion cell function as once was believed. A substantial proportion of the ganglion cells are damaged by the time early visual field defects manifest (Quigley et al, 1982). Consequently, there is interest in developing more sensitive psychophysical measures of ganglion cell functionality.

Temporal modulation transfer functions and related temporal psychophysical tasks offer promise for assisting in the early diagnosis of glaucoma (Tyler, 1981; Johnson, 1995). Data obtained on patients with ocular hypertension (elevated IOPs with normal visual fields) suggest that TMTFs may be a more sensitive indicator of ganglion cell loss than standard visual fields.

The schematic TMTFs in Fig. 8-14 are representative of healthy eyes and certain eyes with ocular hypertension, illustrating that patients with ocular hypertension

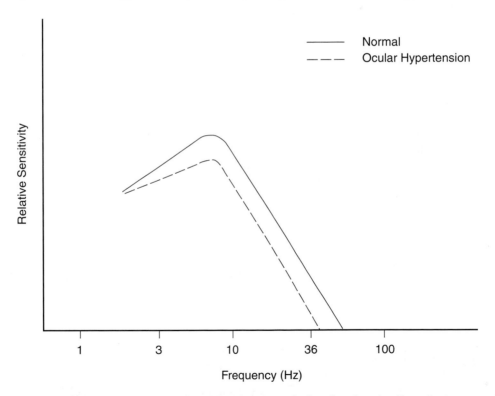

FIGURE 8–14. Expected temporal modulation transfer functions for a healthy patient and a patient with ocular hypertension (Tyler, 1981).

may manifest losses in sensitivity to temporally modulated stimuli. Note that the most obvious losses of sensitivity are at moderate and high temporal frequencies.

Anatomical data reveal that glaucomatous eyes manifest a disproportionate loss of larger axons, presumably parasol axons (Quigley et al, 1987). Because psychophysical and physiological data both suggest that the magno pathway codes high temporal frequencies (see Chap. 13), it is not altogether surprising that patients with glaucoma suffer losses in sensitivity to high temporal frequencies.

As discussed in Chapter 13, the reduced ability of glaucoma patients to perceive frequency doubling is not fully understood at this time. In the clinical determination of frequency doubling thresholds, the patient views a grating presented at a high temporal frequency. The contrast is increased until the patient perceives flicker. It is possible that the threshold determined in a frequency doubling task is actually a measure of the ability to detect high temporal frequencies, not a measure of the ability to detect frequency doubling.

Temporal modulation transfer functions may also provide useful information regarding retinitis pigmentosa and age-related macular degeneration (Tyler et al, 1984; Mayer et al, 1992). Taken together, these findings suggest that measurements of temporal processing may prove to be as useful in the diagnosis of certain eye diseases as are measurements of spatial processing.

SUMMARY

The study of temporal vision involves many of the same concepts associated with spatial vision. Both can be characterized by transfer functions, which show sensitivity as a function of frequency. The low- and high-frequency drop-offs of these functions reflect basic limitations of neural processing. Although not yet commonly used for clinical purposes, tests of temporal vision holds considerable promise.

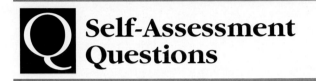

Q Self-Assessment Questions

1. A square wave stimulus has a frequency of 20 Hz. Calculate, in milliseconds, the duration of the on phase of each cycle. (Hint: Draw a diagram of the stimulus and label the duration of a cycle.)

2. A stimulus is on for 20 milliseconds and off for 20 milliseconds. This stimulus is presented continuously. Calculate its temporal frequency in Hz. (Hint: Draw a diagram of the stimulus and label it.)

3. Figure 8–8A shows that relative sensitivity, at low temporal frequencies, remains constant as the background illumination increases. Is this a manifestation of Weber's law? Explain. (Hint: See Chapter 11.)

9

Motion Perception

Changes in the spatial distribution of light, over time, can lead to the perception of motion. Think of a person jogging across your field of vision. The spatial distribution of light that falls on your retina changes from moment to moment, causing the jogger to be perceived as moving.

Consider the jogger in more detail. His or her arms are swinging back and forth, moving in opposite directions. As one leg extends forward, the other leg moves relatively little. The torso is moving slower than the leg that is stepping forward. An analysis of the jogger reveals that various components of his or her body are moving at different rates and in different directions, yet are perceived as a single, unified object moving forward.

A growing body of knowledge provides insight regarding the complex mechanisms underlying motion perception. It is becoming evident that motion is processed along a specialized visual pathway, the dorsal processing stream. This localization of function provides the basis for tests of motion perception that can be useful in the diagnoses of certain neurological disorders. This chapter concentrates on psychophysical aspects of motion perception. Its physiological bases are discussed in Chapter 15.

FIRST-ORDER MOTION STIMULI

When we observe a jogger, we perceive real motion; the image slides across the retina. Much of the motion that we experience, however, can be classified as **apparent**, or **illusory**, **motion.** For instance, when spatially separated lights are sequentially flashed (with an appropriate interval between the flashes) a sense of motion is elicited (Fig. 9–1; Korte, 1915; Bartley, 1963). Referred to as **stroboscopic motion,** or the **phi phenomenon,** this effect is common in lighted signs that create the illusion of motion. A bowling alley sign, for example, might consist of a lighted bowling ball that appears to move down an alley toward the awaiting pins. The sequential flashing, at the proper rate, of the various lights that constitute the sign elicits the illusion of movement.

Movies, television, and computer monitors all create a sense of motion by the use of stroboscopic stimuli. Each frame in a movie has a spatial configuration slightly different from that of the preceding frame. The frames are presented at a temporal rate that creates the illusion of smooth motion.

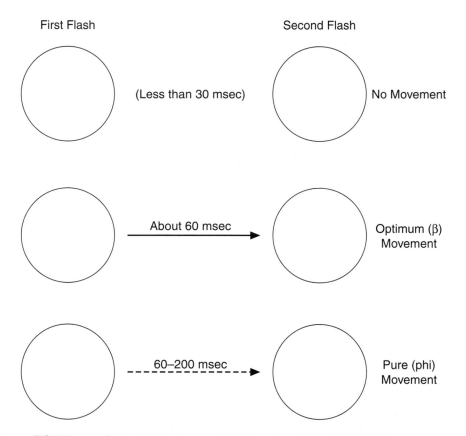

FIGURE 9–1. Stroboscopic movement. Various sensations of movement are produced by different intervals between the two flashes of light. An interval of 60 milliseconds produces a realistic sensation of the spot moving from position A to position B **(optimum or beta movement).** An interval of less than 30 milliseconds produces no sensation of movement, whereas durations of 60 to 200 milliseconds produce a partial illusion of movement **(pure or phi movement).**

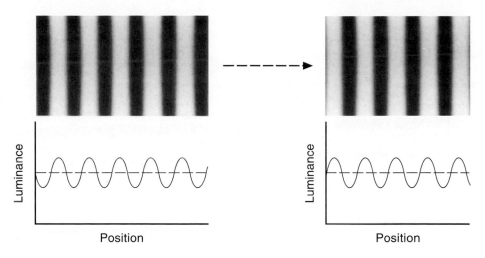

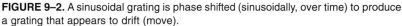

FIGURE 9–2. A sinusoidal grating is phase shifted (sinusoidally, over time) to produce a grating that appears to drift (move).

Although earlier studies of apparent motion used stroboscopic stimuli flashed in sequence, recent investigations frequently use sine wave gratings that undergo a phase shift (Fig. 9–2). The resulting sine wave grating may appear to drift in a given direction.

Since the stroboscopic and sine wave stimuli that we have discussed up to this point are comparatively simple, consisting of a linear exchange of light for dark (or vice versa), they are referred to as **first-order** stimuli for motion. We can, however, extract motion information from more complex stimuli, sometimes referred to as **second-order,** or **global,** stimuli for motion (Logothetis, 1994).

SECOND-ORDER MOTION STIMULI

Figure 9–3 shows how **random dot kinematograms** are used to study global (second-order) motion perception. In panel A, the dots are moving in random directions with respect to each other; by definition, the pattern shows no coherence. As we proceed from panel B to panel C, an increasing percentage of the dots move in a common direction; the percent coherence increases from 50 percent to 100 percent. One measure of a person's ability to detect global motion is the **coherence threshold,** which is defined as the smallest percent coherence that results in the perception of motion in a defined direction (e.g., up, down, left, or right) (Newsome and Paré, 1988; Silverman et al, 1990).

Kinematograms can also be used to study other aspects of motion perception (Fig. 9–4; Nakayama, 1985). The minimum distance that the dots must move in a given direction to elicit the perception of motion is referred to as the **mini-**

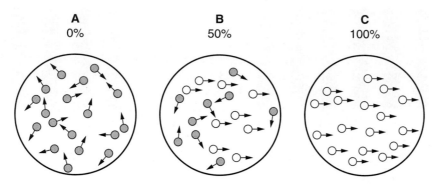

FIGURE 9–3. Random dot kinematograms are used to study global motion perception. **A.** When the dots are moving in random directions, there is no coherence. **B.** At 50 percent coherence, the direction of movement of 50 percent of the dots is correlated. **C.** All the dots are moving in the same direction when the coherence is 100 percent.

mum displacement threshold (D_{min}). Likewise, the maximum distance the dots can move and still elicit motion perception is called the **maximum displacement threshold (D_{max}).**

The processing required to extract motion from random dot kinematograms is more complex than for stroboscopic stimuli (Nakayama and Tyler, 1981). Whereas first-order motion perception can be explained by local luminance changes on the retina, such an explanation will not suffice for second-order motion perception. In order for random dot stimuli to elicit the perception of motion, the visual system must integrate information from many dots over a broad expanse of the retina. This requires sophisticated neural processing that apparently involves higher-level motion centers in the cortex (Newsome and Paré, 1988).

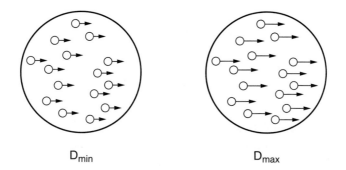

FIGURE 9–4. The minimum movement that elicits the perception of motion is referred to as the minimum displacement threshold (D_{min}), and the maximum movement that elicits the perception of movement is the maximum displacement threshold (D_{max}) (Bullimore, Wood, and Swenson, 1993).

DORSAL PROCESSING STREAM

From the retina to striate cortex, motion information—particularly high-velocity motion—is processed primarily along the magno pathway (see Chap. 15). Although the parvo pathway is not blind to motion cues, it apparently plays less of a role and may be involved in processing low velocity stimuli (Newsome and Wurtz, 1988; Maunsell et al, 1990). Interestingly, amblyopes (see Chap. 17) show reduced sensitivity to low velocities, apparently due to an impairment of the parvo pathway (Steinman et al, 1988).

Motion information is disseminated from striate cortex to neighboring cortical areas, with a convergence of motion information seemingly occurring in **visual area 5**, which is also known as the **middle temporal area, MT, or V5** (see Figs. 14–3 and 15–1). The cortical pathway that originates at striate cortex and continues through visual area 5 to prefrontal cortex is variously referred to as the **parietal** pathway, the **dorsal** processing stream, or the **where** system (Mishkin et al, 1983).

Cells in V5 have features that make them well suited to play a major role in motion perception (Maunsell and Van Essen, 1983). They respond to global stimuli, including random dot kinematograms. Electrical stimulation of cells in V5 of a monkey alters the animal's motion perception (Salzman and Newsome, 1994). Underscoring the centrality of this area to motion perception, damage to V5 can impair the perception of motion (akinetopsia) (Zihl et al, 1983; Barton et al, 1996). The functional physiology of V5 is discussed in more detail in Chapter 15.

We began this chapter with a discussion of the motion perceived when viewing a jogger. This represents a special case of motion perception—**biological motion** perception. There is evidence that the natural movements of humans and other animals may be processed differently than other forms of motion. Functional magnetic resonance imaging (fRMI)[1] reveals that an area of the human cortex, the **posterior superior temporal sulcus (STS)**, is activated when viewing biological motion, but not artificial motion (Grossman and Blake, 2001).

ROLES OF LUMINANCE AND COLOR

Ample evidence suggests that the magno pathway plays an important role in the perception of motion, particularly rapid motion. Can motion perception be elicited by stimuli defined solely by color, such as isoluminant gratings, that are thought to be poor stimuli for the magno pathway (Livingstone and Hubel, 1987, 1988)? These gratings consist of bars of various hues, with each bar having the same luminance (see Chaps. 5 and 13). The grating is visible only because the bars that constitute it have different hues.

---

1. Functional magnetic resonance imaging is discussed in more detail in Chapter 15.

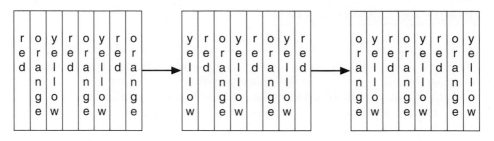

FIGURE 9–5. The bars that constitute an isoluminant grating all have the same luminance. The perception of movement as the bars drift to the right is impaired by the absence of luminance contrast.

Consider the isoluminant grating that is schematically represented in Fig. 9–5. The bars are drifting to the right. Would the bars be seen as moving? The answer is complicated (Cavanagh, 1996). Under certain isoluminant conditions, the perception of motion is impaired—it may be weak or slower than the actual movement of the bars. Adding luminance contrast (i.e., changing the stimulus so that the red and orange bars have different luminances) improves the perception of motion. This psychophysical finding is consistent with a predominant role for the magno pathway in processing motion information. Under certain other isoluminant conditions, however, the perception of motion is robust, pointing to a role for the parvo pathway in coding motion (Cropper and Derrington, 1996).

What do we know about motion perception under scotopic conditions?[2] Psychophysical studies show that objects appear to move slower (about 25 percent slower) under rod-mediated vision than under cone-mediated vision (Gegenfurtner et al, 1999). This raises the possibility that for certain conditions—such as driving at night—objects that are illuminated by the vehicle's headlights and viewed with cone–mediated vision may be perceived as moving faster than objects that are not illuminated by the headlights (i.e., objects falling on the peripheral retina). Such a circumstance could be confusing to a driver, creating the potential for an accident.

DYNAMIC VISUAL ACUITY

Many of the visual stimuli that humans encounter are not stable, but are moving. What effect does the velocity of a moving stimulus have on visual acuity? As stimulus velocity increases, resolution acuity remains relatively constant until the stimulus velocity reaches about 60 to 80 degree/second (Miller and Ludvigh, 1962). Beyond this velocity, the ability to resolve a moving stimulus, commonly referred to as **dynamic visual acuity,** deteriorates (Fig. 9–6). The reduction in

---

2. The magno and parvo pathways are identified and characterized under photopic, not scotopic, conditions.

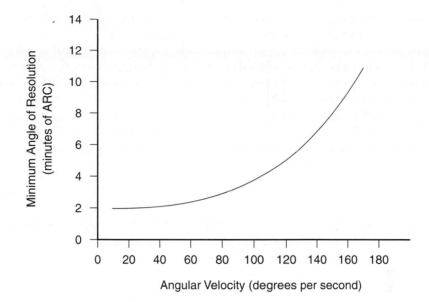

FIGURE 9–6. The minimum angle of resolution remains relatively constant as the velocity of an acuity target increases up to about 60 to 80 degrees per second. Beyond this velocity, there is a degradation in resolution acuity (Miller and Ludvigh, 1962).

dynamic visual acuity at increasing target velocities is apparently due to the inability to accurately follow the stimulus with tracking (or following) eye movements, referred to as **smooth pursuit eye movements** (Barmack, 1970).

SACCADIC SUPPRESSION

Place your two index fingers at arms length, separated by about 1 foot. Now, look back and forth between them. This ballistic eye movement between two fixation points is referred to as a **saccadic eye movement.** Note that as you move your eyes from finger to finger, or from any one object to another object, the visual world remains still and clear. This is in spite of the movement of images across your retinae as you move your eyes.

Vision is suppressed shortly before, during, and shortly after saccadic eye movements. These phenomena, variously referred to as **saccadic suppression** and **saccadic omission,** enable us to look from one object to another without a smearing of our vision that would otherwise be caused by the rapid movement of images across the retina (Matin, 1974; Ciuffreda and Tannen, 1995).

Saccadic suppression is apparently due to a selective inhibition of the magno pathway. This makes sense when you consider that image movement across the retina during saccades is very fast, consisting of high temporal frequencies.

Because the magno pathway is very sensitive to these frequencies, it is presumably suppressed to avoid a smearing of vision (see Chap. 13).

What are the mechanisms underlying saccadic suppression? Neural activity (in cortical motion areas) that would otherwise occur during a saccadic eye movement must somehow be suppressed. Where does the neural signal that is responsible for this suppression originate? Some investigators suggest that image movement across the retina acts as a mask. In this view, the signal for saccadic suppression originates within the retina. Other researchers believe that brain areas associated with the genesis of saccadic eye movements also send signals to cortical areas involved with motion perception. In this latter view, an extraretinal signal (i.e., the signal does not originate in the retina) leads to the suppression of motion perception (Matin et al, 1972; Burr et al, 1994; Schwartz and Godwin, 1996).

To address this interesting question, Thiele et al (2002) recorded the activity of isolated neurons in the monkey cortical area MT and the nearby middle superior temporal area (MST) under two conditions. Under condition one, the monkey viewed a scene on which there were two spots, and made a saccadic eye movement from one of these spots to the other. In condition two, the monkey did not move the eyes, but the scene was shifted so that it moved across the retina as it did during condition one. In both cases, the scene moved across the retina: in condition one, the movement was caused by a voluntary saccade and in condition two, it was due to movement of the scene. If saccadic suppression is caused by an extraretinal signal, one would expect to find neurons in the cortical motion areas (MT and MST) that are activated when the scene moves, but suppressed during saccades. Theile et al (2002) found such neurons, providing strong evidence that a primary contributor to saccadic suppression is an extraretinal signal.

CLINICAL CONSIDERATIONS

As previously discussed, there is evidence that the neural damage in glaucoma is selective for the magno pathway. Given the data in support of a critical role for this pathway in motion perception, it should not be surprising that tests of motion perception have been evaluated to determine if they are useful for the early diagnosis of glaucoma (Trick et al, 1995).

Studies using random dot kinematograms have found that minimum displacement thresholds are elevated in patients with suspected glaucoma (Bullimore et al, 1993). In patients with glaucomatous field defects, motion coherence thresholds are higher in those regions of the visual field showing glaucomatous damage than in comparatively unaffected regions of the visual field (Bosworth et al, 1997). These results suggest that motion deficits occur relatively early in the disease process and that measures of motion perception may prove to be valuable in early diagnosis.

SUMMARY

The perception of motion requires the analysis of spatial displacements over time. Basic (first order) motion perception, which can be elicited with simple stroboscopic stimuli, may be explained by processing that occurs early in the visual system (V1 or earlier). The perception of motion that is elicited by global cues (such as random dot kinematograms), however, apparently depends on an analysis in higher visual centers, in particular, MT. (Additional evidence in support of this view is discussed in Chap. 15.)

MT is part of the dorsal processing stream. This pathway originates in striate cortex, passes through MT, and continues on to prefrontal cortex. The major precortical input to the dorsal processing stream is the magno pathway.

It has been proposed that diseases resulting in selective damage to the magno pathway may lead to deficits in motion perception. This hypothesis has led to studies that demonstrate impaired motion perception in the early stages of glaucoma. The practicality of tests of motion perception for routine clinical practice awaits further study.

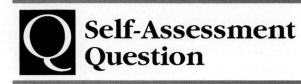

Self-Assessment Question

1. Describe an experiment that would allow you to locate the areas of the human cortex that are most responsible for analyzing motion information. (*Hint:* See Chap. 1.)

Depth Perception

10

It is sometimes assumed that depth perception is predicated on binocular vision. If one eye is covered, however, a strong sense of depth persists, pointing to the importance of monocular depth cues. Although depth is noted monocularly, it is generally enhanced when viewing binocularly, especially at near distances.

In this chapter, we introduce both monocular and binocular cues to depth. Although we touch on some of the processes involved in binocular vision, this discussion is limited to background material sufficient to gain a basic understanding of stereopsis. More detailed information on binocular vision can be found in texts dealing exclusively with this broad topic. Steinman et al (2000) is recommended.

MONOCULAR DEPTH CUES

Monocular depth cues are perceived just as strongly when viewed with one eye as when viewed with both eyes. The major classes of monocular depth cues are pictorial, angular declination below the horizon, motion parallax, and accommodation (Fig. 10–1).

Pictorial Depth Cues

Pictorial depth cues (size, linear perspective, texture, interposition, clarity, and lighting and shadow) can be presented in a two-dimensional representation,

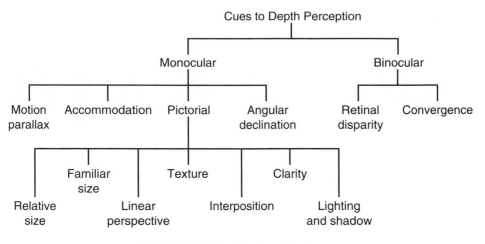

FIGURE 10-1. Classification of depth cues.

such as a photograph or painting.[1] Monocular individuals manifest surprisingly sophisticated depth perception due largely to these cues.

Size. Consider the following experiment. You observe two illuminated balloons in an otherwise pitch-black room. The only visible objects are the balloons. Such a scene may appear similar to that illustrated in Fig. 10–2 (Ittleson and Kilpatrick, 1951). When asked to judge the relative distances of the two balloons, most assume that the larger balloon is closer and the smaller farther away. They do so even if the balloons are the same distance from the observer, with one more inflated than the other.

The aforementioned experiment shows that the perceived distances of objects are often determined by the relative sizes of the retinal images they produce, a cue referred to as **relative size**. If two objects are assumed to be the same size, the object that produces the smaller retinal image size is perceived as farther away. Relative size is an important depth cue when viewing a scene, such as in Fig. 10–2, that includes objects with sizes that can be compared.

Familiar size is a depth cue used when viewing objects of known size. Imagine a barn surrounded by nothing but snow. *Relative* size is not useful for determining the barn's distance; there are no other objects to which it can be compared. In judging its distance; we would probably assume it is the size of a typical barn. If it produces a small retinal image, the barn would be seen as far away.

Linear Perspective. Linear perspective, which is related to relative size, can be experienced by looking down a railroad track or long corridor. When viewing Fig. 10–3, we experience a strong sense of depth because it is assumed that the

---

1. The sense of depth created by pictorial cues can be substantial. Artists are masterful at manipulating them to create a strong sense of depth in a two-dimensional painting.

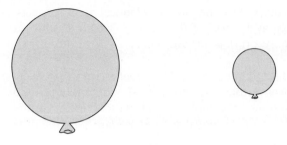

FIGURE 10–2. Imagine that these two balloons are the only illuminated objects in an otherwise dark room. Under these circumstances, the less inflated balloon may appear to be located farther away than the more inflated balloon.

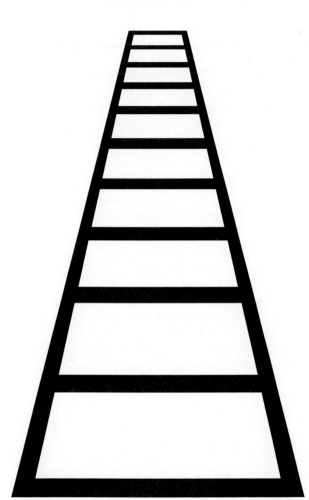

FIGURE 10–3. Linear perspective is a monocular cue to depth. The top of the diagram is perceived to be at a greater distance than the bottom.

horizontal lines on the bottom and top of the picture are identical in all respects, including size. Therefore, the lines at the top of the picture (which produce a smaller retinal image sizes than those on bottom) are perceived as farther away.

Texture. Texture is also related to relative size. The smaller, more densely packed objects in Fig. 10–4A appear farther away than those that are larger and less densely packed because we assume that all objects in the figure are the same size. The objects that produce the smaller retinal image size are perceived as more distant.

Interposition. Interposition occurs when an object blocks the view of another (see Fig. 10–4B). The blocked object appears farther away than the interposed object.

Clarity. Clarity is a form of interposition. Objects seen clearly in a photograph, picture, or actual scene are perceived as closer than those that appear hazy. Fog,

A

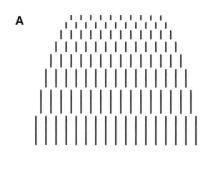

B

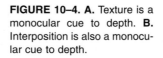

FIGURE 10–4. A. Texture is a monocular cue to depth. **B.** Interposition is also a monocular cue to depth.

smoke, rain, and smog may act as interposing elements that obscure the view of objects, causing them to appear more distant.

Lighting and Shadow. When light falls on an object, the object casts a shadow. The shadow is interpreted as falling behind the object; consequently, a sense of depth is created.

Angular Declination below the Horizon

Consider a monocular observer, standing upright and still in an otherwise empty room, who views an object located on the floor at a distance of, say, 10 ft. Despite the absence of pictorial depth cues, the observer is able to judge correctly the object's distance. How is this done? As indicated in Fig. 10–5, the object makes an angle with the horizon referred to as **angular declination below the horizon**. The visual system apparently uses this angle to determine object distance (Ooi et al, 2001).

Motion Parallax

Motion parallax is a **kinetic monocular depth** cue that results when a moving observer fixates an object while noticing the relative motion of surrounding objects. It can be demonstrated by placing your two index fingers directly in line with each other, with one located 15 cm, and the other 30 cm, in front of your right eye. Close your left eye. Fixate on the distant finger while moving your head sideways. Without changing your fixation, notice that the near finger appears to move in the opposite direction of your head (against-motion). Now fixate the near finger and again move your head sideways. This time, notice that the far finger appears to move in the same direction as your head (with-motion). In both cases, relative motion provides information regarding relative distance.

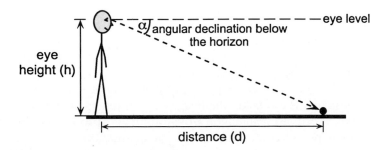

FIGURE 10-5. Angular declination below the horizon is a monocular cue used to determine distance. (*Diagram kindly provided by Dr. Teng-Leng Ooi.*)

Motion parallax has useful clinical applications when viewing ocular structures with a monocular instrument. Consider a small, dot-like opacity that is observed during monocular ophthalmoscopy. If the clinician fixates on the pupil and moves his or her head sideways, the opacity shows against-motion if located anterior to the iris, whereas with-motion is noted if the opacity is located posterior to the iris.

Accommodation

During accommodation, the dioptric power of the crystalline lens increases, allowing near objects to be focused clearly on the retina. Although the signal to accommodation contains information that could be used to determine the distance of viewed objects, the extent to which this information is utilized is not known.

BINOCULAR DEPTH CUES

Stereopsis

Figure 10–6 depicts an observer viewing a ball centered between two other balls. While fixating the central ball, the observer is able to judge the relative distances of the three balls even if all monocular depth cues (e.g., relative size, interposition) are eliminated. How is this accomplished?

Consider the retinal images produced by the most distant ball. Light rays emanating from it strike the retinas nasal to the foveas, giving rise to **retinal disparity**, a binocular depth cue that allows the visual system to determine that the ball is distant to the fixated object. When the images fall nasal to the foveas, as in this example, the retinal disparity is said to be **uncrossed.**

Now take the case of the nearest ball, which is imaged temporal to the foveas. Here, the disparity is **crossed**, signaling that the ball is located closer than the fixated object.

The perception of depth that is produced by retinal disparity is referred to as **stereopsis**, an important contributor to finely tuned depth perception at near distances (particularly within arm's length when other depth cues are absent). Stereopsis is less important when viewing objects at far distances because the threshold for retinal disparity, which is specified as an angle at the eye, requires such objects to be separated by great distances.

Retinal disparity produces stereopsis only if it is sufficiently small to allow fusion. If the disparity is too large, the images fall on retinal positions that signal grossly different directions, resulting in **physiological diplopia** (double vision).

You can experience physiological diplopia by holding one index finger about 15 cm from your nose, and your other index finger directly behind it at arm's

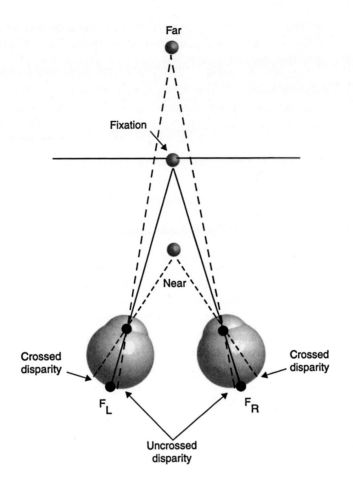

FIGURE 10–6. Uncrossed disparity results in an object being perceived as farther away than the fixation point, whereas crossed disparity results in an object being perceived as closer than the fixation point. (*From Steinman SB, Steinman BA, Garzia RP. Foundations of Binocular Vision: A Clinical Perspective. Copyright 2000. Reprinted by permission of McGraw-Hill, Inc.*)

length. Fixate on the near finger. Notice that the distant finger is doubled. Now slowly move the distant finger toward your nose while maintaining fixation on the near finger. Note that before you reach the near finger, the physiologic diplopia disappears and only the sense of depth is noted. At this point, the retinal disparity is sufficiently small to allow fusion and stereopsis.

As discussed in Chapter 14, certain binocular cortical neurons are maximally responsive when a stimulus is located at a specific distance from the eyes (see Fig. 14-10). The same stimulus, when positioned at other distances, elicits a less vigorous neural response. By encoding disparity, these neurons may contribute to the physiological basis for stereopsis.

Convergence

The eyes converge when we view near objects and diverge when we view distant objects. Although the degree of convergence can potentially provide information regarding distance, the manner in which this information is incorporated into the conscious perception of depth, if at all, is unresolved (Brenner and Van Damme, 1998).

SIZE ILLUSIONS

Visual illusions are erroneous perceptions. We limit the discussion to those illusions that can result when pictorial depth cues are used to determine object size.

In spite of changes in retinal image size, the apparent size of an object does not normally change with viewing distance. Although an automobile that is nearby produces a larger retinal image than when it is farther away, it is not perceived as larger. Our visual system compensates for differences in retinal image size by taking into account the relative distance of an object, a phenomenon referred to as **size constancy.** When judgments of distance are erroneous, such as occurs when viewing a flat picture, size constancy may fail, resulting in a **size illusion.**

In the **corridor illusion**, size constancy fails because monocular depth cues provide incorrect information regarding the relative distances of the circles (Fig. 10–7). Although the two circles are at the same distance from you, the top circle is perceived as farther away. This leads to the illusion that the top circle is larger. In fact, the two circles have the same dimensions.

When viewed on the horizon, the moon appears larger than when viewed on the zenith, even though its angular subtence is the same under both conditions. This well-known **moon illusion** is considered by some to be a size illusion (Kaufman and Rock, 1962). Because trees, houses, fields, and other interposing objects cause the moon to be seen as farther away when viewed on the horizon, it appears larger (Fig. 10–8).

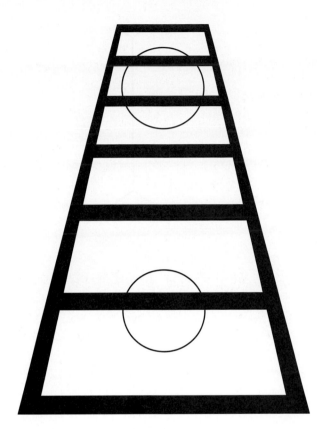

FIGURE 10–7. Corridor illusion. Both circles are the same size, but the top circle appears larger than the bottom circle.

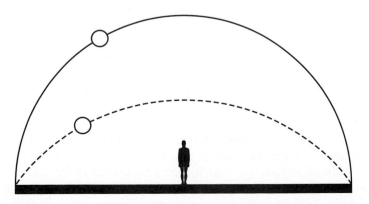

FIGURE 10–8. The actual trajectory of the moon is given by the solid line and the perceived trajectory by the dashed line. When viewed on the horizon, the moon is judged as farther away than when viewed overhead. Because the angular subtense of the moon is the same under both conditions, the moon looks larger on the horizon.

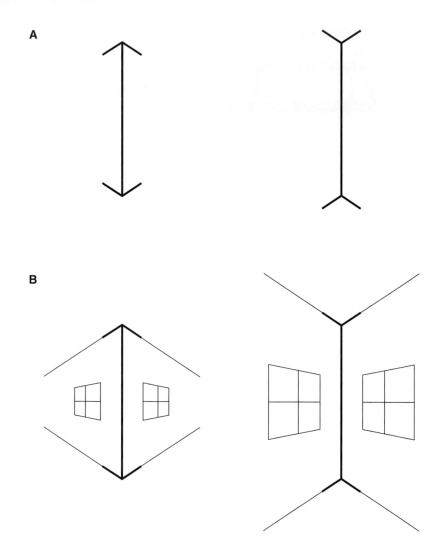

FIGURE 10–9. A. The Müller–Lyer illusion. The two lines are the same length. **B.** One explanation for the illusion is that the arrows may be likened to outgoing and ingoing corners of a room.

The famous **Müller–Lyer illusion** (Fig. 10–9) can be understood by considering the vertical lines to be corners of a room (Gregory, 1978). The line that appears to form an outgoing corner is judged as farther away than the line that appears to form an ingoing corner. Because the lines are equal in length, the line that is judged to be farther away is perceived as longer.

CLINICAL CONSIDERATIONS

Stereopsis and Visual Development

The measurement of a patient's degree of stereopsis provides important information regarding the status of his or her visual system. Stereopsis is measured clinically by asking a patient to view a flat surface that has two identical figures separated by a very small distance. Using Polaroid or red and green glasses, only one object is presented to each eye. The separation of the images is designed to produce retinal disparity, and this disparity results in stereopsis. In a typical stereopsis test, the minimum amount of disparity required for the patient to perceive depth is determined. This threshold disparity is referred to as the patient's **stereoacuity** (a form of hyperacuity), and it can be as small as 3 seconds of arc.

For there to be highly developed stereoacuity, the visual cortex must contain a normal complement of binocular neurons. This can only occur if the visual system is exposed to a normal visual environment during its development. Disorders of binocular vision, such as anisometropia and strabismus, may alter an infant's visual environment and retard the development of binocular cortical neurons, resulting in a reduction in stereoacuity (Birch and Stager, 1985).[2] Consequently, the clinical measurement of stereoacuity provides important information regarding a patient's visual development and current binocular status.

Monovision

Monovision is the common clinical practice of correcting one eye of a presbyope for distance and the other eye for near, thereby enabling the patient to alternate between the two eyes to see both distant and near objects clearly.[3] Because the unused eye is largely suppressed, diplopia does not typically occur. Monovision may, however, interfere with stereopsis because the patient's binocularity is reduced at all distances. Nonetheless, these patients may retain a substantial amount of depth perception because many important cues to depth are monocular. In fact, a patient with only one eye manifests excellent depth perception. Although stereopsis is an important depth cue for near distances, especially within arms length, it is less important at greater distances.

Will monovision correction cause a reduction in stereopsis that interferes with driving safety? This is not an easy question to answer because each individual adapts to monovision at a different rate and to a different extent. Some patients perform well with monovision; others do not. Although many of the judgments required in driving are for far distances, where stereopsis is less important, other judgements are for relatively near distances.

At a minimum, monovision patients should be advised of a reduction in depth perception that could potentially interfere with driving. When driving, spectacle or contact lens correction of the eye that is used for near vision should be considered.

---

2. See Chap. 17 for a more detailed discussion of visual development.

3. Monovision is most often used in conjunction with contact lenses or refractive laser procedures. Whenever a monovision laser procedure is contemplated, it is advisable for the patient to first undergo a monovision contact lens trial to see if he or she can successfully adapt to it.

SUMMARY

The cues for depth perception are both monocular and binocular in nature. Stereopsis, a form of binocular depth perception, is dependent on normal visual development. For this reason, the clinical measurement of stereoacuity provides important information regarding visual development.

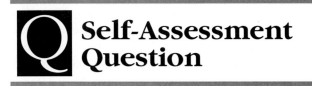

Self-Assessment Question

1. Could monovision contact lenses interfere with a pilot's ability to safely fly an airplane? Explain.

11

Psychophysical Methodology

Many of the routine procedures used in eye care, including the determination of a patient's visual acuity, refractive status, visual fields, and color vision status, are psychophysical in nature. Knowledge of psychophysical theory and methodology better enables the clinician to properly perform these procedures and interpret their results in a meaningful manner.

The past several decades have seen substantial progress in the understanding of basic visual processes. These insights are now being applied to the diagnosis and treatment of clinical conditions. Clinical applications largely take the form of noninvasive psychophysical tests that enable the clinician to diagnose disease at an early stage and to monitor the effectiveness of treatment.

THRESHOLD

Psychophysical experiments and psychophysically based clinical procedures frequently involve the determination of a threshold, the minimum quantity of a stimulus that can be detected. For example, in a visual acuity test, the threshold is the minimum angle of resolution (MAR). For a visual field test, the threshold is the minimum light intensity that can be detected (Fig. 11–1A).[1]

---

1. A distinction can be made between psychophysics and perception. In psychophysical experiments, a physical aspect of a stimulus is adjusted until a threshold is reached. For instance, the intensity of a stimulus is increased until the observer detects it. Alternatively, the observer could be asked to report when a stimulus appears colored, flickers, moves, etc. Perceptual experiments, in comparison, may require the observer to describe what he or she perceives. An observer could be presented with a complex scene, and asked to describe certain aspects of that scene.

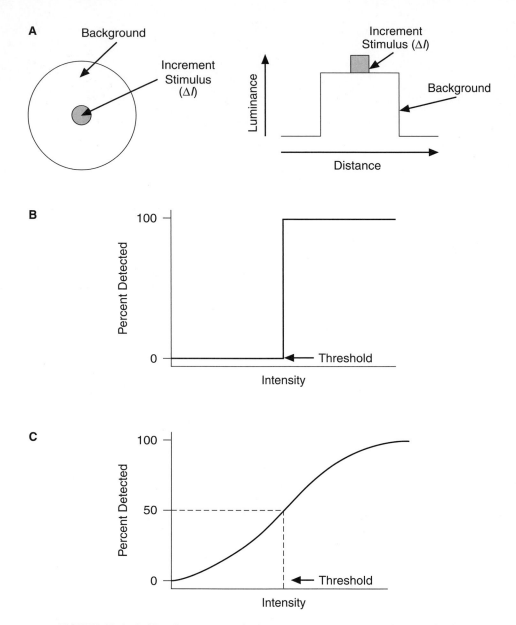

FIGURE 11–1. **A.** The diagram on the left shows an increment stimulus on a background. This is how the stimulus appears to the observer. The diagram on the right is a luminance profile of the stimulus and background. **B.** A psychometric function for a hypothetical ideal observer. Such observers do not actually exist. **C.** A typical psychometric function for a real observer.

The determination of a threshold is complicated by the fact that humans (and other animals) are not perfect observers. A perfect observer would give the same threshold each time it is measured. In practice, the threshold varies on repetition of the measurement.

Figure 11–1 shows the results of a psychophysical experiment conducted with a hypothetical ideal (perfect) observer and real observer. It involves the determination of an increment threshold, such as when performing visual field testing. The observer is required to detect a light (stimulus) that is flashed on a surrounding background. The task is repeated for a range of stimulus intensities, from dim to intense, and the percentage of stimuli detected is plotted as a function of stimulus intensity to produce a **psychometric function.**

An ideal observer manifests a perfect threshold (see Fig. 11–1B). Below the threshold intensity, T, this observer never sees the stimulus. Above the threshold intensity, the observer always sees the stimulus. In comparison, a real observer produces results similar to those in Fig. 11–1C. As the intensity of the stimulus is increased, the probability of seeing the stimulus increases. There is no clearly defined intensity, however, below which the stimulus is never seen and above which it is always seen.

Since there are no perfect observers, threshold is based on theoretical considerations. It is usually defined as the intensity that results in detection of the stimulus on one half of the presentations. This value is read off the psychometric function, as indicated in Fig. 11–1C.

Humans are not perfect observers because they are complex biological systems, not simple mechanical devices. A stimulus results in neural activity. If this neural activity is sufficiently strong, the stimulus is seen. Random neural noise is inherent within the visual system, however, and the signal produced by the stimulus must be perceived as different than this neural noise. As discussed later in this chapter, neural noise can be thought of as varying over time. At any given moment, the amount of neural noise is unpredictable. Therefore, the threshold is variable. Attention, motivation, and fatigue can also affect threshold.

DETERMINATION OF THRESHOLD

The scientist or clinician may choose among several methods to measure a threshold, with the most suitable method determined by the nature of the experiment or clinical procedure. In the following discussion, we introduce the primary methods of threshold determination and discuss some of their advantages and disadvantages.

Method of Ascending Limits

Consider an increment threshold procedure. In the method of ascending limits, the stimulus is initially below threshold. It is not visible. During a trial, which consists of a number of stimulus presentations, the stimulus intensity is increased systematically until the observer reports that it is visible. Several trials may be performed. The results are averaged to obtain a threshold.

The method of ascending limits is particularly advantageous in dark adaptometry, where it is important that the state of retinal adaptation be minimally affected by the stimulus (see Chap. 3).[2] A potential disadvantage of ascending limits, which may lead to an artificially low threshold, is observer anticipation. If the stimulus starts at the same intensity on each trial, the observer may anticipate when he or she "should" see the stimulus based on when he or she saw it on the previous trial. Beginning each trial at a different intensity can mitigate this disadvantage.

Method of Descending Limits

The method of descending limits is essentially the reverse of the method of ascending limits. A trial commences with a clearly visible stimulus (i.e., the stimulus is above threshold)[3] and the visibility is decreased systematically until it can no longer be seen. In the method of ascending limits, the stimulus is initially not visible and becomes visible; in the method of descending limits, the reverse occurs.

Descending limits is commonly used to determine visual acuity. The patient is asked to read down the Snellen eye chart, which consists of optotypes that become progressively smaller from top to bottom (and more difficult to resolve). The threshold MAR is determined when the optotypes are too small to be resolved (see Chap. 7).

When using descending limits, the initial stimulus presentations are visible, serving to familiarize the patient with the task. Consider the clinical determination of visual acuity. The patient obtains practice by reading the large optoypes at the top of the chart, thereby increasing the clinician's confidence that the patient understands the task.

Similar to the method of ascending limits, the method of descending limits may be contaminated by observer anticipation. In an increment threshold experiment where each trial commences at the same intensity, the observer may anticipate when he or she "should" no longer see the stimulus. This can be addressed by starting each trial at a different intensity.

Staircase Method

The staircase method of determining a threshold is a combination of the methods of ascending and descending limits. A stimulus is presented in discrete

---

2. Consider the determination of one point on a dark adaptation curve (see Fig. 3-9). If this threshold were obtained by the method of descending limits (our next topic), the initial stimulus presentations might be intense, bleaching substantial amounts of photopigment. This could lead to an inaccurate threshold measurement—the measured threshold would be higher than the actual threshold.

3. A stimulus that is above threshold is sometimes referred to as suprathreshold stimulus.

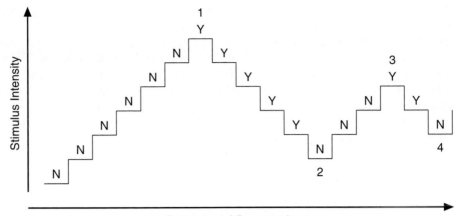

FIGURE 11–2. Staircase method for threshold determination. The stimulus intensity is increased from nonseeing (N) to seeing (Y). A reversal occurs at point 1 and, subsequently, the intensity is decreased until another reversal occurs at point 2. Threshold is taken as the intensity at reversal 4.

steps of increasing visibility called an ascending staircase (Fig. 11–2). Eventually, the observer reports seeing the stimulus. At this point, the staircase is reversed and the visibility of the stimulus is reduced until the observer reports that it cannot be detected (descending staircase). The staircase is again reversed and the stimulus intensity is increased until it is visible. Threshold is taken to be the stimulus intensity at one of the reversals—for example, the fourth reversal.

This strategy provides a quick and reliable method of determining a threshold. It is commonly used in psychophysical experimentation and automated visual field testing.

Method of Constant Stimuli

In the method of constant stimuli, the stimulus visibility is varied randomly from presentation to presentation. Because the observer is typically asked whether or not he or she sees the stimulus, this method is often referred to a "yes-no" procedure. Blank trials, in which no stimulus is presented, are typically included. The number of times that the observer reports seeing the stimulus during a blank trail (so-called false positive or false alarm responses) is an indication of the reliability of the data.

Consider the determination of an increment threshold. Suppose there are 220 trials, with the stimulus presented numerous times at each of 10 intensities. Twenty of the trials are blanks. Stimuli are presented in random order with the blanks randomly interspersed. On each presentation, the observer is asked whether or not he or she sees the stimulus. A psychometric function is plotted and 50 percent visibility is taken as the threshold.

Let us take this a step further. Suppose the subject reports seeing a stimulus on 145 trials. The stimulus is present, but not seen (misses) on 60 trials. How many times was the stimulus present and seen (hits), falsely seen in a blank trial (false positives), and not seen during a blank presentation (correct rejects)? Figure 11–3 shows how these values can be calculated by completing a chart that contains cells for hits, misses, false positives, and correct rejects.

The method of constant stimuli is so named not because the stimulus is kept constant from presentation to presentation, but because the procedure is designed to maintain the observer's expectations at the same level from presentation to presentation. The observer has no valid basis on which to anticipate the visibility of an upcoming presentation; consequently, there is little variation in expectations. Because of this, the method of constant stimuli provides valuable information for laboratory experiments. It is, however, time consuming and not typically indicated for clinical applications.

Method of Adjustment

In the method of adjustment, the subject adjusts the stimulus intensity until it is barely visible, allowing for a relatively quick threshold determination. This method suffers, perhaps more than those previously mentioned, from anticipation and variations in the observer's threshold criterion.

Forced Choice Method

The previously discussed methods of determining a threshold share a common flaw: not all observers use the same criteria when deciding whether or not they see a stimulus. For example, observers with **strict** threshold criteria do not report seeing a stimulus until they are absolutely certain they see it. This results in a relatively high threshold (low sensitivity). Other observers that have **lax** criteria report seeing a stimulus even though they may have a great deal of uncertainty regarding their decision. The result is a relatively low threshold (high sensitivity).

Not only may the threshold criteria vary from observer to observer, it may vary from trial to trial for the same observer. At certain times during an experiment, an observer may be more willing to guess that he or she sees a stimulus than at other times. Moreover, an observer may use one set of criteria for one type of stimulus and another set for a different stimulus. For example, the criteria used by an observer to detect stimuli under photopic conditions could be different than those applied under scotopic conditions. These variations in threshold criteria potentially complicate the interpretation of experimental results.

Stimulus
(*n* = 220)

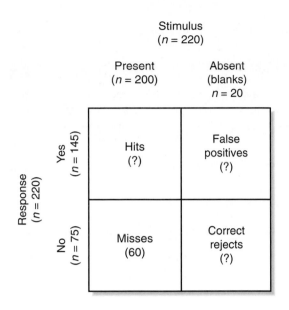

Present
(*n* = 200)

Absent
(blanks)
n = 20

FIGURE 11-3. Outcome matrix for the yes-no experiment discussed in the text. Using this matrix, the number of hits, false positives, and correct rejects can be calculated to be 140, 5, and 15, respectively.

In forced choice methodology, the effects of the observer's criteria are minimized by forcing him or her to choose between several alternative choices, one of which contains the stimulus. In the example shown in Fig. 11–4A, the stimulus is randomly presented in one of the two windows. The other window does not contain a stimulus. It is blank. The observer is forced to choose which window contains the stimulus. Because a response of "I cannot see the stimulus" is not acceptable, the role of the observer's threshold criterion is reduced.

To construct a psychometric function, a large number of trials are presented using stimuli of various visibilities.[4] If the experiment forces the observer to choose between two alternatives, as in the previous example, it is referred to as a two-alternative forced choice (2AFC) experiment. A psychometric function for a 2AFC experiment is given in Fig. 11–4A. Note that the lowest percentage correct is 50 percent (chance performance). It is not 0 percent, as is the case with the method of constant stimuli, because even when the observer cannot see the stimulus, he or she is expected to guess correctly 50 percent of the time.[5] The threshold value is typically taken as the point midway between chance performance and perfect performance. As indicated in Fig. 11–4A, the threshold for a 2AFC experiment is 75 percent.

Forced choice experiments can present the participant with more than two choices. Consider Fig. 11–4B, which shows a four-alternative forced choice (4AFC) stimulus array in which the stimulus is randomly presented in one of the four windows. The observer is forced to choose the correct window. Note that the psychometric function for this experiment shows chance performance of 25

4. In forced choice experiments, a trial consists of the stimulus and the blank (or blanks).

5. Because there are two windows and the stimulus must be in one of the two windows, the observer guesses correctly on one half of the trials.

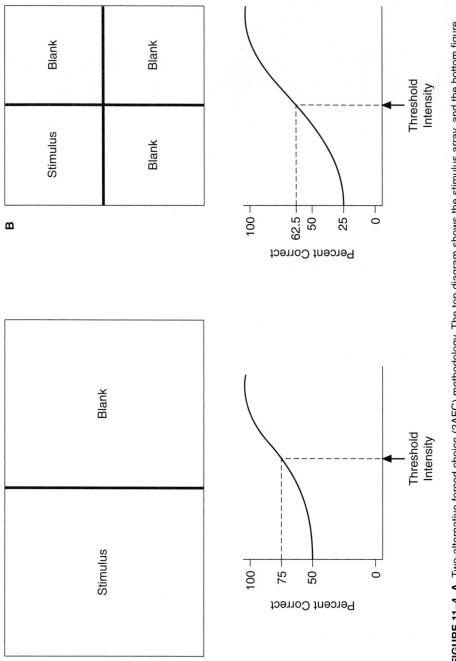
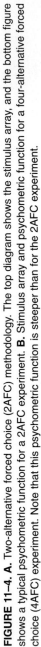

FIGURE 11–4. A. Two-alternative forced choice (2AFC) methodology. The top diagram shows the stimulus array, and the bottom figure shows a typical psychometric function for a 2AFC experiment. **B.** Stimulus array and psychometric function for a four-alternative forced choice (4AFC) experiment. Note that this psychometric function is steeper than for the 2AFC experiment.

percent. Threshold is taken as the point midway between chance performance and 100 percent, which is 62.5 percent.

Increasing the number of choices typically increases the complexity of the experiment and causes it to take longer to perform. Is there an advantage to using more than two choices? The answer can be seen by studying Fig. 11–4. Note that the psychometric function is flatter for 2AFC compared to 4AFC. This increases the chance of error when reading the threshold off the graph because there are many points on the flat function that fall close to 75 percent correct— any noise in the data can make it difficult to choose accurately the stimulus that corresponds to the 75 percent point. Because the psychometric function for 4AFC is steeper, the threshold can be ascertained with more confidence.

Compared to other psychophysical methods, forced choice typically results in lower thresholds. When observers are forced to guess, they often do remarkably well despite claims that they cannot see the stimulus.

Forced choice preferential viewing techniques have been successfully used to determine the visual acuity and other visual capabilities of infants (see Chap. 17) (Teller et al, 1974). In these procedures, the experimenter observes the infant's gaze as the infant views a 2AFC display (see Fig. 17–9). The experimenter is forced to choose the location of the stimulus based on observation of the infant's eyes. By using a forced choice methodology, the criterion (i.e., strict or lax) used by the experimenter is less of a confounding factor.

SIGNAL DETECTION THEORY

The threshold that is determined in an experiment or clinical procedure may be influenced by a number of factors, including decision criteria, attention, motivation, and internal neural noise. Signal detection theory can be used to predict the effects of certain of these factors (Swets et al, 1961). Although signal detection theory presents a useful predictive model, it is, nonetheless, only a model.

Signal detection theory assumes that within the visual system there is a randomly fluctuating level of background neural activity—so-called noise. A stimulus produces a neural signal that is superimposed on this neural noise. The observer's task is to differentiate the signal and noise combination from the background noise alone. An analogy would be listening to white noise (static) and attempting to distinguish a discrete increase in the level of noise (i.e., the signal) from the white noise itself.

A key element of this model is that the neural noise is randomly distributed over time. Figure 11–5A shows the probability of a given level of neural activation at any instant in time. At some times, there is much noise, and at other times, there is little noise. Returning to the white noise analogy, one can think of the level of static as randomly fluctuating over time.

The signal produced by a stimulus is a constant that can be added to a noise distribution (N) to produce a noise plus signal distribution (N + S) (see Fig.

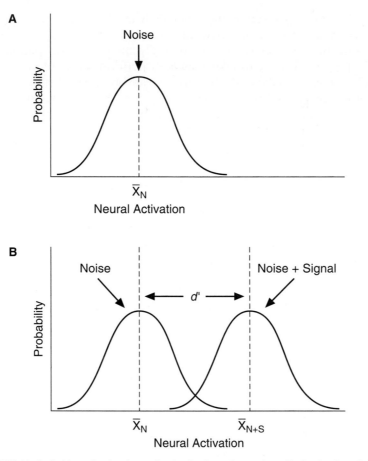

FIGURE 11–5. A. Neural noise is randomly distributed over time. **B.** A stimulus elicits a signal that can be added to the noise distribution to produce a noise + signal distribution. The detectability, *d′*, is a measure of the strength of the stimulus.

11–5B). It is important to keep in mind that neural noise is present in the absence of the signal, and the signal is superimposed on this noise. The observer's task is to determine if what he or she is seeing (or hearing) is noise or signal plus noise.

The larger the signal, the easier it is for the observer to distinguish the signal plus noise from noise alone (Fig. 11–6A). As the signal becomes larger, the distributions of N and N + S become further apart, and the detectability (*d′*) of the stimulus increases.[6] With a very large *d′*, there is no overlap of the distributions; therefore, there is no uncertainty regarding whether a stimulus is present.

---

6. Detectability refers to the difference between the means of the N and N + S distributions.

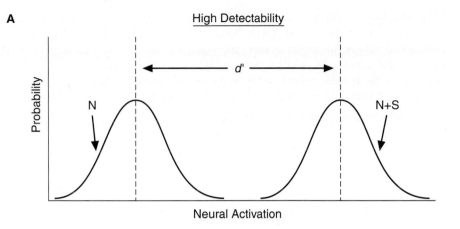

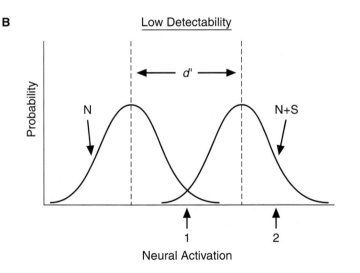

Figure 11–6. A. The larger the detectability of a stimulus, the greater the separation of the noise and noise plus signal distributions. For the high detectability illustrated, it is easy for the observer to determine if the level of neural activation is due to noise alone or signal plus noise. **B.** When the detectability is low, a stimulus may result in a level of neural activity that could be produced by noise or stimulus plus noise (indicated by point 1). If the stimulus is delivered at a time when the noise level is high, the resultant neural activation is unambiguously due to signal plus noise (point 2).

The situation is not so clear-cut when the stimulus is weak, resulting in substantial overlap of the N and N + S distributions (see Fig. 11-6B). If the stimulus is delivered when the noise is low, the resulting level of neural activation (for example, the level indicated by *point 1*) is ambiguous. There is no way for the observer to be certain whether the stimulus is absent or present because this level of neural activation can be produced by either the signal plus noise or noise alone. If, however, the stimulus is delivered at a point in time when the noise is very high, the resulting level of neural activation (for example, the level indicated by *point 2*) is unambiguous. This level of neural noise occurs only when the stimulus is present.

Effect of Observer Criterion

Signal detection theory allows us to predict how the observer's criterion affects stimulus detection. To understand this, consider Fig. 11–7A, which shows the results of a yes-no experiment. The dashed line represents a lax criterion, such as may be adopted by, for example, an intern or resident, who when learning to examine a patient's retina, wishes to be certain that he or she detects any deviation from the norm, no matter how small. Any level of neural activation above the lax criterion line alerts the clinician to a possible abnormality, whereas levels of activation below this line do not elicit a response.

The observer's responses fall into the four categories labeled in Fig. 11–8. According to signal detection theory, if the stimulus results in neural activity that exceeds the threshold criterion, the result is a **hit.** If the activity resulting from the stimulus does not exceed the criterion, there is a **miss**. On those occasions that no stimulus is present (i.e., a blank trial), but the neural activity exceeds the criterion, there is a **false positive** (or **false alarm**). Finally, if the neural noise is below the criterion during a blank trial, the result is a **correct reject**.

Returning to the example of the intern or resident, note that a lax criterion results in very few misses, but many hits and a substantial number of false positives (see Fig. 11–7A). This is the outcome we would expect if a lax criterion were employed when examining the retina. There may be few misses of retinal disease, yet there may be many false alarms.

Now consider the case of a strict criterion, such as that adopted by a deer hunter who wishes to be absolutely certain that the target in his or her sights is indeed a deer (see Fig. 11–7B). Note that d' is the same as for the previously discussed lax criterion. The only difference between the two examples is the location of the criterion line. The strict criterion results in fewer hits than does a lax criterion. A practical implication of this, with regard to the example, is that some deer will not be shot. The payoff, however, is the low number of false positives. By employing a strict criterion, the hunter rarely shoots at targets other than deer.

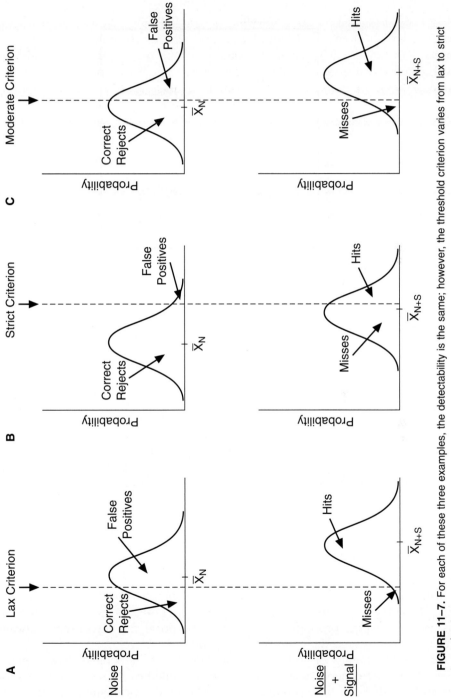

FIGURE 11–7. For each of these three examples, the detectability is the same; however, the threshold criterion varies from lax to strict to moderate.

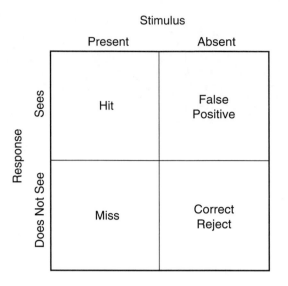

FIGURE 11–8. Possible outcomes for a signal detection experiment.

Receiver Operating Characteristic Curves

A receiver operating characteristic (ROC) curve, which shows the probability of a hit as a function of the probability of a false positive, allows us to predict the effect of the observer criteria for a given detectability (d'). Consider Fig. 11–9A, which shows a ROC curve where $d' = 1$, and L represents a lax criterion, S a strict criterion, and M a moderate criterion. This graph summarizes nicely what we have already learned. For a lax criterion, the probability of a hit is high, but so is the probability of a false positive. For a strict criterion, the probability of a hit is low, but so is the probability of a false positive.

As illustrated in Fig. 11–9B, the ROC is a straight line when $d' = 0$, and becomes more curved as the detectability increases. In the special case of $d' = 0$, the stimulus is so weak that it produces virtually no signal. The straight-line function tells us that no matter what the criteria, lax or strict, the proportion of hits matches the proportion of false positives.

Now consider the other extreme, where the stimulus produces an infinitely large signal (i.e., $d' = \infty$). As can be seen in Fig. 11–9B, the observers' criterion has no effect on the proportion of hits and false positives. The observer always sees the stimulus, and there are never false positives.

How is the family of ROC curves in Fig. 11–9B generated? For a given detectability, the observer's criterion can be controlled by providing rewards for hits and penalties for false positives (a payoff matrix). For example, participants

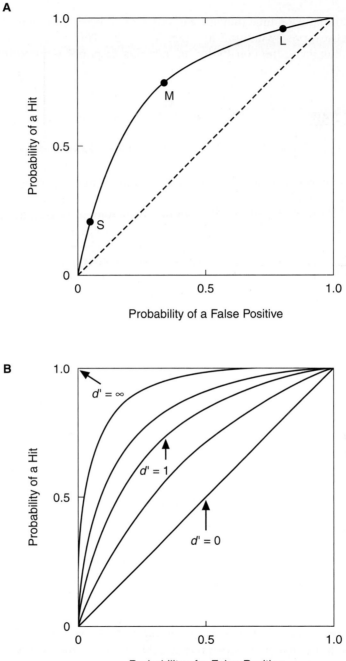

FIGURE 11–9. A. Receiver operating characteristic (ROC) curve, where $d' = 1$ (solid curve). *S*, *M*, and *L* represent strict, moderate, and lax criteria, respectively. **B.** ROCs for various levels of detectability.

may be told that each time they answer correctly, they will receive $5; however, an incorrect response will result in a penalty of $20. This would produce a strict criterion. Minimizing the penalty for an incorrect response would produce a lax criterion.

WEBER'S LAW

Up to now, we have discussed threshold without consideration of the background against which the stimulus is detected. In many psychophysical procedures and experiments, however, the task is to discriminate between the combination of the stimulus and the background, and the background alone.

This can be understood by considering an increment threshold experiment, as illustrated in Fig. 11–10A. The observer's task is to detect the increment stimulus, ΔI, which is flashed on the background, I_b. The threshold increment is often referred to as a **just noticeable difference (JND).** (A JND is also called a **difference limen, or DL.)** Another way of thinking of this task is that the observer must discriminate between the combined stimulus and background, and the background itself.

The JND is not a constant, but changes as the background changes. As the background intensity increases, the JND also increases such that the ratio of the JND to the background intensity remains constant (see Figs. 11–10B and 11–10C). This is referred to as Weber's law, and it is expressed mathematically as

$$\Delta I = KI_b$$

or

$$K = \frac{\Delta I}{I_b}$$

where

ΔI = increment threshold (JND)
I_b = background illumination
K = Weber's constant or fraction

Weber's law applies not only to vision, but to other senses as well. Consider the task of discriminating between two weights. Suppose the observer can barely tell the difference a dumbbell that weighs 10.0 lb (let us call it the background weight) and one that weighs 11.0 lb. In this case, the JND (or increment threshold) is 1 lb. Weber's constant is calculated as (11.0 − 10.0)/10.00 = 0.10.

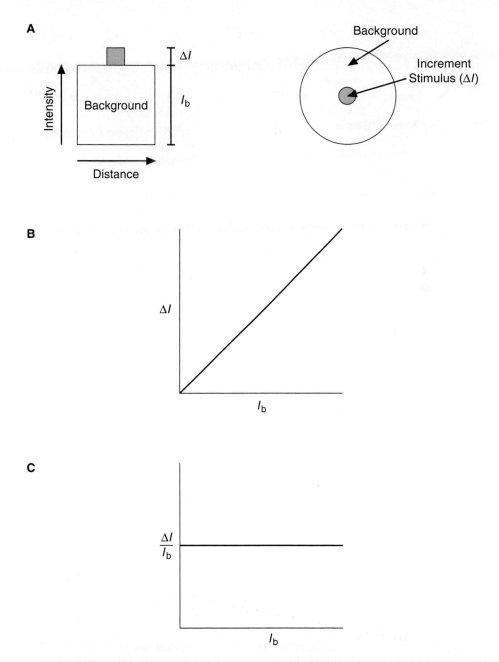

FIGURE 11–10. A. Increment threshold arrangement that can be used to demonstrate Weber's law. A luminance profile is on the left, and the observer's view of the stimulus is on the right. **B.** Graphical representation of Weber's law showing that the ratio of ΔI to I_b is a constant. **C.** Figure B replotted to show $\Delta I/I_b$ as a function of I_b.

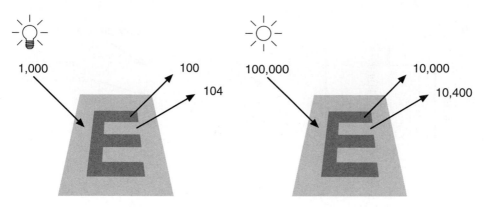

FIGURE 11–11. The optotype **E** reflects 10.00 percent of the light incident upon it, and the gray background reflects 10.40 percent. Whether under dim illumination (1000 units of light) or bright illumination (100,000 units of light), the ratio of the optotype to background luminance (contrast) is the same. Because the visual system has evolved to detect contrast, rather than absolute luminance, the appearance of the **E** is the same under both dim and bright lighting conditions. This phenomenon is referred to as lightness constancy.

If the background weight were 50 lb, what would now be the JND?

$$\Delta I = KI_b$$
$$(X - 50 \text{ lb})/ X = 0.10$$
$$X = 55 \text{ lb}$$

where X is the combination of the increment and background weights. The increment threshold is calculated as follows:

$$\Delta I = X - 50 \text{ lb}$$
$$\Delta I = 5 \text{ lb}$$

To maintain a constant Weber's fraction of 0.10, the JND is 5 lb rather than the original 1 lb. The observer will barely be able to tell the difference between weights of 50 and 55 lb (and certainly will not be able to distinguish between 50 and 51 lb).

As discussed in Chapter 3, the visual system follows Weber's law over much (but not all) of its operational range, with different fractions for scotopic and photopic vision.[7] As the background becomes more intense (within the Weber regions), the increment threshold increases. Consequently, absolute sensitivity decreases, while relative sensitivity remains constant. This process, sensitivity

---

7. Recall that the Weber's fraction for scotopic vision is 0.14 and for photopic vision is 0.015.

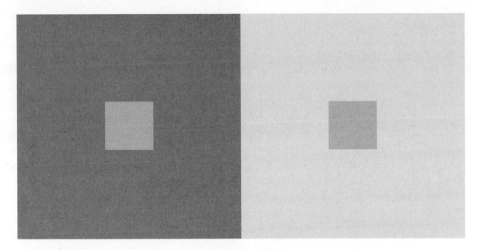

FIGURE 11–12. Although the central squares are physically identical (i.e., they have the same luminance), each has a different brightness. As the background becomes darker, the central square appears brighter. This phenomenon is referred to as simultaneous contrast.

regulation, results in a constant contrast threshold regardless of the background brightness. For scotopic vision, this contrast threshold is 0.14 (or 14 percent); for photopic vision it is 0.015 (or 1.5 percent).

An important result of sensitivity regulation is illustrated by Fig. 11–11, which shows a dark optotype on a gray background under dim and bright photopic illumination. The optotype reflects 10.00 percent of the light that falls on it, and the background reflects 10.40 percent: consequently, the optotype's contrast is approximately 2 percent. When the illumination increases, contrast remains constant because the amount of light reflected from both the dark and gray surfaces increases at the same rate, resulting in a constant ratio of optotype to background luminance. Because Weber's fraction for photopic vision is about 0.015, the optotype is at threshold (barely detectable) under both lighting conditions.[8] The optotype does not become more visible when more light is reflected from it. Rather, because the contrast remains constant, the appearance remains the same, a phenomenon referred to as **lightness constancy**.[9]

What is the appearance of a stimulus of constant luminance when viewed against backgrounds of various luminances? Figure 11–12 demonstrates that brightness depends on the background, a phenomenon referred to as **simultaneous contrast.** Consistent with Weber's law, the contrast of the stimulus, not its luminance, is the key factor in predicting its appearance.

---

8. This is true only at those light levels where Weber's law is followed.

9. Another example of lightness constancy is the appearance of a black and white striped shirt viewed indoors under dim photopic conditions and outdoors under bright photopic conditions. The shirt appears the same under both conditions.

MAGNITUDE OF SENSATION

The discussion thus far has been limited to threshold stimuli. It is of interest, however, to quantify the growth in magnitude of sensation as the intensity of a stimulus is increased to suprathreshold levels. If the intensity of a light bulb is doubled, will it appear twice as bright? What is the relationship between magnitude of sensation and stimulus intensity?

Fechner (1860) attempted to answer this question by assuming that Weber's law applies to suprathreshold stimuli. According to Fechner's model, if the intensity of a light were to increase by 5 JNDs, it would appear five units brighter. This would result in a log relationship between intensity and sensation, as illustrated in Fig. 11–13A. **Fechner's log law** is mathematically expressed as

$$S = c \log I$$

where

S = magnitude of sensation (e.g., brightness)
I = stimulus intensity
c = constant related to Weber's constant

Fechner provided empirical evidence for this law by **indirect scaling.** Essentially, Fechner determined JNDs and assumed that all JNDs produce equal differences in the magnitude of sensation. This assumption is incorrect.

Stevens (1957) applied a remarkably simple paradigm to address this problem—he simply asked observers to directly assess the intensity of suprathreshold stimuli. This is referred to as **direct scaling,** or **magnitude estimation.** When investigating brightness, lights of various intensities are presented, and the observer is asked to assign a number to the perceived brightness of each of the stimuli. For example, a very dim light may be labeled 1, and a very bright light may be labeled 10. Sensation, indicated by the numerical values assigned by the observer, is plotted as a function of light intensity.

The results of such an experiment, plotted on linear coordinates, are given in Fig. 11–13A. When plotted on log–log coordinates, the relationship is seen to be a power function (see Fig. 11–13B). Mathematically, these results are expressed as **Stevens' power law:**

$$S = I^c$$

where

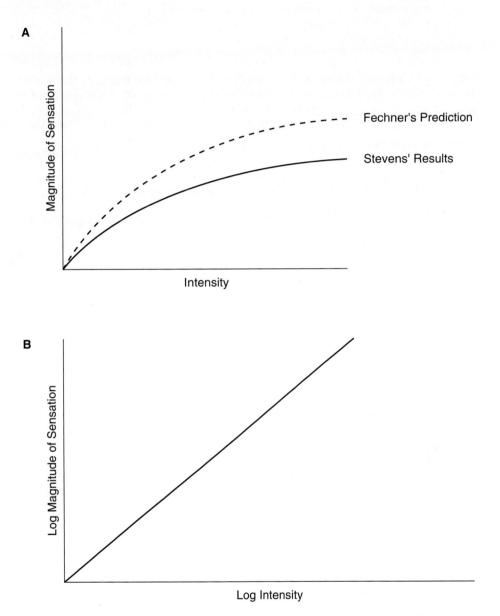

FIGURE 11–13. A. Fechner's log law and Stevens' power law plotted on linear coordinates. **B.** Stevens' power law plotted on log–log coordinates.

S = magnitude of sensation (e.g., brightness)
I = stimulus intensity
c = constant

By magnitude estimation, Stevens was able to show that the growth in magnitude of sensation follows a power relationship, rather than a log relationship as postulated by Fechner. This means that a constant ratio of sensation is produced by a constant ratio of stimulation.

Stevens' law shows that there is a compression (i.e., saturation) of sensation as stimulus intensity increases. Consider a three-way light bulb that can be set at 0, 50, 100, or 150 watts. The physical difference between each of these settings is the same (50 watts), yet turning the light on (going from 0 to 50 watts) is much more noticeable than adjusting the setting from 100 to 150 watts.

SUMMARY

The determination of thresholds plays a large role in vision research and clinical eye care. The specific methodology used to determine a threshold may significantly affect the value obtained.

There is frequently a trade-off between the ease of determining a threshold and its validity. For clinical purposes, the repeatability (reliability) of a threshold measurement may be more important than its validity. Consequently, psychophysical procedures that are not unduly taxing for patients, such as the staircase method or method of limits, may provide clinically useful information.

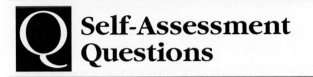

Q Self-Assessment Questions

1. **A.** For a three-alternative forced choice experiment, what is the percentage correct used to determine the threshold? **B.** Answer the same question for a five-alternative forced choice experiment.

2. An experiment is conducted where thresholds for the detection of temporally stable gratings are compared to thresholds for gratings that are temporally modulated. What would be the best methodology for determining these thresholds? Explain.

12

Functional Retinal Physiology

This and the following three chapters emphasize data obtained through single-unit electrophysiological investigations, where single neurons located within the visual system of an anesthetized experimental animal are isolated and their electrical activity recorded. The recordings can be either extracellular or intracellular.

In **extracellular recording,** a microelectrode, placed in extremely close proximity to a neuron, records action potentials generated by the neuron. For **intracellular** recording, a microelectrode pierces the membrane of a neuron and records the membrane potential (i.e., the neuron's degree of depolarization or hyperpolarization). This technique, which is more technically challenging than extracellular recording, is necessary when studying neurons that produce **graded (slow) potentials** (but not action potentials). This includes several classes of retinal cells.

Intracellular recording provides other advantages. The microelectrode (a glass micropipette) can be used to inject a dye into a neuron after recording its electrical activity (Fig. 12–1). When the experimental animal is subsequently sacrificed, the neuron is located and examined histologically, thereby allowing correlations to be made between the electrophysiological properties of the neuron and its morphology.

The generation of a neural potentials involves the opening and closing of various ion channels. The channels are voltage-sensitive, meaning that their opening and closing is triggered by the membrane potential. By combining intracellular

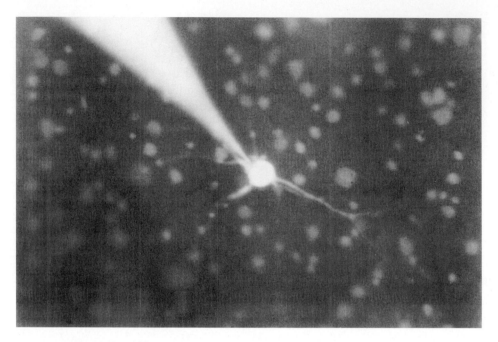

FIGURE 12–1. A micropipette (foreground) fills a rabbit ganglion cell with dye following intracellular recording. Note the dendrites that emerge from the neuron's soma. *(Photograph is courtesy of Dr. Ralph Jensen.)*

recording with a technique called patch-clamping, where a probe that is similar to an extracellular electrode is used to control the membrane potential, it is possible to isolate the various ion channels and study their dynamics in detail.

THE RETINA

The retina is a multilayered tissue containing several distinct classes of neurons that communicate with each other through a multitude of synaptic connections rich in both their diversity and complexity. The retina, a part of the brain, is not a passive receiver of information. Rather, the optical image that falls on the retina is analyzed and encoded into a complex neural signal that is transmitted to higher visual centers.

In this chapter, basic retinal processing is examined. The discussion begins by studying the receptive field characteristics of the neurons that represent the *final stage* of retinal processing, the ganglion cells. We then examine the receptive field characteristics of the major classes of retinal cells that are distal to the ganglion cells.

RECEPTIVE FIELDS OF GANGLION CELLS

Consider the electrophysiological experiment illustrated in Fig. 12–2. The fovea of an anesthetized animal, such as a monkey or a cat, is aligned with a point on a screen. A microelectrode is placed in close proximity to a single ganglion cell, such that it records action potentials from this one cell (extracellular single-unit recording). If a spot of light is directed onto various areas of the screen, an area is found that influences the neural activity of the cell, the so-called the **receptive field** of the cell.

Even when a spot of light is not shining on the receptive field, the cell spontaneously generates action potentials. These action potentials, which occur in the absence of a stimulus, are referred to collectively as the **spontaneous activity,** or **maintained discharge,** of the neuron.

A stimulus positioned within a neuron's receptive field can either increase or decrease its discharge rate (Fig. 12–3). A small light located within the center of this receptive field causes an increase in the frequency of action potentials, as indicated by the plus signs. The same small light positioned in the surround of the receptive field produces a reduction in the frequency of action potentials, as indicated by the minus signs.

The receptive fields of mammalian ganglion cells often have a **center–surround** organization, meaning that light falling on the receptive field's center has the opposite effect of light falling on the surrounding area of the receptive field. This is often referred to as **spatial antagonism** or **lateral inhibition** (Kuffler, 1953). For the ganglion cell in Fig. 12–3, light falling on the receptive field center causes the frequency of action potentials to increase—the cell is excited. In contrast, light falling on the receptive field surround inhibits the cell and there is a reduction in the frequency of action potentials. This ganglion cell is said to have an on-center and off-surround. (Other ganglion cells have the reverse arrangement, an off-center and on-surround. Light falling on the receptive field center produces a decrease in the frequency of action potentials, whereas light falling on the surround produces an increase in frequency.)

The preceding discussion may be confusing if this is your first exposure to this concept. Let us approach it from a slightly different perspective. Consider an experiment in which we record extracellularly from an on-center, off-surround ganglion cell in a cat retina (Fig. 12–4). Using a projector, we shine a very small light onto the center of the cell's receptive field, eliciting an increase in the frequency of action potentials (as compared with the maintained discharge). If the experiment is repeated with a slightly larger spot of light, there is a greater increase in the frequency of action potentials due to spatial summation that occurs within the receptive field's center.

This result can be represented graphically by plotting the frequency of action potentials as a function of the diameter of the spot of light (see Fig. 12–4). As the diameter of the spot increases, the cell's firing rate increases (area B). A diam-

A

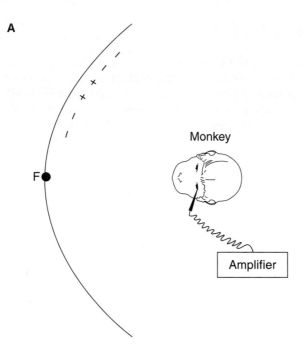

B

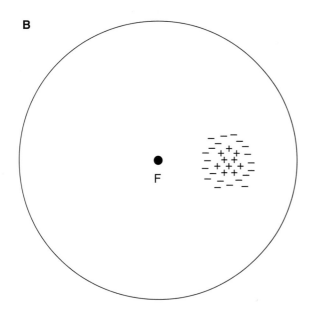

FIGURE 12–2. A. Determination of a ganglion cell's receptive field. The animal's eye is aligned with the fixation point, F, and small spots of light are projected onto a screen. Light falling on a circumscribed region of the screen affects the activity of the neuron. This is the neuron's receptive field, indicated by the plus and minus signs. Light falling on the area indicated by plus signs causes the neuron to become excited, whereas light falling on the area indicated by minus signs causes it to be inhibited. **B.** Face-on view of the screen and receptive field.

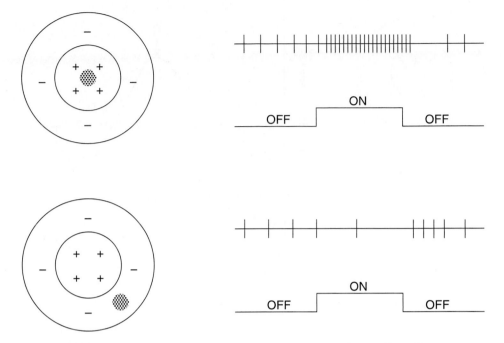

FIGURE 12–3. A spot of light falling on the excitatory center of a ganglion cell receptive field causes an increase in the frequency of action potentials. The same spot of light falling on the inhibitory surround causes a reduction in the frequency of action potentials.

eter is eventually reached, however, where the response is maximum (point C), and any further increase in stimulus diameter produces a decrease in the rate of firing (area D) because the stimulus is now falling on the inhibitory surround, which is antagonistic to the excitatory center.

As the stimulus encroaches on more and more of the inhibitory surround, the response diminishes because of spatial summation within the surround. Eventually, a point is reached where further increases in the stimulus diameter have no effect on the cell's response. This point, indicated by E, represents the termination of the cell's receptive field. Any light falling beyond this point does not influence the activity of the neuron. Note that the response to a stimulus that fills the entire receptive field is about the same as when there is no stimulus (point A), illustrating that spatially antagonistic ganglion cells do not respond well to diffuse illumination (Fig. 12–5).

What is a strong stimulus for a ganglion cell? Consider the response to a sine wave grating (Fig. 12–6). The bright bar falls on the receptive field's excitatory center, resulting in an increased frequency of action potentials. The dark bars fall on the receptive field's inhibitory surround, also increasing the frequency of

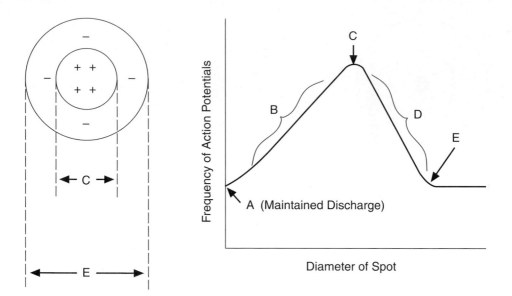

FIGURE 12–4. As the diameter of a spot of light is increased, a ganglion cell manifests spatial summation up to the perimeter of its receptive field center, *C*, resulting in an increase in the frequency of action potentials. Beyond this diameter, light also falls on the antagonistic surround, producing a decrease in the frequency of action potentials. For the graph on the right, point *A* represents the cell's maintained discharge, area *B* represents the receptive field center, point *C* represents the border between the center and surround, area *D* represents the receptive field surround, and point *E* represents the termination of the cell's receptive field.

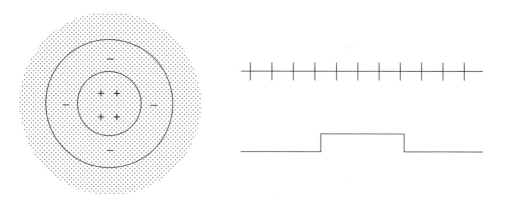

FIGURE 12–5. A ganglion cell is not responsive to diffuse illumination. There is no change in the frequency of action potentials from the baseline maintained discharge.

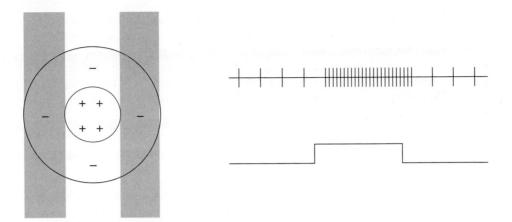

FIGURE 12–6. A spatial grating is a strong stimulus for a ganglion cell. Because light falls on the excitatory center and darkness on the inhibitory surround, the neural response is vigorous.

action potentials.[1] The result is that the spatial grating vigorously excites the cell.

This illustrates a critical point. Ganglion cells are selective for spatial contrast, not diffuse illumination. Very early in the visual system, within the retina itself, contrast information is extracted from the visual scene.

In the remainder of this chapter, we examine the transfer of information in the retina, starting with the activation of the photoreceptors and culminating with the signal that is transmitted out of the eye along the optic nerve. The receptive field properties of photoreceptors, horizontal cells, bipolar cells, and amacrine cells are discussed along with additional characteristics pertaining to the receptive fields of ganglion cells.

RECORDING FROM RETINAL NEURONS

Before further discussing the neurophysiological properties of retinal cells, let us address a procedural problem. Photoreceptors and several classes of retinal neurons generate only graded (slow) potentials, not action potentials. Because extracellular microelectrodes can record only action potentials (but not graded potentials), intracellular recording techniques, in which the microelectrode impales the cell, must be used. This is problematic because many of the retinal cells in the mammalian retina are very small, making it technically difficult to insert an electrode into these cells.

---

1. If light were to fall on the inhibitory surround, the frequency of action potentials would be decreased. The dark bars, by blocking light from falling on the inhibitory surround, lead to an excitatory response.

Werblin and Dowling (1969) overcame this obstacle by recording membrane potentials from the unusually large retinal cells of an aquatic salamander, the mudpuppy *(Necturus maculosus)*. The large cells are a result of an aborted metamorphosis in which the cells undergo mitosis without division. By recording from the various classes of retinal cells, Werblin and Dowling (1969) were able to determine the basic outline of information transfer within the retina. Their results are summarized in Fig. 12–7.[2]

PHOTORECEPTORS

Photoreceptors are specialized sensory receptors containing a photosensitive pigment that absorbs light quanta, converting this radiant energy into electrical activity. This is the first step in vision.

Both rods and cones are slightly depolarized relative to a typical neuron. Rather than manifesting a resting membrane potential of −70 mV, the potential is about −50 mV. When exposed to light, photoreceptors *hyperpolarize*—their potential goes from −50 mV to a value closer to −70 mV (Tomita, 1970). You may find this surprising because stimulation is typically thought to cause depolarization rather than hyperpolarization.

The degree of photoreceptor hyperpolarization is related to the intensity of the stimulus, with an intense stimulus causing greater hyperpolarization than a less intense stimulus. This is one reason that the potentials produced by photoreceptors are referred to as graded potentials.

A summary of the steps that lead to the hyperpolarization of a rod are outlined in Fig. 12–8 (Lamb, 1986; Pugh and Cobbs, 1986; Stryer, 1986). In the dark, sodium ions (Na^+) flow into the rod outer segment through pores (channels), the so-called **dark current,** producing a slight depolarization. The absorption of light by rhodopsin initiates a series of events that result in the blockage of the Na^+ pores and the resultant hyperpolarization of the outer segment.

A molecule of rhodopsin consists of two portions: **opsin** and a **chromophore.** Opsin is a visually inert chain of amino acids that is interlaced into the disk membranes of the rod outer segment. As discussed in Chapter 5, opsin determines the absorption profile of the photopigment. The chromophore, which is responsive to light, consists of retinal, an altered form of retinol (vitamin A).

When unbleached, retinal is in the 11-*cis* state. (There is a bend at carbon number 11 of the molecule.) Absorption of a quantum of light transforms the retinal molecule to the all-*trans* isomer. Subsequently, the protein transducin activates the protein phosphodiesterase (PDE). PDE breaks down cyclic GMP (cGMP) into ordinary GMP. A decrease in cGMP levels leads to the closing of the Na^+ channels of the rod outer segment. This results in rod hyperpolarization.

The number of sodium channels located in the rod outer segment is limited, constraining the potential magnitude of rod hyperpolarization (Baylor et al, 1984).

---

2. Modern techniques now allow intracellular recordings from smaller mammalian neurons.

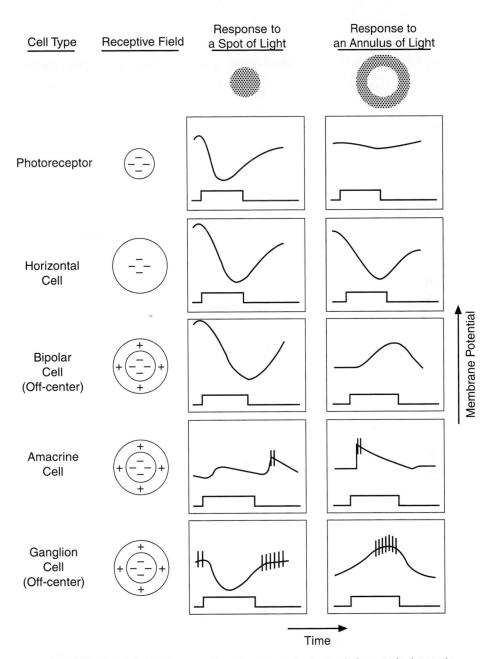

FIGURE 12–7. Intracellular recordings from the various neural elements in the mud-puppy retina. Only amacrine cells and ganglion cells generate action potentials; all other retinal neurons generate graded potentials. Note that the spot and annulus elicit responses of opposite signs from the bipolar cell. This is because the spot falls on the bipolar cell receptive field center, whereas the annulus falls on its antagonistic surround. The same effect is also found for the ganglion cell (Werblin and Dowling, 1969).

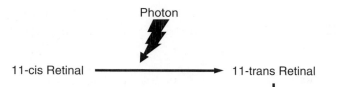

Photon

11-cis Retinal ───────────────▶ 11-trans Retinal

│ Activates

Transducin (a Protein)

│ Activates

Phosphodiesterase (PDE)(a Protein)

│

▼

Breaks Up cGMP into GMP

│

▼

Na$^+$ Pores Close

│

▼

Rod Hyperpolarizes

FIGURE 12–8. Flow diagram showing the stages that lead to rod hyperpolarization.

When about only 10 percent of a rod's rhodopsin is bleached, a critical number of sodium channels are closed and further bleaching of rhodopsin does not result in further hyperpolarization. This helps to explain the psychophysical phenomenon of rod saturation (see Chap. 3). After about 10 percent of rhodopsin is bleached, rods cannot hyperpolarize any further. They are saturated.

HORIZONTAL CELLS

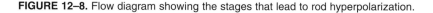

A large number of photoreceptors, distributed over a relatively large area of the retina, synapse with the widely dispersed dendritic tree of a single horizontal cell (Fig. 12–9). Because light falling on any of these photoreceptors may affect the neural activity of the horizontal cell, it manifests substantial spatial summation.

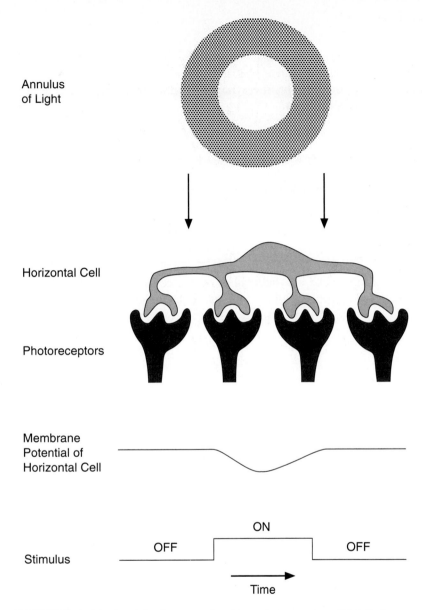

Annulus
of Light

Horizontal Cell

Photoreceptors

Membrane
Potential of
Horizontal Cell

ON

OFF   OFF

Stimulus

Time

FIGURE 12–9. A horizontal cell sums up input from photoreceptors distributed over a large area of the retina. Because of this high degree of spatial summation, an annulus elicits a strong response from a horizontal cell, causing it to hyperpolarize. This figure is a schematic.

There are two classes of horizontal cells—H1 and H2 cells (Dacheux and Raviola, 1990; Dacey et al, 1996; Martin, 1998). The H1 cells receive input primarily from the M- and L- cones, and little input from the S-cones. In comparison, H2 cells show strong connectivity with S-cones and also receive input from M- and L-cones.

Like photoreceptors, horizontal cells show graded responses and do not generate action potentials. Because photoreceptors and horizontal cells both hyperpolarize in response to light, the synapses connecting them are referred to as **sign-conserving synapses.**

BIPOLAR CELLS

Bipolar cells are the first (i.e., most distal) retinal cells to display spatial antagonism. Like the photoreceptors and horizontal cells that precede them, bipolar cells do not generate action potentials. The receptive fields of two different types of bipolar cells, along with schematic illustrations of their synaptic connections with photoreceptors and horizontal cells, are given in Fig. 12–10. The receptive field on the left is similar to the on-center ganglion cell receptive fields that were discussed earlier in this chapter: light falling on the center of the cell's receptive field cause excitation (depolarization), whereas light falling on the surround causes

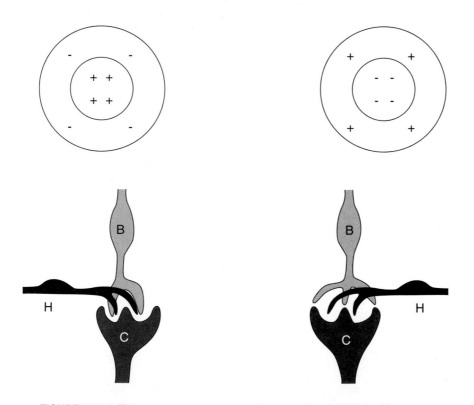

FIGURE 12–10. The on-center bipolar cell on the left makes an invaginating synapse with the photoreceptor, whereas the off-center bipolar cells makes a flat synapse.

inhibition (hyperpolarization). As indicated in Fig. 12–10, on-center bipolar cells are characterized by an **invaginating** synapse that they make with photoreceptors in the outer plexiform layer (Famiglietti and Kolb, 1976; Stell et al, 1977).

Another class of bipolar cells, also illustrated in Fig. 12–10, shows an inhibitory off-center bordered by an excitatory on-surround. Unlike on-center cells, off-center bipolar cells form a **conventional flat synapse** with photoreceptors.

Both on- and off-center bipolar cells synapse with ganglion cells in the inner plexiform layer (IPL). As illustrated in Fig. 12–11, they synapse at different sub-layers within the IPL, with off-center cells forming synapses in the outer sub-layer and on-center cells synapsing in the inner sub-layer (Nelson et al, 1978; Peichl and Wassle, 1981).[3]

What occurs within the outer plexiform layer that causes some bipolar cells to have an on-center arrangement and others to have an off-center configuration? The answer appears to be that the neurotransmitter **glutamate,** released by the photoreceptors, has different effects on the two classes of bipolar cells (Slaughter and Miller, 1985).

Under dark conditions, photoreceptors continuously release neurotransmitter. Light stimulation causes hyperpolarization of the photoreceptors and a consequent reduction in the release of neurotransmitter. It is thought that for on-center bipolar cells, glutamate is inhibitory. Therefore, a reduction in its release causes a relative excitation (depolarization) of the bipolar cell. For off-center bipolar cells, the same neurotransmitter has the opposite effect; it is excitatory, and a reduction in its release, secondary to the hyperpolarization of a photoreceptor, causes a relative inhibition (hyperpolarization) of the bipolar cell.

In addition to being categorized as on- or off-center, bipolar cells are also characterized as **midget** or **diffuse** (Boycott and Wassle, 1999).[4] Compared to diffuse bipolar cells, midget bipolar cells have smaller soma and less extensive dendritic trees.

The receptive field centers of those primate midget bipolar cells that are located in the central and midperipheral retina manifest input from a single M- or L-cone cone (Wassle et al, 1994). Such an arrangement accounts for the high level of visual acuity seen in primates. In the periphery, the receptive field centers of midget bipolar cells receive input from more than one photoreceptor, consistent with the reduced visual acuity associated with the peripheral retina.

Recall from Chapter 5 that certain cells in the dorsal lateral geniculate nucleus are color opponent, whereas others are noncolor opponent. This dichotomy is present

---

3. As will be discussed, bipolar cells can be categorized as midget or diffuse. Either cell type can manifest an on- or off-center receptive field. Whereas the synapses made in the IPL by on- and off midget cells are clearly stratified into two sub-layers, the stratification of the synapses made by diffuse cells is not as obvious.

4. An on-center bipolar cell may be a midget or diffuse cell. The same is true for an off-center bipolar cell.

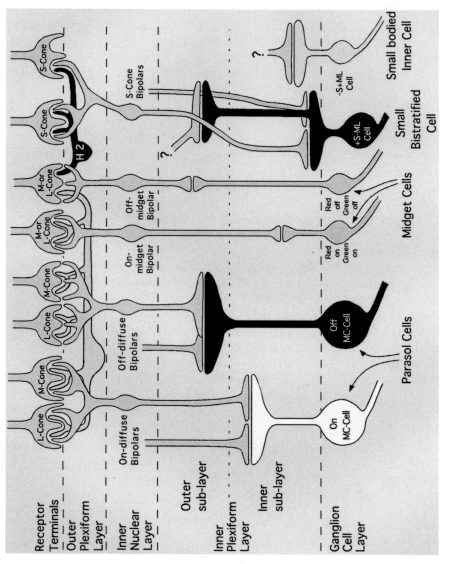

FIGURE 12-11. Schematic showing the organization of the primate retina. (*Diagram kindly provided by Dr. Barry B. Lee.*)

at the level of the bipolar cells, with midget bipolar cells (both on- and off-center) manifesting color opponency. Diffuse bipolar cells are noncolor opponent.

What accounts for the color opponency of midget bipolar cells? A single cone forms the receptive field center (in the central and midperipheral retina), and the surround is apparently formed by input from H1 horizontal cells. Because H1 horizontal cells receive input from both M- and L- cones, the midget bipolar cell manifests a different spectral sensitivity in its surround than its center, hence color opponency (Martin, 1998).

The receptive field centers of the midget bipolar cells are formed by either M- or L-cones. S-cones apparently communicate with a distinct class of bipolar cells, referred to as S-cone bipolar cells (Dacey and Lee, 1994).

A diffuse bipolar cell's receptive field center is formed by 5 to 10 cones (Boycott and Wassle, 1999). Because more than one cone type may form the center, its spectral sensitivity is very similar to the surround, which also reflects a mixture of different cone types. (The surround is formed by H1 cells that receive input from many M- and L-cones.)

Midget bipolar cells help to account for both the excellent visual acuity and color vision found in primates.[5] Which of these functions evolved first? Many scientists believe that a receptive field center formed by only a single cone evolved first to provide for high-resolution acuity (e.g., Boycott and Wassle, 1999). Although visual acuity is maximized by this arrangement, it also creates the basis for color opponency, which occurs because the surround is composed of a combination of different cone types, giving it a different spectral sensitivity than the center. According to this view, there may have been subsequent evolution of certain of the brain's visual areas to more fully take advantage of the color opponency displayed in the retina, permitting our ancestors to manifest highly developed color vision. This capability presumably provided a competitive advantage, leading to the survival and further development of color vision capabilities through natural selection (Osorio et al, 1996).[6]

Figure 12-11 summarizes much of what we discussed regarding bipolar cells, showing the synaptic connections involved in the formation of diffuse on-center, diffuse off-center, midget on-center, midget off-center, and S-cone bipolar cells. There are at least four other classes of bipolar cells that are not discussed.

---

5. The view that midget bipolar cells transmit both chromatic and acuity information is controversial. Some investigators believe that one class of retinal cells transmits a pure color signal, while another class of cells processes acuity information. See Calkins and Sterling (1999) for a review of this subject.
6. Detecting ripe, red fruit against the background of green leaves is one example where highly developed color vision capabilities would provide monkeys and apes with a competitive advantage.

AMACRINE CELLS

Many amacrine cells, like bipolar cells, show a center–surround organization. An important feature that distinguishes them from bipolar and other more distal retinal cells is the time-related characteristics of their neural response. Amacrine cells tend to respond briefly—transiently—at the stimulus onset and offset. Because of this characteristic, they are thought to play a critical role in coding movement.

Amacrine cells are the first retinal neurons to display action potentials. Photoreceptors, horizontal cells, and bipolar cells show graded potentials, not action potentials (Barnes and Werblin, 1986).

GANGLION CELLS

The receptive field properties of ganglion cells reflect the collective properties of the neurons that precede them. A primary focus of contemporary retinal research is directed toward determining the precise synaptic connections that result in the receptive field properties of ganglion cells and of other retinal neurons.[7]

This chapter started with a discussion of the receptive field properties of ganglion cells. As you may have surmised, the center-surround organization found in ganglion cells has its origin in the bipolar cells. On-center midget bipolar cells synapse with on-center **midget ganglion cells**, and off-center midget bipolar cells synapse with off-center midget ganglion cells.[8] Midget ganglion cells are sometimes referred to as **retinal parvo** cells.

Likewise, on-center diffuse bipolar cells synapse with on-center **parasol ganglion cells**, and off-center diffuse bipolar cells synapse with off-center parasol ganglion cells (Fig. 12–12). Parasol ganglion cells are sometimes called **retinal magno** cells.

S-cone bipolar cells synapse onto a distinct class of ganglion cells, the **small bistratified cells** (Fig. 12–13). The receptive fields of these neurons have an on-center that is formed exclusively by S-cones (Dacey and Lee, 1994).

As discussed previously, a key feature of central and midperipheral midget bipolar cells is the contribution of only one cone to the formation of the receptive field center. This also holds true for midget ganglion cells located in the fovea (Fig. 12–14). These cells receive input from only one midget bipolar cell, hence only one cone (Kolb and DeKover, 1991). This limited spatial summation accounts for the exquisite visual acuity of central vision. In the peripheral retina, more than one bipolar cell feeds into a midget ganglion cell, increasing spatial summation and accounting for the periphery's reduced visual acuity. The increased spatial summation of peripheral midget ganglion cells is reflected in their larger receptive fields (compared to foveal cells) (Rodieck, 1991).

---

7. The roles of the myriad neurotransmitters associated with these synapses are also of great interest.
8. Recall that on- and off-center midget bipolar cells synapse in different sub-layers of the IPL.

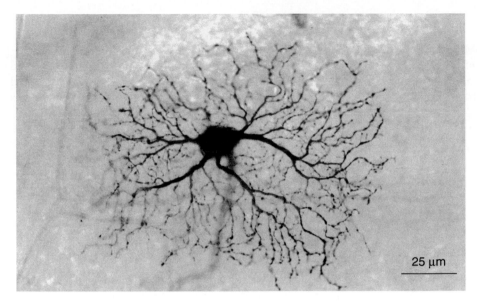

25 µm

FIGURE 12-12. Macaque parasol cell. (*Photomicrograph kindly provided by Drs. Barry B. Lee and Dennis M. Dacey*).

Parasol cells have large dendritic trees and presumably synapse with more than one diffuse bipolar cell. This contributes to the extensive receptive field that typifies these cells (Fig. 12–14).

Similar to amacrine cells, ganglion cells generate action potentials. Action potentials, unlike graded potentials, do not decay over distance. This is critical because ganglion cell axons must traverse a substantial distance before they reach their primary destination, the dorsal lateral geniculate nucleus (dLGN). The speed of conduction of action potentials, however, is slow. Conductance speed is increased by the myelin sheath along the ganglion cell axons, giving rise to saltatory transmission.[9] The axons of ganglion cells become myelinated as they leave the eye at the disk to form the optic nerve.

As discussed in the following chapter, parasol ganglion cells respond transiently to a flash of light, and midget ganglion cells manifest a sustained response (see Fig. 13–5) (DeMonasterio and Gouras, 1975). This difference may be due to the nature

---

9. Retinal cells distal to the amacrine cells communicate with each other through so-called slow potentials, also referred to as electrotonic conduction or decremental spread. The term, slow potentials, is a misnomer—these potentials spread very rapidly, allowing for fast communication between cells. A problem with slow potentials is that they decay as they move away from their origin, eventually dissipating. In comparison, action potentials do not decay, but they are very slow. When a myelin sheath is present along an axon that generates action potentials, there is rapid electrotonic transmission under the sheath, with the action potential being regenerated at the gaps within the myelin sheath (nodes of Ranvier). This form of transmission—saltatory transmission—allows for the rapid transmission of information over long distances without decay of the signal.

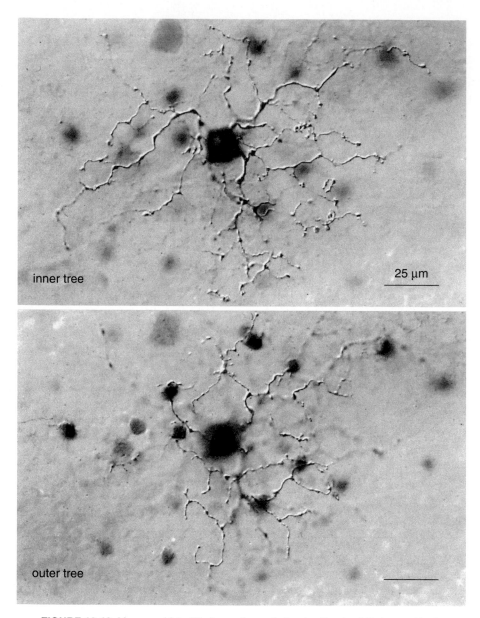

FIGURE 12-13. Macaque bistratified ganglion cell showing the dendritic trees at both levels of stratification. (*Photomicrograph kindly provided by Drs. Barry B. Lee and Dennis M. Dacey.*)

of the amacrine cell input, with parasol ganglion cells presumably receiving substantial input from transient amacrine cells and midget ganglion cells receiving a large input from sustained amacrine cells (Werblin and Dowling, 1969).

The axons of midget and parasol ganglion cells synapse in the dLGN, forming the first leg of the parvo and magno retinocortical pathways. A third pathway,

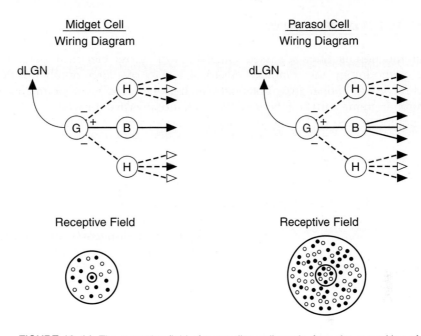

FIGURE 12–14. The receptive field of a ganglion cell results from the apposition of central photoreceptors to surrounding photoreceptors. In the case of an on-center midget cell, the receptive field center is constituted of a single cone and the surround by a mixture of M- and L-cones. In comparison, the receptive field center of an on-center parasol cell is constituted of a mixture of M- and L-cones, as is the surround.

the konio pathway, is formed by the axons of the bistratified ganglion cells, which also synapse in the dLGN. Less is known about this pathway. After the dLGN, the parvo and magno pathways maintain various degrees of independence through the striate cortex, visual area 2, and specialized higher cortical centers (Fig. 14–16) (Livingstone and Hubel, 1988).

Not all ganglion cells project to the dLGN—certain ganglion cells project to the superior colliculus, a midbrain structure involved with control of eye movements (see Chap. 2). Recent work has led to the discovery of a subset of ganglion cells that contain the photopigment melanopsin (Hattar et al, 2002). In the rat, these cells project to the suprachiasmic nucleus (SCN) of the hypothalamus, a structure that is responsible for the circadian rhythm (Berson et al, 2002; Provencio et al, 2002).[10] The melanopsin-containing ganglion cells found in the macaque monkey retina manifest peak sensitivity at about 483 nm (Smith et al, 2003).

---

10. The circadian rhythm refers to bodily functions that follow a pattern of activity that is based on a 24-hour clock.

CLINICAL CONSIDERATIONS

Retinal function is often assessed clinically with gross electrical potentials. In this methodology, the combined electrical activity of a large number of neurons is recorded. Retinal gross potentials, such as the electrooculogram and the electroretinogram, can be obtained through noninvasive procedures. These gross potentials and their clinical application are described in Chapter 16.

SUMMARY

The photoreceptors have simple requirements for activation: diffuse light falling on their receptive fields elicits a response. At more proximal locations within the retina, the requirements for neural activation are more stringent. Ganglion cells, for example, are responsive only to stimuli that manifest spatial contrast.

From a teleological point of view, the retina is designed largely to extract contrast information from the visual world. This is consistent with the singular role that spatial contrast plays in our visual experience.

Q Self-Assessment Questions

1. In Chapter 7, we discussed the concept of the visual system as a Fourier analyzer. Explain how the receptive field properties of ganglion cells could be considered consistent with this hypothesis.

2. Foveal visual acuity is 20/20, whereas peripheral visual acuity is on the order of 20/200. How can this be explained in terms of the receptive field properties of ganglion cells?

3. Psychophysical experiments show that the human visual system manifests greater spatial summation under dark-adapted conditions than under light-adapted conditions. How could the receptive fields of ganglion cells change to account for this psychophysical finding?

Parallel Processing

13

Figure 13–1 shows a coronal section of the dorsal lateral geniculate nucleus (dLGN) of a monkey. The axons of most retinal ganglion cells synapse on the neurons that constitute this laminated structure. The dLGN, in turn, sends its primary projection to the visual cortex.

A striking feature of the dLGN is its division into three distinct sections, each constituted of a different type of neuron. The two most ventral layers in Fig. 13–1 consist of large neurons referred to as **magno cells,** and the dorsal four layers consist of smaller neurons referred to as **parvo cells.** In between these principal layers, in the interlaminar regions (intercalated layers), are collections of yet smaller cells called **konio cells** (Hendry and Yoshioka, 1994). These cells are hardly visible in Fig. 13–1.

Extracellular recordings reveal that parvo and magno cells manifest different visual sensitivities (Schiller and Malpeli, 1978). For instance, parvo cells are selective to color contrast, but not to fast movement. In comparison, magno cells are largely monochromatic and very sensitive to movement. Because of their anatomical segregation and different visual sensitivities, parvo and magno cells can be considered to be components of parallel retinocortical visual pathways. The less-well studied konio cells appear to be part of yet another visual pathway (Fig. 13-2). Although the division of the visual system into parallel pathways may be most apparent at the level of the dLGN, this division is also found in the retina (i.e., midget and parasol ganglion cells) and, to a lesser extent, in the striate cortex and higher cortical areas (DeMonasterio and Gouras, 1975; Livingstone and Hubel, 1987, 1988).

Dorsal

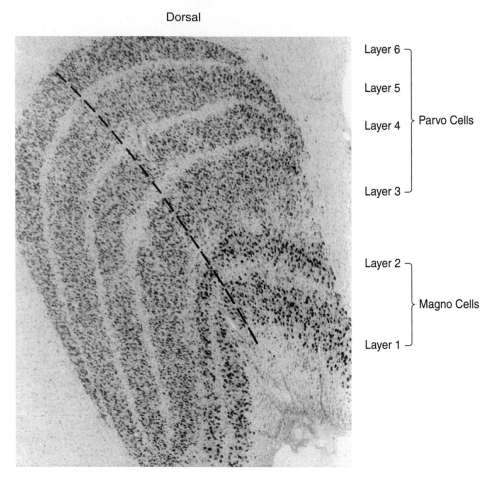

Layer 6 ⎤
Layer 5 ⎥
Layer 4 ⎬ Parvo Cells
Layer 3 ⎦

Layer 2 ⎤
⎥ Magno Cells
Layer 1 ⎦

Ventral

FIGURE 13–1. Coronal section of a monkey dorsal lateral geniculate nucleus. Note the division into two ventral magnocellular layers (bottom layers) and four dorsal parvocellular layers (upper layers). Konio cells are found in between these principal layers. The dashed line represents a microelectrode track. (*From Hubel DH.* Eye, Brain, and Vision. *New York: Scientific American Library; 1988. Reprinted with permission of Dr. David Hubel.*)

WHAT THE FROG'S EYE TELLS ITS BRAIN

The concept of parallel processing received much impetus from the identification of feature detectors in the frog retina (Lettvin et al, 1959).[1] Frogs prey on small, airborne bugs. Curiously, one class of frog ganglion cells responds best to

---

1. Lettvin et al (1959) recorded extracellularly from frog ganglion cells.

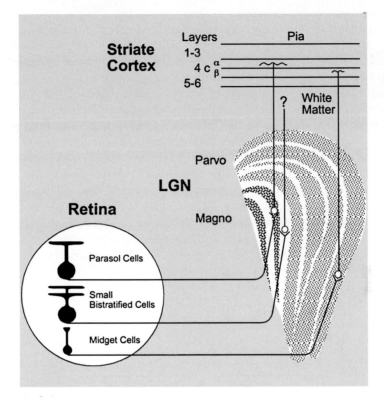

FIGURE 13-2. Schematic showing the retinogeniculate parvo, magno, and konio pathways. *(This diagram was kindly provided by Dr. Barry B. Lee.)*

small black spots of the same visual characteristics as an airborne bug. These cells, which do not respond well to other stimuli, are called bug detectors. Another class of ganglion cells responds best to large moving shadows, making them well adapted to signal the presence of a predator, such as a hawk.

It appears that certain ganglion cells in the frog's retina, so-called **feature detectors,** have evolved to detect particular facets of the visual world. Feature detection is a manifestation of **parallel processing,** whereby specific aspects of visual information are processed along specialized visual pathways (channels).

X- AND Y-CELLS

Strong evidence for parallel processing in the mammalian retina was first found by scientists examining the responses of cat ganglion cells to spatial stimuli, specifically sine wave gratings (Enroth-Cugell and Robson, 1966). This experiment was performed at a time when linear system analysis (Fourier analysis) was initially used to study the visual system (see Chap. 7). Because this model requires spatial linearity, scientists were eager to determine if ganglion cells had this property. The results were surprising—whereas some cat ganglion were spatially linear, others were nonlinear. To avoid any connotation of function, the linear cells were named **X-cells** and nonlinear cells, **Y-cells**.

To obtain a better understanding of spatial linearity, refer to Fig. 13–3. For an X-cell, a spatial grating can be positioned within the cell's receptive field such that no response is elicited. At this position, referred to as the **null position**, excitation and inhibition are linearly summed and cancel each other. The excitation is equal to the inhibition.

The nonlinear Y-cell behaves differently. A null position cannot be found for this neuron. No matter where the grating is positioned, the cell responds. The lack of a null position indicates that this cell does not sum spatial information in a linear fashion.

Because of differences in linearity and other response properties, it is clear that X- and Y-cells play different roles in vision. One can think of them as forming parallel visual pathways.

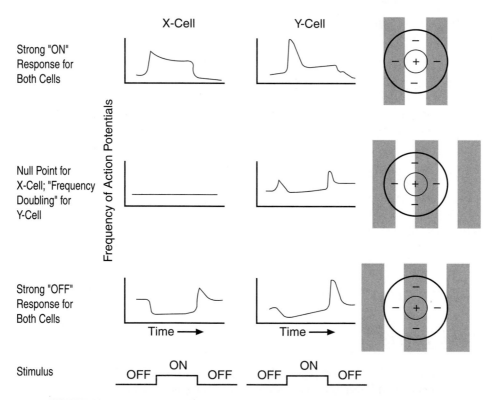

FIGURE 13–3. A spatial grating can be positioned within the receptive field of X-cells such that a null position is located (left). This indicates that X-cells manifest linear spatial summation. For Y-cells, which are nonlinear, a null position is not found (Enroth-Cugell and Robson, 1966).

TABLE 13–1. CHARACTERISTICS OF PARVO AND MAGNO NEURONS LOCATED IN THE PRIMATE RETINA AND DORSAL LATERAL GENICULATE NUCLEUS

Characteristic	Parvo Neurons	Magno Neurons
Color coding	Color opponent	Weak or no color opponency
Temporal responsiveness	Sustained	Transient
Speed of transmission	Slow	Fast
Spatial linearity	Linear	Linear or nonlinear
Spatial sensitivity	High frequencies	Low frequencies
Response to contrast	Weak	Strong, but saturates
Cortical projection (V1)	$4C\beta$	$4C\alpha$

PARVO AND MAGNO CELLS

Based on the results found in cats, scientists studied the primate visual system looking for comparable findings (DeMonasterio and Gouras, 1975; Dreher et al, 1976; Schiller and Malpeli, 1978; Shapley, 1990). Extracellular recordings were made in the retina and dLGN of rhesus monkeys, Old World monkeys that manifest essentially the same visual capabilities as humans and serve as a valuable animal model for human vision (DeValois et al, 1974). These experiments reveal that the primate retinocortical visual system is organized into two major pathways, the parvo and magno pathways (Fig 13–2).[2] The neurons that constitute these pathways manifest different sensitivities to chromatic, temporal, and spatial stimuli.[3] Features of these neurons are summarized in Table 13–1.[4] Note that the results discussed in this chapter were obtained under photopic conditions, where rods make little or no contribution.

Parvo neurons are characterized by color opponency, meaning that such a cell is excited by certain wavelengths and inhibited by others (Fig. 13–4). The sign of the response (excitatory or inhibitory) presumably serves as a basis for encoding the stimulus wavelength (DeValois et al, 1966; Wiesel and Hubel, 1966). Color-opponent neurons are thought to play a critical role in wavelength-based discrimination.

In comparison, magno neurons show weak color opponency (Lee et al, 2003). Regardless of the stimulus wavelength, these cells generally give a response of the same sign (Fig. 13–5). They are apparently not capable of contributing significantly to wavelength-based discriminations (see Chap. 5).

---

2. The konio cells are part of a less-studied third pathway. These neurons receive input from retinal small bistratified cells, which are fed by the S-cone bipolar cells. See Figs. 12–11 and 13–2.

3. Parallel processing apparently continues on into the cortex, but the division into distinct parvo and magno pathways may no longer hold. While the parvo pathway may be the predominant input to the ventral processing stream and the magno pathway to the dorsal stream, there appears to be significant cross talk between the streams (see Chap. 15).

4. Retinal midget (parvo) and parasol (magno) ganglion cells manifest properties similar to their counterparts in the dLGN.

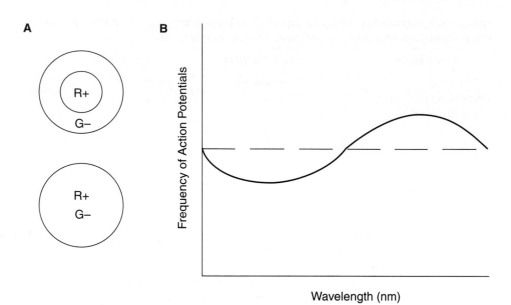

FIGURE 13–4. A. The receptive fields of parvo cells show color opponency. The color opponent regions can be spatially segregated (top) or spatially coincident (bottom). **B.** For this color-opponent neuron, short wavelengths cause inhibition, whereas longer wavelengths cause excitation.

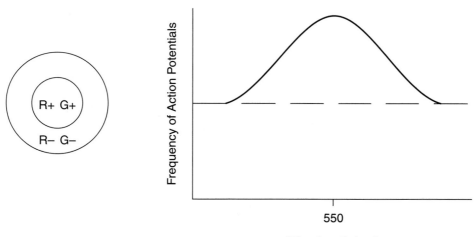

FIGURE 13–5. Magno neurons show approximately the same spectral sensitivity in their center and surround. This neuron manifests spatial antagonism, but not color opponency. Because all wavelengths cause this neuron to increase its rate of firing, it is essentially monochromatic.

A parvo neuron manifests a sustained response when presented with a long-duration stimulus—it responds to the stimulus for a relatively long period of time (Fig. 13–6). Magno neurons respond to the same stimulus in a transient manner, with only a brief burst of activity at stimulus onset and offset. The transient nature of magno neurons may be due to a substantial input from transient amacrine cells (Werblin and Dowling, 1969).

Transient responses to rapid changes in illumination give magno neurons the capability to resolve high temporal frequency stimuli (see Fig. 8–6). Because sustained neurons respond to a stimulus for a longer period of time, they are better suited to code low temporal frequencies. Consistent with this, temporal modulation transfer functions (TMTFs) show that magno cells respond best to high temporal frequencies and parvo neurons respond best to low temporal frequencies (Lee et al, 1990).

Parvo cells manifest smaller receptive fields than magno cells, making them more sensitive to higher spatial frequencies. Recall from Chapter 12 that the receptive field centers of centrally located midget (parvo) ganglion cells are constituted of a single cone, contributing to the highly developed visual acuity manifested by primates. Parvo cells make up the great majority of retinal ganglion cells, both foveal and nonfoveal (Lennie et al, 1990).

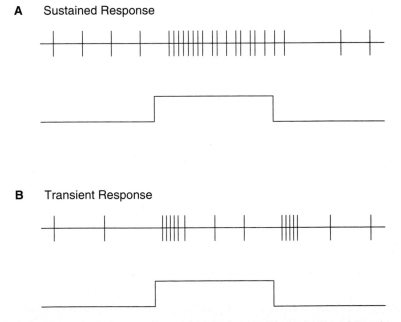

A   Sustained Response

B   Transient Response

FIGURE 13–6. **A.** This parvo neuron responds throughout the duration of the stimulus. Note that the frequency of action potentials is greatest soon after the stimulus comes on and then diminishes. **B.** In comparison, this magno neuron responds only to the onset and offset of the stimulus.

Cable properties dictate that the larger diameter axons of magno neurons transmit action potentials faster than the smaller diameter axons of parvo neurons. As a result, stimuli that isolate the magno pathway are expected to result in a shorter visual latency than those that isolate the parvo pathway.

As discussed in Chapter 15, the parvo pathway is the predominant input to the ventral cortical processing stream, and the magno pathway is the predominant input to the dorsal processing stream (Livingstone and Hubel, 1987, 1988). There seems to be significant communication between the two cortical processing streams.

FUNCTIONS OF THE PARVO AND MAGNO PATHWAYS

Given their anatomical segregation and dissimilar visual sensitivities, it is reasonable to suspect that the parvo and magno retinocortical pathways play different roles in perception. Evidence to support this notion comes from animal studies in which lesions are made in the pathways and human psychophysical investigations.

Behavioral Studies in Monkeys

When a lesion is made in the parvocellular region of the monkey dLGN, the animal's vision is altered in a dramatic, yet predictable, manner (Merigan, 1989; Schiller et al, 1990a,b). These animals manifest a substantially reduced ability to make wavelength-based discriminations and poor contrast sensitivity for high spatial frequencies. Other visual capabilities, such as the detection of high-frequency flicker, remain unaltered.

Lesions in the magno pathway have very different effects (Merigan and Maunsell, 1990; Schiller et al, 1990a,b). The animals retain normal wavelength-based discrimination and high-frequency contrast sensitivity. There is, however, a profound reduction in the ability to resolve high-frequency flicker, as well as a reduction in low-frequency contrast sensitivity.

These results are consistent with the notion that the parvo pathway is key to color discrimination and visual acuity, visual capabilities that are so well developed in primates. The magno system, in comparison, encodes movement and low spatial frequencies.

As discussed previously, the magno pathway appears to feed primarily into the dorsal cortical **"where"** system, and the parvo system to the ventral cortical **"what"** system (Livingstone and Hubel, 1987, 1988). Most visual events that deserve attention are associated with movement, and the magno system, being sensitive to high temporal frequencies, detects this movement and its location. Because the magno system is fast, this information rapidly reaches the cortex. The details of the alerting visual event are then analyzed by the "what" system, which processes information that the "where" system does not encode, such as color and spatial detail.

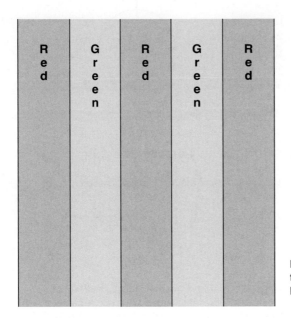

FIGURE 13–7. The red and green bars that constitute an isoluminant grating have equal luminance.

At the risk of oversimplifying this issue, consider a monkey that is stalked by a leopard. The "where" system alerts the monkey to the danger, and the "what" system allows the danger to be identified.

Psychophysical Studies in Humans

With the proper choice of stimuli, it may be possible to isolate the magno and parvo pathways in human observers. This strategy helps to elucidate the precise functions of the pathways and provides opportunities for clinical applications.

Isoluminant gratings, which are composed of bars all of the same luminance, but varying chromaticities, are often used to isolate the parvo system (Fig. 13–7). If there were no variation in chromaticity (chromatic contrast), the individual bars of the grating would not be discernible.

The spectral sensitivity of a magno neuron is similar to the photopic luminance function (see Chap. 5). Therefore, a green bar of the isoluminant grating in Fig. 13–7 activates a magno cell to the same extent as a red bar, making the border formed by the bars invisible to the cell. In essence, the magno pathway is "silenced" by isoluminant stimuli, leaving the isolated parvo system to detect these stimuli (Livingstone and Hubel, 1987, 1988).[5]

---

5. The bars of an isoluminant grating would not be discernible by a hypothetical observer who was missing his or her parvo pathway.

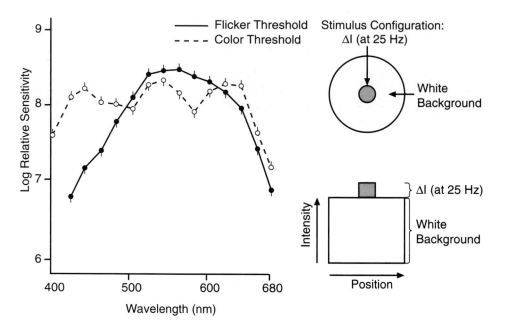

FIGURE 13–8. Increments, modulated at 25 Hz, are used to obtain color and flicker spectral sensitivity functions. The dashed curve represents thresholds for color detection, and the solid curve represents thresholds for flicker detection (Schwartz, 1993).

This strategy is controversial because, among other considerations, the spectral sensitivity of magno cells varies slightly from cell to cell. This makes it unlikely that isoluminant stimuli silence all magno neurons. Consequently, perceptions obtained using isoluminant stimuli may reflect predominantly the parvo system, but probably not the system in isolation (Cavanagh, 1991; Logothetis et al, 1990).

Increment threshold stimuli have also been used to isolate the parvo and magno pathways (Fig. 13–8). Spectral increments, which are temporally modulated at a high rate, are presented on a white background. For each wavelength, two thresholds are determined—a threshold for flicker detection (solid curve) and a threshold for color detection (dashed curve). At some wavelengths (e.g., 440 nm), sensitivity is greater for detection of color. Only after the stimulus intensity is increased beyond the color threshold is a flicker threshold reached. At other wavelengths (e.g., 580 nm), the opposite effect is noted: sensitivity is greater for flicker than for color.

Discrete thresholds for color and flicker suggest the existence of two independent physiological pathways (Schwartz, 1993). The color curve presumably represents thresholds for the color-coding sustained parvo pathway, and the flicker curve represents thresholds for the transient magno pathway.[6]

---

6. Although the flicker threshold curve in Fig. 13-8 is similar to the photopic luminosity curve, this does not necessarily mean that the magno pathway encodes luminance. Spectral sensitivity for the magno pathway could have a form similar to the photopic luminosity function regardless of the veracity of the double-duty hypothesis (see Chap. 5).

CLINICAL CONSIDERATIONS

Glaucoma

In this chapter, we learned that visual information is transmitted along two major retinocortical pathways that are constituted of neurons with different morphologies and physiological sensitivities. In the dLGN, the pathways are anatomically segregated.

It is possible that a given disease process may impact one of the pathways more than the other. For instance, a certain ocular disease may affect primarily the parvo pathway, whereas another disease may affect primarily the magno pathway. If this is the case, noninvasive psychophysical procedures that isolate the pathways could be useful for the early and differential diagnosis of these eye diseases.

Although work in this area is in its early stages, there are encouraging results. Consider primary open angle glaucoma (POAG), a condition in which an elevation in the intraocular pressure often, but not always, precedes optic nerve damage. The disease is progressive and can lead to blindness. The diagnosis is usually made on the basis of standard visual field loss and the appearance of the optic nerve head (Fig. 13-9). Unfortunately, the disease cannot be detected with these diagnostic procedures until a substantial proportion of the optic nerve fibers have been destroyed (Quigley et al, 1982). It would be preferable to make the diagnosis earlier in the disease process so that treatment could be initiated. Early treatment delays the progression of visual loss (Heijl et al, 2002).

Autopsies of patients with POAG reveal that the axons of large neurons are apparently damaged prior to the axons of smaller neurons, leading to the suggestion that the magno pathway is more vulnerable to glaucomatous damage

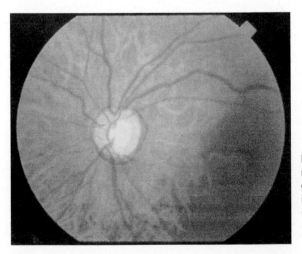

FIGURE 13-9. Glaucomatous optic nerve head. Note the vertical elongation of the optic cup, particularly inferiorly, indicating nerve fiber loss. (*This photograph was kindly provided by Dr. Mitchell Dul.*)

than the parvo pathway (Quigley et al, 1987). Based on this model, psychophysical studies have been performed on glaucoma patients and glaucoma suspects (persons with ocular hypertension) using stimuli that are intended to reveal magno function. This line of investigation has led to the development of clinical instrumentation that is based on the phenomenon of **spatial frequency doubling** (Maddess and Henry, 1992).

Consider a healthy patient viewing a flickering sine wave grating. As the temporal rate is increased, the patient will note that the apparent *spatial* frequency of the grating doubles, hence the term, spatial frequency doubling.[7] If the magno pathway mediates spatial frequency doubling, and it is susceptible to glaucomatous damage, one would predict that the perception of the phenomenon would be impaired in the early stages of POAG. This appears to be the case.

What is the physiological basis of spatial frequency doubling? Some investigators suggest that it results from nonlinearities found in certain magno cells (Maddess and Henry, 1992). Utilizing stimuli that elicit spatial frequency doubling in human observers, however, White et al (2002) found no characteristic of the magno cell neural response (in monkey retina) that could account for spatial frequency doubling. Although clinical spatial frequency doubling procedures have proven effective in the early diagnosis of glaucoma, the physiological underpinnings of this finding are not understood.[8]

Tremendous progress has been made over the past three decades in understanding basic visual processes, but routine clinical application of this knowledge has occurred at a comparatively slow pace. Many of the psychophysical procedures routinely utilized in clinical eye care are over a century old. Frequency doubling highlights the potential benefits of applying new basic science knowledge to clinical problems, while also cautioning us to carefully examine our assumptions regarding the linkage between physiological pathways and perceptual phenomenon.

Reading Disability

Developmental dyslexia is a selective impairment of reading skills in spite of normal intelligence, vision, hearing, instruction, and motivation. The origins of this condition remain controversial. Some believe that it is due to sensory defects, whereas others consider it to be primarily a cognitive disorder.

There are data suggesting that developmental dyslexics manifest deficits in the processing of temporal information (Lovegrove et al, 1990). In particular, individuals with this condition display abnormalities in flicker fusion rates and the ability to

---

7. Although the term "frequency doubling" is in common use in the scientific and clinical literature, we will use the term "spatial frequency doubling" because it more accurately describes the phenomenon.

8. See Chap. 8 for an alternative hypothesis for clinically determined spatial frequency doubling.

temporally resolve two consecutive stimuli (Slaghuis and Lovegrove, 1985; Brannan and Williams, 1988). These and other findings have led some investigators to propose that developmental dyslexia is associated with a defect in the pathway most responsible for processing high-frequency temporal information, the magnocellular pathway (Livingstone et al, 1991). Other researchers, however, contend that this view is overly simplistic (Hill and Raymond, 2002; Ramus, 2001).

SUMMARY

A fundamental characteristic of the human visual system is its organization into parallel retinocortical pathways that play different roles in visual perception. The magno pathway is best suited to encode motion and low spatial frequencies, and the parvo pathway enables highly developed color discrimination and visual acuity. Less is known about the role of the konio pathway. It appears to play a role in processing chromatic information transmitted by S-cones.

Certain disease processes are believed to preferentially affect one of the pathways. By designing psychophysical tests that isolate them, it may be possible to diagnose disease at an earlier stage. Such methodologies hold substantial promise.

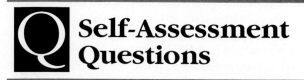

Self-Assessment Questions

1. Provide an example of a commonly encountered animal that appears to have an exceptionally well-developed magno system and a less-developed parvo system. Justify your answer.

2. A disease is thought to have a predilection for the parvo system. What would you expect the increment threshold functions in Figure 13-8 to look like in a patient with this disease?

3. If glaucoma does indeed affect primarily the magno pathway, what effect would you expect early stages of this disease to have on visual acuity. Explain.

4. Isoluminant gratings are thought by some investigators to "silence" the magno pathway. Because all the bars are of equal luminance, the grating is thought not to activate magno neurons. Present an argument against this hypothesis.

Striate Cortex

14

It is within the cerebral cortex that visual information is organized and integrated with memory and other senses to produce visual perception as we experience it. Although recent decades have seen significant progress in ascertaining the neural processes that underlie perception, a more complete unraveling of these processes remains one of the greatest challenges facing scientists in the 21st century.

The first stage of cortical processing occurs within striate cortex, the primary target for projections from the dLGN. Fundamental aspects of visual analysis occur within this structure. Visual information is then disseminated widely throughout the cortex along two major processing streams, the ventral and dorsal streams.

BASIC ORGANIZATION OF THE CORTEX

As illustrated in Fig. 14–1, cortex tissue consists of superficial gray matter (cell bodies) and underlying white matter (myelinated axons). Although the gray matter is rather thin (about 4 mm thick), the cortical surface area is substantial, on the order of 2200 cm^2 in humans, contributing to its spectacular operational capacities.[1] The human cortex, which weighs about 3 pounds, contains about 10^{10} cells, 10^{15} synapses, and 2000 miles of axonal connections (Tovée, 1996; Young and Scannel, 1993).

The cortex is constituted of four lobes: frontal, parietal, temporal, and occipital (Fig. 14–2). These are separated from one another by particularly deep sulci. Striate cortex is located within the occipital lobe.

---

1. This tissue can fit within the skull because it is folded into numerous ridges (gyri) and furrows (sulci).

Surface

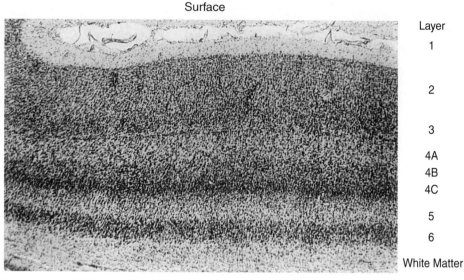

Layer

1

2

3

4A
4B
4C

5

6

White Matter

⊢————⊣ 1 mm

FIGURE 14–1. Cross section of monkey striate cortex showing its layered nature. The surface of the cortex is at the top of the picture. Axons from the dorsal lateral geniculate nucleus tend to synapse in the middle layers. (*Reprinted with permission from Hubel DH, Wiesel TN. Functional architecture of the macaque monkey visual cortex. Proc R Soc Lond [Biol]. 1977;198:1–59.*)

Upon gross inspection, the tissue of the cortex appears mostly to be uniform. However, neurophysiological and brain imaging studies and anatomical tracings reveal that each of the lobes is organized into many different functional areas, or modules. Certain of these areas (approximately 20) are predominantly devoted to analyzing visual information (DeYoe and Van Essen, 1988; Van Essen et al, 1992).

Striate cortex is so named because of the dense plexus of geniculate axons that forms a distinctive stria, referred to as the **line of Gennari,** in layer 4B. It also referred to as primary visual cortex, visual area 1, V1, and Brodmann area 17. As is the case for all of cortex, striate cortex is a layered tissue (see Fig. 14–1).

Although striate cortex contains a representation of the entire visual field, it is dominated by the fovea. This so-called **cortical magnification of foveal vision** is apparently due primarily to the large area of cortex devoted to the fovea, rather than the high density of ganglion cells found in the fovea (Popovic and Sjostrand, 2001). Striate cortex projects to **extrastriate cortex,** the region of visual cortex that is not distinguished by the line of Gennari. Among extrastriate areas that we refer to are visual area 2 (V2 or Brodmann area 18), visual area 4 (V4), inferotemporal cortex (IT), and visual area 5 (V5), also referred to as middle temporal cortex or (MT).[2]

---

2. Certain of these labels are best applied to the human cortex, while others are best applied to the monkey cortex. We do not distinguish between the two species in this text.

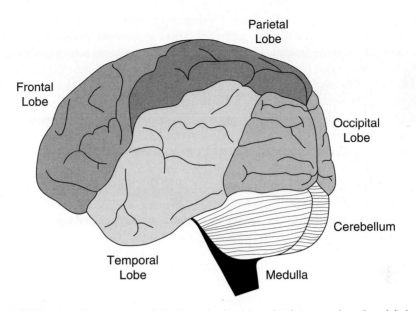

FIGURE 14–2. The cortex is divided into the frontal, parietal, temporal, and occipital lobes. Striate cortex is located in the occipital lobe.

Figure 14–3 shows the basic flow of information within the cortex. In general, visual information appears to travel along two processing streams, or pathways (Mishkin et al, 1983). The **ventral processing stream** (also referred to as the

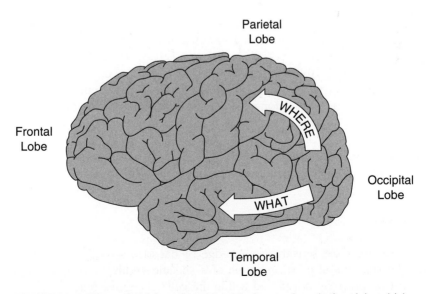

FIGURE 14–3. The ventral (also referred to as the temporal or what) and dorsal (also referred to as the parietal or where) processing streams emanate from striate cortex (Mishkin, Ungerleider, and Macko, 1983).

temporal pathway, or "what" system) is thought to receive its predominant input from the parvo retinogeniculate pathway, and the **dorsal processing stream** (also referred to as the **parietal** pathway, or "where" system) is thought to receive its predominant input from the magno pathway. There is significant communication between the two processing streams; they are not independent.

Striate cortex projects not only to extrastriate cortex, but also sends a major reciprocal projection to the dLGN, as well as a projection to the pulvinar, a thalamic nucleus thought to be associated with visual attention, motion processing, and visually guided movement (Merabet et al, 1998). As a general rule, projections to lower visual centers (e.g., dLGN, pulvinar) originate from the deeper layers of striate cortex (in particular, layer 6), whereas those to extrastriate cortex originate from more superficial layers (particularly, layers 2/3) (Lund et al, 1979; Miller, 2003). It is important to note that information also flows back toward striate cortex from extrastriate cortex via reciprocal pathways (i.e., feedback loops). These feedback loops, which in some ways are analogous to the retinal centrifugal pathway and the reciprocal projection from striate cortex to the dLGN, may be involved in the gating of information.

This chapter concentrates on striate cortex. The subsequent chapter emphasizes visual processing distal to striate cortex, in regions of extrastriate cortex frequently referred to as higher visual areas.

SIMPLE AND COMPLEX CELLS

Forearmed with the knowledge that retinal ganglion cell receptive fields are concentrically organized, scientists initially looked for similar cells in the cortex. Yet, when striate cortex was studied using stimuli appropriate for concentric receptive fields (small spots of light), visually responsive cells were not found.

Then in the late 1950s, David Hubel and Tortsen Wiesel, who later won the Nobel prize for their work on vision, unexpectedly found neurons in cat striate cortex that were sensitive to elongated stimuli, such as bars and edges (Hubel and Wiesel, 1959, 1962). Making certain assumptions regarding cortical organization that are discussed later in this chapter, Hubel and Wiesel divided these cells into two general categories: simple and complex cells. They later found comparable cells in monkey cortex (Hubel and Wiesel, 1968).

Simple Cells

Simple cells are most sensitive to an edge or bar of a specific orientation (Fig. 14–4). The stimulus, if a bar, must be of a specific width. Moreover, the bar or edge must be properly positioned within the cell's receptive field.

Simple cell receptive fields can be mapped out with small spots of light. When this is done, it is apparent that the receptive fields are divided into antagonistic excitatory and inhibitory regions (Fig. 14–5).

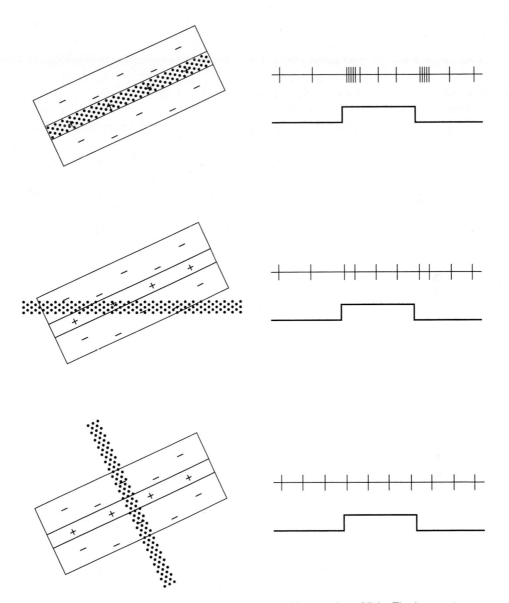

FIGURE 14–4. This simple cell is maximally sensitive to a bar of light. The bar must be at a specific orientation to activate the neuron maximally (top diagram). When the stimulus is presented at other orientations, as indicated in the bottom two diagrams, the response is diminished.

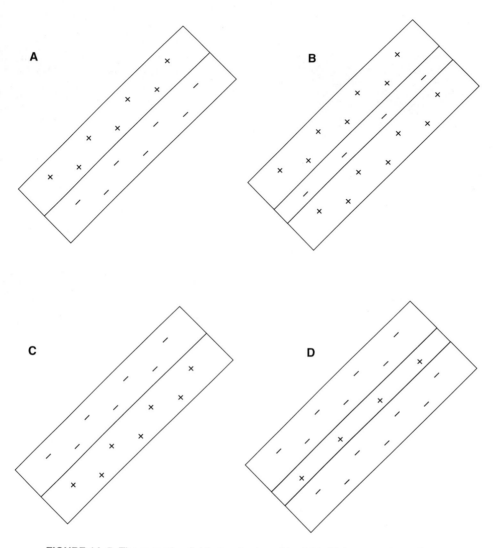

FIGURE 14–5. The receptive field of a simple cell is divided into separate excitatory and inhibitory regions. Some cells are maximally sensitive to dark or light bars **(B** and **D)**; others respond best to edges **(A** and **C)**.

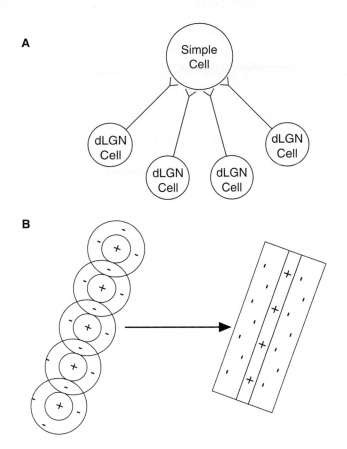

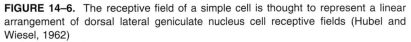

FIGURE 14–6. The receptive field of a simple cell is thought to represent a linear arrangement of dorsal lateral geniculate nucleus cell receptive fields (Hubel and Wiesel, 1962)

It has been suggested that the receptive fields of simple cells result from input of dLGN neurons whose receptive fields lie along a straight line (Fig. 14–6). The formation of increasingly complicated receptive field arrangements (e.g., simple cells) from less complicated arrangements (e.g., concentric dLGN cells) is referred to as **serial**, or **hierarchical**, **processing** (Hubel and Wiesel, 1962, 1965a). This process occurs in the retina where, for example, the comparatively simple receptive fields of distal retinal elements (i.e., photoreceptors and horizontal cells) give rise to the spatially antagonistic receptive fields of bipolar cells.

Complex Cells

Like simple cells, complex cells respond best to an elongated stimulus of a specific orientation (Fig. 14–7). However, the receptive field properties of simple and complex cells differ in several important respects. Whereas stimulus position

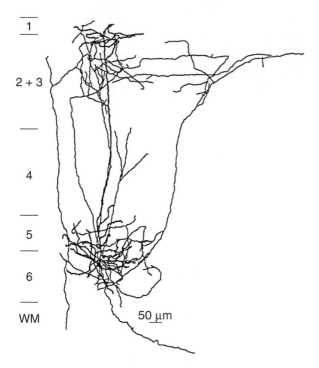

1

2 + 3

4

5

6

WM

50 μm

FIGURE 14–7. Trace of a complex cell in cat striate cortex. Note the projections to the superficial cortical layers. (*Photomicrograph kindly provided by Dr. Judith Hirsch. Reprinted with permission from Hirsch JA, Gallagher CA, Alonso J-M, Martinez LM. Ascending projections of simple and complex cells in layer 6 of the cat striate cortex.* J Neurosci. *1998;18:8086-8094. Copyright 1998 by the Society for Neuroscience*).

within the receptive field of a simple cell is critical, the stimulus can be positioned anywhere within a complex cell's receptive field. Many complex cells are characterized by direction selectivity—for the cell to be stimulated, the stimulus must move in a specific direction. A stimulus moving in the opposite direction, even if of the proper orientation, does not elicit a response (Fig. 14–8). Unlike simple cells, the receptive fields of complex cells cannot be divided into separate excitatory and inhibitory regions.

It has been suggested that the receptive fields of complex cells are the result of hierarchical processing (Hubel and Wiesel, 1962, 1965a). Just as the signals of dLGN cells are combined to produce a simple cell's receptive field, the signals of simple cells are thought to be combined to produce a complex cell's receptive field. The manner in which these signals are combined is not fully understood. If there were linear addition of simple cells, complex cells would manifest separate excitatory and inhibitory areas. This is not the case. Perhaps the summation is nonlinear. Or perhaps nonlinear dLGN cells (magno cells) play a larger role in the formation of the receptive fields of complex cells than they do for simple cells (Hoffman and Stone, 1971; Stone et al, 1979).

Hubel and Wiesel (1965a) found that certain cortical neurons are sensitive to the length of the stimulus (Fig. 14–9). These **end-stopped neurons** were originally classified as **hypercomplex cells.** Subsequent examination of visual cortex revealed that sensitivity to stimulus length is a feature common to many cortical

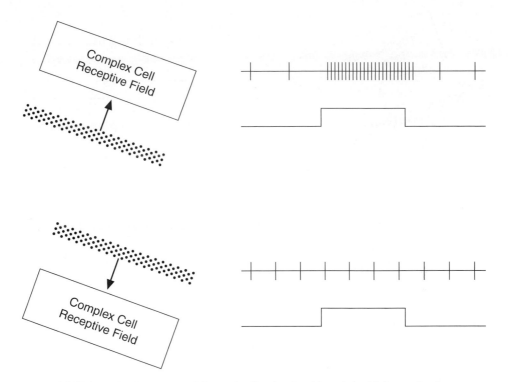

FIGURE 14–8. A complex cell is maximally stimulated by a bar of light moving in a specific direction (top). When moving in the opposite direction, the stimulus is not effective at driving the complex cell (bottom).

cells (Schiller et al, 1976; Gilbert, 1977). Consequently, hypercomplex cells are generally not considered to be a separate category of cortical neurons.

Hubel and Wiesel's model of hierarchical processing holds that the receptive fields of higher neurons are constructed from those of preceding neurons. This would explain why the stimulus paramaters required to activate a neuron become more specific at progressively higher stages in the visual system. A cone responds to diffuse light, a ganglion cell to a spot of light of a specific diameter, a simple cell to a bar of light of a specific orientation, and a complex cell to this same bar of light moving in the proper direction. The higher up in the visual system, the more stringent are the requirements to drive a visual neuron.

In the previous chapter, we developed the concept of parallel processing. The concepts of parallel processing and hierarchical processing are compatible. Hierarchical processing occurs along each of the parallel pathways. For example, the first elements in the parvo pathway are cones, which are followed by color opponent horizontal cells, followed by spatially and chromatically antagonistic bipolar cells, and so forth. Likewise, hierarchical processing also occurs along the magno pathway.

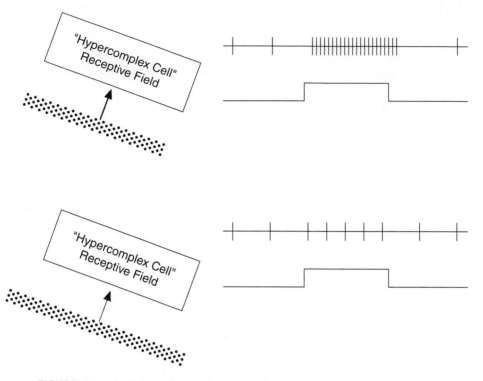

FIGURE 14–9. End-stopped cortical neurons show a maximal response to a bar of light of a specific length (top). A stimulus longer than this optimal length elicits less of a response (bottom).

EDGES OR GRATINGS

Cortical neurons respond well to sine wave gratings, and are selective for a particular spatial frequency (DeValois et al, 1982). One cell may be finely tuned to stimuli of 3 cycles/degree, whereas another cell is tuned to 6 cycles/degree. Although this is consistent with the hypothesis that the visual system operates as a Fourier analyzer, it does not prove that it is its primary operating principle (see Chap. 7).

STRIATE CORTICAL ARCHITECTURE

Many cortical neurons are binocular, receiving input from both eyes. This can be demonstrated by recording from a cortical cell while stimulating one eye, and subsequently recording from the same cell while stimulating the other eye. The proper stimulus, presented to either eye, will activate a binocular neuron.

Binocular cortical cells may mediate stereopsis (see Chap. 10). At a given distance from the eye (for example, at the fixation distance in Fig. 14-10) the receptive field that is determined by stimulating the right eye may be in a slightly different position than for the left eye. The cortical receptive fields do, however, over-

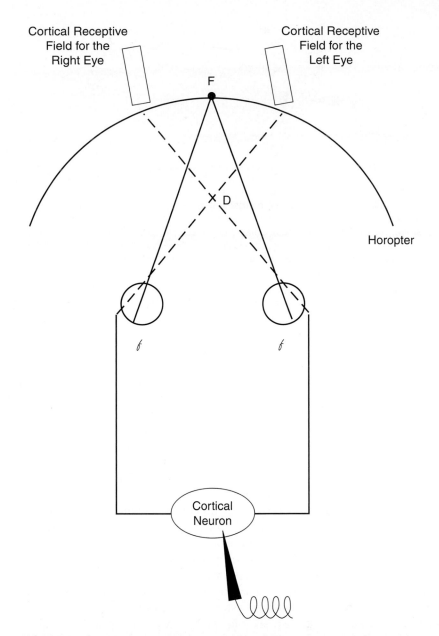

FIGURE 14–10. When measured at the fixation distance, the monocular receptive fields of this cortical cell do not overlap. They do overlap, however, at point *D*. Stimuli presented binocularly at this distance maximally excite the cortical cell. This is presumably the physiological mechanism whereby stimulus distance is encoded by cortical cells and is the basis for stereopsis. The solid curve represents the Veith–Müller horopter. See Steinman, Steinman, and Garzia (2000) for a discussion of horopters and other aspects of binocular vision.

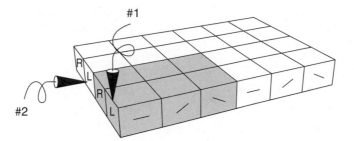

FIGURE 14–11. Striate cortex is organized into ocular dominance slabs (R and L) and orientation slabs. All cells encountered in an electrode penetration of an ocular dominance slab—perpendicular to the cortical surface—are of the same ocular dominance (electrode 1). Likewise, all cells in an orientation slab manifest the same orientation sensitivity. An electrode penetration *parallel* to the cortical surface reveals a systematic organization of the orientation slabs (electrode 2). The shaded region shows a hypercolumn, which consists of a complete set of orientation columns for both eyes.

lap at a critical distance from the eyes (at point D in Fig. 14–10). Because the inputs from the two eyes are summed, a stimulus located at this critical distance maximally activates the cortical neuron. The stimulus distance can thereby be encoded, presumably providing the physiological basis for stereopsis (Barlow et al, 1967).

Although the majority of striate cortical neurons are binocular, most are dominated by one eye. Stimulation of the neuron through the so-called **dominant eye** causes a stronger response than stimulation through the fellow eye.[3] Ocular dominance is laid out in a regular pattern of alternating right and left ocular dominance slabs, sometimes called ocular dominance columns ("R" and "L" in Fig. 14–11 and 14–14; also see Fig. 14–12) (Hubel and Wiesel, 1965b, 1968). Because the slabs run through the substance of the cortex, perpendicular to its surface, an electrode that penetrates the cortex perpendicular to its surface (e.g., electrode 1 in Figure 14–11) encounters neurons that are all dominated by the same eye.

Striate cortex is organized into orientation slabs as well as ocular dominance slabs. An electrode that penetrates the cortex perpendicular to its surface encounters neurons all tuned to the same orientation (Hubel and Wiesel, 1962, 1974). If withdrawn and subsequently reinserted perpendicular to the surface at another location, the electrode encounters neurons that may be tuned to a different orientation. When a penetration is made parallel to the cortical surface, however, the orientation sensitivity may change systematically from one neuron to the next (electrode 2 in Fig. 14–11; also see Fig. 14–13). A complete set of ocular dominance columns (both eyes) and orientation columns (all orientations) forms a **hypercolumn** (Figs. 14–11 and 14–14) (Hubel and Wiesel, 1977; Hubel et al, 1978). Each hypercolumn has dimensions of approximately 1 x 1 mm.

The development of normal cortical architecture requires normal visual input early in life (Hubel and Wiesel, 1965b). As discussed in Chapter 17, cortical archi-

---

3. The term "dominant eye" can be confusing because it is also used clinically to refer to the eye with which the patient prefers to view.

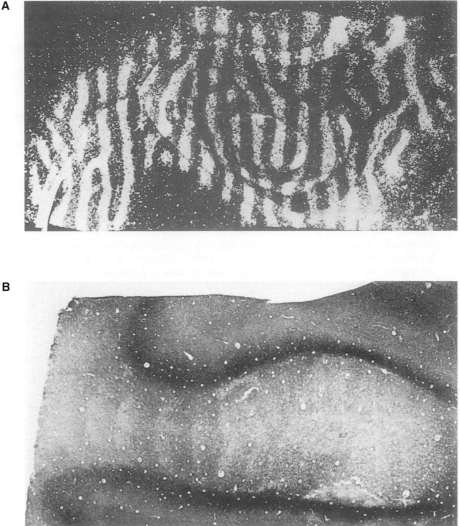

FIGURE 14–12. A. Ocular dominance columns in striate cortex of a monkey. (*Reprinted with permission from Hubel DH, Wiesel TN. Functional architecture of macaque monkey visual cortex. Proc R Soc Lond [Biol]. 1977;198:1–59.*) **B.** Ocular dominance columns in the human striate cortex. (*Reprinted with permission from Hitchcock PF, Hickey TL. Ocular dominance columns: Evidence for their presence in humans. Brain Res. 1980;182:176–179. Photograph kindly provided by Dr. Peter F. Hitchcock.*)

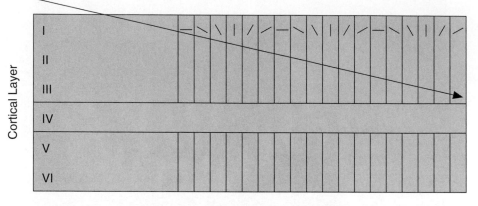

FIGURE 14–13. As an electrode (indicated by the arrow) transverses the orientation columns in striate cortex, the orientation selectivity of the encountered neurons systematically changes. In this case, there is a systematic shift in the clockwise direction. Orientation columns do not extend through layer IV; cells in this layer tend to have a center-surround organization (Hubel and Wiesel, 1977).

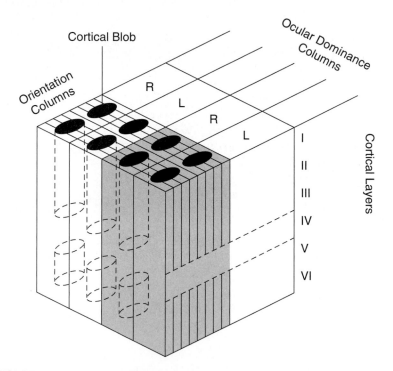

FIGURE 14–14. This simplified diagram shows the relationship of the cytochrome oxidase blobs to the functional architecture of striate cortex. Note that the orientation columns do not extend through layer IV. The lightly shaded area is a cortical hyper-column (Hubel, Weisel, and Stryker, 1978).

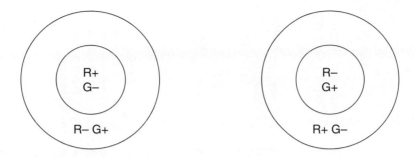

FIGURE 14–15. Examples of double color opponent neurons found in striate cortex blobs.

tecture can be altered by environmental manipulations early in life, such as the occlusion of one eye.

The segregation of the visual system into parallel pathways continues, to some extent, into striate cortex and beyond (Livingstone and Hubel, 1987, 1988). Staining striate cortex for cytochrome oxidase reveals an irregular pattern of **blobs** within its superficial layers (see Fig. 14–14) and a regular pattern of stripes in adjoining visual area 2 (Wong-Riley, 1979).[4] Striate blobs are rich with concentrically organized, double-color opponent neurons that presumably result from parvo input (Fig. 14–15) (Ts'o and Gilbert, 1988). The superficial region of striate cortex between blobs, the **interblob** region, also appears to receive substantial parvo input. The magno pathway apparently bypasses blobs and the interblob regions. As illustrated schematically in Fig. 14-16, the parvo and magno pathways give rise to the ventral and dorsal processing streams, which are discussed in the following chapter. As mentioned previously, there may be significant communication between these processing streams.

CLINICAL CONSIDERATIONS

A patient with **blindsight** presents as blind secondary to a lesion that has destroyed all of striate cortex. Under certain circumstances, however, the patient will respond to a visual stimulus although he or she claims that no stimulus is seen. Blindsight can be demonstrated with a forced-choice methodology (see Chap. 11). A stimulus is flashed on one of two spatially adjacent panels, and the

---

4. Cytochrome oxidase staining reveals that visual area 2 contains so-called thin, pale, and thick stripes. These stripes may be specialized to code color, orientation, and retinal disparity, respectively (Ts'o et al, 2001).

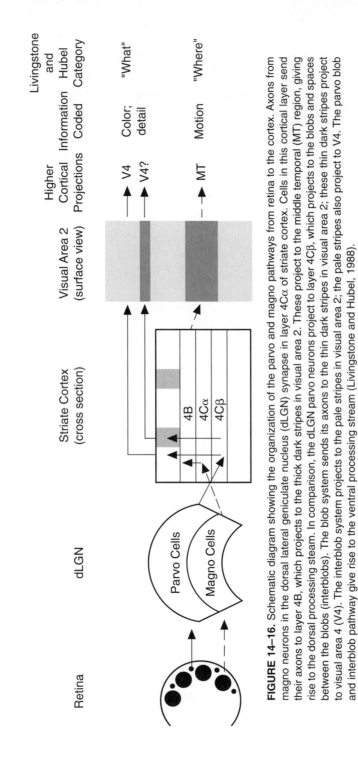

FIGURE 14–16. Schematic diagram showing the organization of the parvo and magno pathways from retina to the cortex. Axons from magno neurons in the dorsal lateral geniculate nucleus (dLGN) synapse in layer 4Cα of striate cortex. Cells in this cortical layer send their axons to layer 4B, which projects to the thick dark stripes in visual area 2. These project to the middle temporal (MT) region, giving rise to the dorsal processing steam. In comparison, the dLGN parvo neurons project to layer 4Cβ, which projects to the blobs and spaces between the blobs (interblobs). The blob system sends its axons to the thin dark stripes in visual area 2; these thin dark stripes project to visual area 4 (V4). The interblob system projects to the pale stripes in visual area 2; the pale stripes also project to V4. The parvo blob and interblob pathway give rise to the ventral processing stream (Livingstone and Hubel, 1988).

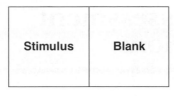

FIGURE 14–17. In a two-alternative forced choice task, the performance of a patient with blindsight is above chance. Although the patient is by all standard measurements blind, he or she can use visual information to locate a target.

patient is forced to choose which panel contains the stimulus (Fig. 14–17). The patient may object to performing this task, claiming that he or she is blind and not able see where the stimulus. Nonetheless, he or she is encouraged to choose the panel that contains the stimulus.

The result is surprising; performance at locating the stimulus is above chance (Weiskrantz, 1986). Visual information is presumably processed along pathways that bypass striate cortex, but activate extrastriate cortex (Goebel et al, 2001). The activation of extrastriate cortex, in the absence of striate cortex, is not sufficient to result in conscious vision. It is, however, sufficient to permit nonconscious vision—blindsight.

SUMMARY

The receptive fields of striate cortical neurons are more complicated than those of neurons situated earlier in the visual system, largely due to hierarchical processing. Parallel processing occurs in concert with hierarchical processing.

Striate cortex is organized into ocular dominance and orientation slabs. The parvo and magno pathways feed into different areas of striate cortex, which projects to higher visual areas (extrastriate cortex) that are specialized to analyze specific visual attributes. The manner in which these cortical areas process visual information is discussed in the following chapter.

Self-Assessment Questions

1. Ocular dominance columns are not present at birth, but develop early in life secondary to normal visual experience. Devise an experiment that would allow you to determine the time course of development of ocular dominance columns in an animal model such as the cat.

2. Describe the stimulus that would maximally excite each of the double color opponent cells in Fig. 14–15.

3. Beginning with photoreceptors, draw the receptive fields of all visual neurons up through complex cells.

Information Streams and Extrastriate Processing

Although basic analysis of visual information occurs in striate cortex, considerably more processing is required to produce the rich visual world that we perceive. This analysis occurs in visual areas outside of striate cortex, collectively referred to as extrastriate cortex.

INFORMATION DIVERGES BEYOND STRIATE CORTEX

Beyond striate cortex there is a substantial divergence of information through projections to neighboring cortical visual areas, which in turn send projections to numerous other higher visual areas, and so forth (Figs. 2–11 and 14–3) (Van Essen et al, 1992). In addition to this feed-forward distribution of information, there is feedback (through reciprocal connections) from the higher cortical areas to lower areas.

The cortex contains at least 20 distinct visual areas, each containing a map of the visual field called a **retinotopic map**. It appears that these various areas, which can be conceptualized as specialized modules, play different roles in processing visual information.

Visual information appears to flow along distinct, but not independent, processing streams (Mishkin et al, 1983; Maunsell and Newsome, 1987; Merigan and

Maunsell, 1993). One of these streams (variously referred to as the **temporal, ventral,** or **"what"** stream) is apparently critical for identifying and recognizing objects, whereas the other major stream (the **parietal, dorsal,** or **"where"** stream) plays a central role in motion perception and localization in visual space (see Fig. 14–3). Although the ventral and dorsal processing streams are adapted to analyze different aspects of visual information, there is communication between the two pathways. The ventral and dorsal processing streams are commonly considered to be extensions of the parvo and magno pathways, respectively (Chap. 13).

CORTICAL MODULARITY

Numerous lines of evidence support the notion that certain higher visual areas are specialized modules that analyze specific attributes of the visual world (Fig. 15–1). Extracellular recordings in the macaque **visual area 4 (V4)** reveal an abundance of cells with chromatic sensitivities, making this area well adapted to play an important role in color perception (Zeki, 1983). Cells in the **inferotemporal cortex (IT)** respond to complex forms, including faces, indicating a role in form perception (Gross, 1973; Tovée and Cohen-Tovée, 1993; Rolls and Tovée, 1995). Both V4 and inferotemporal cortex are considered part of the ventral processing stream. Cells in **V5** (also called **middle temporal cortex, or MT),** a component of the dorsal processing stream, are well suited for the encoding of motion (Rodman and Albright, 1989).

Additional compelling evidence for cortical modularity comes from imaging studies in which brain activity is monitored while a subject (human or monkey) performs a task (such as looking at a moving object) (Posner, 1993; Ungerleider,

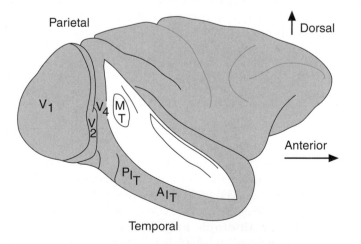

FIGURE 15–1. In this lateral view of the right hemisphere of the macaque cortex, the superior temporal sulcus (unshaded region) has been opened to reveal visual areas that are normally hidden from view, such as MT. Other labeled areas discussed in the book are V1 (striate cortex), V2, V4, and inferotemporal cortex (AIT and PIT)(Maunsell, 1995).

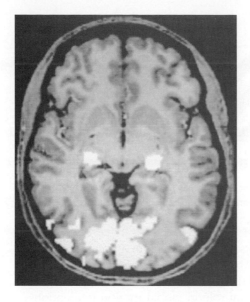

FIGURE 15-2. Axial section of the human brain showing activity, as indicated by fMRI, in the left and right dLGN and visual cortex. The stimulus was a checkerboard. Activation is indicated by white. (*This figure was kindly provided by Dr. Sabine Kastner.*)

1995). In **positron emission tomography (PET),** a radioactive tracer is used to observe changes in blood flow that are indicative of increased cortical metabolism. **Functional magnetic resonance imaging (fMRI)**, which has better resolution, apparently reveals cortical activity by detecting levels of oxygenation (Fig. 15–2).

Imaging studies reveal that the region of the brain that is most active depends on the task (Corbetta et al, 1990). If a human subject views an array of variously colored, moving objects (for example, red and green objects) and is asked to attend to the green object, areas in the ventral stream shows the most activity. In comparison, when the subject views the same array, but is asked to pay attention to the movement of the objects, the dorsal stream manifests the most activity. If shape (or form) of the object becomes the focus, activity is greatest in the ventral processing stream.

VISUAL AREA 5

Cells in V5 have properties that enable them to perform a comparatively sophisticated analysis of motion information, perhaps due to substantial input from the magno pathway (Albright, 1984; Maunsell et al, 1990). Consider the dilemma posed by the stimulus illustrated in Fig. 15–3C (Adelson and Movshon, 1982; Stoner and Albright, 1996). This stimulus, which is perceived as a plaid moving in the direction indicated, is composed of two drifting gratings as illustrated in A and B of the figure. Whereas each of the two component drifting gratings would appear to move in the directions indicated, the plaid (a **global stimulus** composed of two components) appears as a single object moving in an intermediate direction.

Extracellular recordings in rhesus monkeys reveal that direction selective neurons in striate cortex tend to respond strongly to the movement of the individual grating components of the plaid, but weakly well to the movement of the plaid

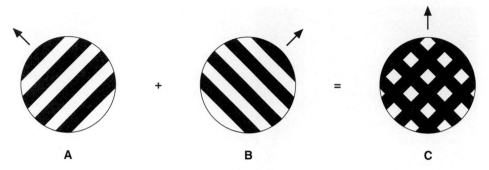

FIGURE 15–3. The gratings in **A** and **B** are combined to produce the plaid in **C.** The plaid is perceived as a unified figure moving in the indicated direction (Stoner and Albright, 1996).

itself (Movshon et al, 1985). In comparison, certain cells in V5 respond best to the movement of the plaid as a whole. These neurons encode what we perceive (i.e., the integrated movement of the plaid rather than the individual grating components) and apparently play an important role in global motion perception.

Global motion perception in monkey V5 has also been studied with random dot kinematograms (see Fig. 9–3). Extracellular recordings show that certain of the neurons that constitute this region manifest coherence thresholds that are very similar to those measured psychophysically in the same animal (Newsome and Paré, 1988).

Additional support for V5 involvement in motion perception comes from human PET and fMRI studies. V5 is more active when a human subject views a moving object than when he or she views a stationary object (Watson et al, 1993).

Transcranial magnetic stimulation (TMS) provides evidence that fast backprojections from V5 to striate cortex are necessary for visual awareness of movement (Pascual-Leone and Walsh, 2001). In this noninvasive experimental technique, neural activity can be induced in targeted cortical areas of alert human subjects by applying magnetic stimulation to the cranium. Induced neural activity in V5 results in the perception of moving phosphenes.[1]

Application of TMS to striate cortex prior to stimulation of V5 does not affect the perception of moving phosphenes. However, when TMS is applied to V5 about 5 to 45 msec prior to its application to striate cortex, the perception of movement is disrupted, suggesting that stimulation of striate cortex interferes with a signal presumably transmitted along a fast backprojection from V5.

Motion Aftereffects

Is V5 active while a subject experiences a **motion aftereffect (MAE)**, a motion illusion that occurs in the absence of motion? A commonly experienced MAE is

---

1. Phosphenes are images induced by mechanical or electrical stimulation of the visual system. If you close an eye and apply gentle pressure to the temporal part of the globe, you will see a phosphene located nasally.

the waterfall illusion, which is induced by staring at downward rushing water for several minutes. When gaze is changed from the waterfall to the surrounding landscape, the landscape appears to rise.

MAEs are presumably due to the adaptation of direction-specific motion detectors. The adapting stimulus reduces sensitivity to its direction of movement, and subsequently viewed stationary stimuli appear to move in the opposite direction. It has long been suspected that the motion detectors are located in the cortex, the first site of substantial interaction between the two eyes, because adaptation of one eye elicits a MAE in the other eye (Mitchell et al, 1975).

Suppose that a human subject views concentric rings moving in an outward direction (Fig. 15–4). These moving rings activate V5. The rings suddenly become stationary and the individual experiences a MAE (i.e., the illusion of the stationary rings moving inward). Although there is no moving stimulus, fMRI

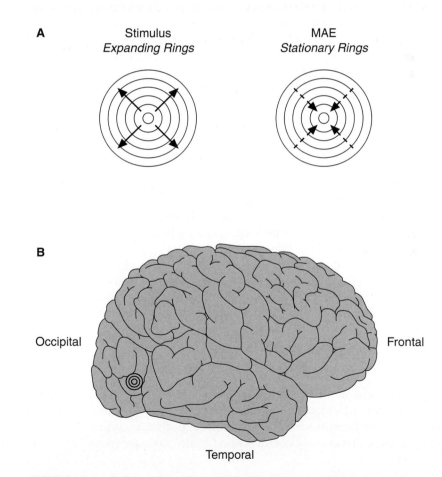

FIGURE 15–4. **A.** Prior adaptation to outwardly moving concentric rings leads to a MAE, in which stationary rings appear to move inward. **B** While a human subject is experiencing the MAE, fMRI reveals activity in the visual area MT. In this schematic, the activity is indicated by the concentric circles (Tootell et al, 1995).

shows that V5 is active, providing additional evidence for its role in motion perception (Tootell et al, 1995).

VISUAL AREA 4 AND INFEROTEMPORAL CORTEX

Visual area 4 (V4) and inferotemporal cortex (IT) belong to the ventral processing stream, and contain cells that are responsive to color and sophisticated forms, respectively. Although a simplification, V4 is sometimes said to analyze color information (Zeki, 1983), while IT is thought to analyze form information (Fuster and Jervey, 1981; Tanaka et al, 1991).

The receptive fields of cells in IT are large, thereby providing the basis to integrate information over an extensive area and analyze complex patterns (Gross, 1973; Rolls and Tovée, 1995). Certain of the shapes to which cells in IT respond are given in Fig. 15–5. Whereas cells in striate cortex respond best to bars, edges, and gratings, cells in IT respond best to comparatively sophisticated, albeit basic, shapes (e.g., circles, squares, and ovals) that could serve as building blocks to construct even more complex forms (Gallant et al, 1993).

The area of monkey cortex that is called IT is probably equivalent to the lateral occipital complex (LOC) in humans[2]. Based on fMRI studies in human subjects, it appears that the LOC responds well to objects, but not to scrambled objects or object fragments (Grill-Spector et al, 2001). It seems to respond to all objects, not showing selectivity for a particular type.

Compare this to the more specialized properties of two nearby areas, the fusiform face area (FFA) and the parahippocampal place area (PPA) (Tong et al, 1998). The FFA responds well to faces, but not other objects, and may be involved in face detection and/or recognition. In comparison, the PPA is strongly activated by objects (e.g., a house) and places—but not by faces—indicating a possible role in perceiving scenes.

The cortical areas that process faces and color are in close proximity to each other. Consequently, patients who suffer from **prosopagnosia** (the inability to recognize faces) frequently manifest achromatopsia, the inability to distinguish hues (Tovée, 1996).

VISUAL AGNOSIAS

The specialization of the cortex into so-called modules (cortical modularity), which has been elucidated with extracellular recordings and brain imaging studies, had long been suspected based on the distinctive visual deficits that are manifested by patients with circumscribed brain damage secondary to trauma,

---

2. Although the monkey and human cortex are anatomically similar, there are differences that make it challenging to identify cortical areas in one species (e.g., IT in monkey) that are equivalent to areas in the other species (e.g., LOC in humans).

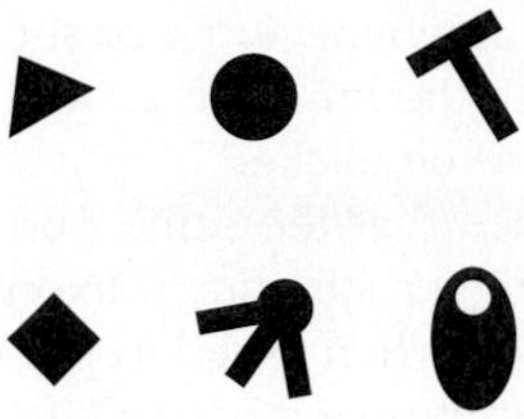

FIGURE 15–5. Certain neurons in IT respond well to basic shapes, which could serve as the building blocks to construct more complex forms (Tanaka et al, 1991).

infarcts, or tumors. Whereas lesions in striate cortex produce simple blind spots (scotomas), extrastriate lesions can lead to the inability to recognize objects, **visual agnosia** (Damasio et al, 1980). This condition can take many different forms, as indicated in Table 15–1, depending on the area of the brain that is compromised.

Certain lesions can lead to **visual neglect.** A patient with this condition may, for example, shave only the left side of his face and ignore the right side (Bisiach and Rusconi, 1990; Tovée, 1996). Although long associated with lesions in the parietal lobe, recent research suggests that visual neglect is secondary to lesions in the superior temporal lobe (Graziano, 2001). The neglect is apparently accentuated when a patient is presented with objects in both the affected and non-affected regions of his or her visual field. It is for this reason that clinicians, when performing a confrontation visual field test, sometimes present objects simultaneously to both the patient's left and right visual fields (Newman, 1992). Presentation of an object in the normal visual field *extinguishes* visualization of the object in the field affected by the lesion, thereby facilitating detection of the abnormality.

In patients with the rare condition of **synaesthesia**, cortical modules appear to be abnormally linked to each other such that stimulation of one sense results in the activation of another. In one form of synaethesia, the presentation of a letter or a number results in the perception of a color (Mattingley et al, 2001).

TABLE 15–1 VISUAL AGNOSIAS

Classification	Deficiency
Form and Pattern	
Object agnosia	Recognition of real objects
Agnosia for drawings	Recognition of drawn objects
Prosopagnosia	Recognition of faces
Color	
Color agnosia	Association of colors with objects
Color anomia	Naming colors
Achromatopsia	Distinguishing hues
Depth and Movement	
Visual spatial agnosia	Stereoscopic vision, topographical relations
Akinetopsia	Motion perception

For instance, the patient may report the perception of green whenever he or she is presented with the number "6," red when presented with the number "2," and so on. Not only can the effect (e.g., the perception of green) be elicited by physical presentation of a stimulus (e.g., "6"), there is evidence that the same perception can result without external presentation of the trigger stimulus (Dixon et al, 2000). The patient may, for example, experience green when asked to perform a mental calculation whose answer is the trigger stimulus (e.g., "4 + 2").

ARE THERE GRANDMOTHER CELLS?

When thinking about specialized higher cortical centers and the hierarchical processing that results in these centers, you might conclude that visual information is continuously processed until it reaches a high-level cortical cell whose activity results in visual consciousness. In this scenario, there might be a cell so specialized that it responds only to the face of your grandmother—a so-called **grandmother cell.**

Brain imaging studies are inconsistent with the existence of grandmother cells. When participants are asked to visualize a specific object (e.g., their grandmother's face), activity is distributed over a fairly wide expanse of cortex. Interestingly, the activity does not seem to be confined to higher cortical areas, but also occurs in the lower centers including striate cortex (Kosslyn and Oschner, 1994). Apparently, the visualization of a remembered object results in a pattern of activity that is similar to that elicited by actually viewing the object (Ishai and Sagi, 1995).

Information from the various cortical areas must be combined to result in an integrated percept (Schiller, 1993). For instance, to perceive a red automobile that is traveling along a highway, the motion and position information that is processed along the dorsal stream must be integrated with color and form information that is processed along the ventral stream. Information from these two streams must be combined with memory. This integration is apparently coordinated in **prefrontal cortex,** an area that has long been thought to play a role in cognition (Rao et al, 1997).

BINOCULAR RIVALRY AND NEURONAL ACTIVITY

Consider the stimuli displayed in Fig. 15–6A. If the left-tilted bars are viewed exclusively by the left eye and the right-tilted bars exclusively by the right eye, the observer—at any given instance—will perceive either the left or right-tilted bars. His or her perception will alternate between the left and right-tilted bars—he or she never fuses the disparate stimuli. This alternating perception of non-fusible images is referred to as **binocular rivalry.**

Macaque monkeys perceive binocular rivalry and can be trained to indicate (by pushing a button) which stimulus they see (i.e., the left or right-tilted bars).

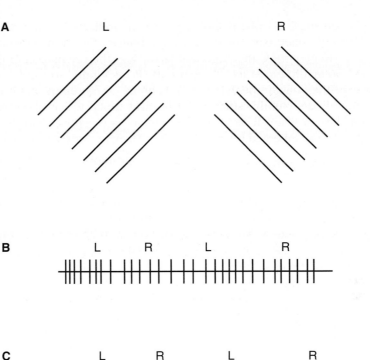

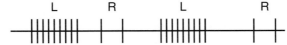

FIGURE 15–6. A. Stimulus used to induce binocular rivalry. When left-tilted gratings are viewed by the left eye and right-tilted gratings by the right eye, the observer experiences an alternating perception of left and right-tilted gratings: one of the gratings (e.g., the left-tilted grating) is seen, followed by the right-tilted grating, followed by the left-tilted grating, and so forth. **B.** Idealized recording from a neuron in a macaque monkey's striate cortex taken while the animal is experiencing binocular rivalry. This neuron is tuned (optimally sensitive) to left-tilted gratings, which are continuously present in the cell's receptive field. (If the gratings were stable, the neuron would adapt to them and stop responding. Therefore, the gratings are made to drift.) The "L" and "R" designate which orientation (left or right-tilted) the animal *experiences.* Note that the neuron continues to fire regardless of whether the animal perceives a left or right-tilted grating. **C.** Idealized recording from a neuron located in V4 measured under the same conditions. Note that this neuron's response is modulated; it only responds when the animal reports that it perceives a left-tilted grating. Other neurons show a response that is linked to perception of a right-tilted grating. Although modulated neurons are found in both striate cortex and V4, a higher percentage of neurons in V4 show modulated responses than is the case for striate cortex (Leopold and Logothetis, 1996.)

An important question regards the responses of single neurons in striate cortex and higher cortical areas to bars that elicit binocular rivalry. Does the activity of these neurons correspond to the stimulus that is falling within their receptive fields or does their activity reflect the animal's perception?

To answer the question posed above, Leopold and Logothetis (1996) made extracellular recordings from neurons in striate cortex and V4 while monkeys were experiencing binocular rivalry. The animals indicated which stimulus they saw (left or right-tilted bars) by depressing a button. For most orientation selective cells in striate cortex, the important factor was the orientation of the bars. If a cell was optimally tuned to left-tilted bars, it responded to the left-tilted bars regardless of the animal's perception. The animal could report that it was *seeing* the right-tilted bars, yet this striate cell (that was tuned to left-tilted bars) would respond as long as the left-tilted bars fell within its receptive field (Fig. 15–6B).

A different story emerged for area V4. Whereas many orientation selective cells responded the same as those in striate cortex, other cells responded only when the animal reported seeing a stimulus of a given orientation. For instance, such a cell would respond when the monkey reported that it was seeing the left-tilted bars, but would not fire when the monkey reported seeing the right-tilted bars (Fig. 15–6C). Keep in mind that the stimulus did not change—what changed was the monkey's perception. These results show that cells in higher cortical areas are more likely to code what the animal is actually seeing than are cells in lower visual areas (i.e., striate cortex).

A similar explanation may hold for ambiguous figures that produce bistable percepts, such as the **Necker cube** and **Rubin's face-vase** reversible figure (Leopold and Logothetis, 1996) (Fig. 15–7). Cells in lower visual areas may respond to the physical characteristics of the stimulus, and activity in the higher centers may reflect which of the two equally plausible perceptions the observer experiences. This hypothesis awaits empirical investigation.

Binocular rivalry and ambiguous figures are sometimes said to be manifestations of **bottom-up** visual attention. The untrained observer presumably does not choose which perception he or she experiences. A more classic example of bottom-up attention is an observer's response to a sudden flash of light or movement

A   **B**   **C**

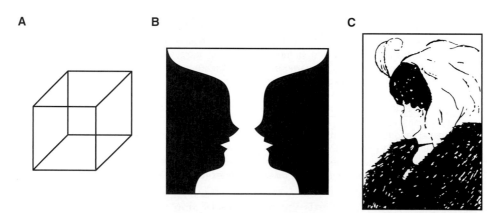

FIGURE 15–7. Examples of ambiguous figures. **A.** The Necker cube is seen as either projecting into or out of the page. **B.** The Rubin face–vase figure is perceived as either two faces or a vase. **C.** This ambiguous figure is seen as either an older or younger woman. You may need to stare at this figure for a few minutes to visualize both images.

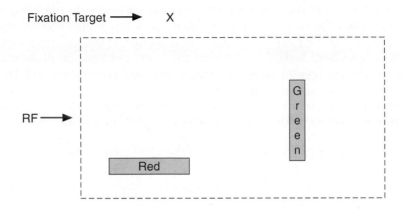

Fixation Target ⟶ X

RF ⟶

Red

Green

Figure 15–8. To study top-down attention, red and green bars are presented within the receptive field (RF) of a neuron located in V4. The activity of certain neurons depends on the bar to which the animal is paying attention. For instance, a neuron may only respond when the animal is attending to the red bar. The same neuron may not respond when the animal attends to the green bar although neither the stimulus nor the animal's eye position (i.e., fixation) have changed (Moran and Desimone, 1985).

in the periphery of the visual field. The attention that is induced by these stimuli is not voluntary or conscious, and can be considered as resulting from bottom-up processes (Steinman and Steinman, 1998; Steinman et al, 1995). This form of attention is to be contrasted with top-down visual attention, our next topic.

TOP-DOWN ATTENTION AND NEURONAL ACTIVITY

We perform better on certain tasks when we are attentive to the demands of these tasks. If you are a batter in a baseball game and you suspect that the pitcher is about to throw you a curve ball, you are more likely to hit the pitch than if you were not attending to this likelihood.

Do cortical cells reflect this conscious choice of attention, a process sometimes referred to as **top-down** attention? This question can be addressed by performing extracellular recordings on cortical visual neurons while a monkey chooses to attend to a specific aspect of a stimulus.

The stimulus array in Fig. 15–8, which consists of a red and green bar, is positioned so that it falls within the receptive field[3] of a red-sensitive neuron in V4. When the animal is required to attend to the red stimulus, the neuron responds vigorously. However, when the animal is required to attend to the green stimulus, the response is diminished (Moran and Desimone, 1985; Motter, 1994). Note

---

3. The receptive fields of neurons in higher visual centers tend to be larger than those in lower centers, making it possible to study them with large, complex stimulus arrays.

that the stimulus and the monkey's eye position are precisely the same under both conditions. The only thing that has changed is the animal's focus of attention, which affects the response of the cell. Because the choice of which object to attend comes from higher areas within the brain, perhaps the prefrontal cortex, this is an example of top-down visual attention (Desimone and Duncan, 1995).

In comparison to the results found in V4, cells in striate cortex apparently do not demonstrate top-down attentional influences (Moran and Desimone, 1985). This suggests that there is a filtering of visual information from striate cortex to V4 that is at least partially dependent on the stimulus to which the animal is attending.

CAN VISION BE TRAINED?

It has been the practice among certain eye care practitioners to train the vision of their patients. This visual training is often directed at improving performance in particular visual skills, such as awareness of the peripheral field of vision. Although there have been numerous reports of the efficacy of this form of visual skill training, the underlying mechanisms have not been fully elucidated.

The mechanisms underlying attention may provide the basis for improvement in visual skills that results from visual training. We know that top-down attention leads to temporary modifications in the receptive field sensitivities of visual neurons. With practice, it is conceivable that these changes in receptive field properties become ingrained, leading to improved task performance.

Psychophysical studies reveal that the visual performance of adults can be improved with practice, so-called perceptual learning (Goldstone, 1998). This seems to be the case for stereoscopic, orientation, and vernier tasks, but not for resolution tasks (Westheimer, 2001). The learning of certain tasks appears to be selective (e.g., specific to retinal location or the trained eye), suggesting that the neural learning occurs early in the visual system (Fiorentini and Berardi, 1980; Ball and Sekuler, 1982; Sowden et al, 2002). The learning of other tasks, however, is generalizable (Beard et al, 1995; Levi et al, 1997). For example, a vernier acuity task that is practiced at one orientation may lead to improved performance at other orientations. The generalizable nature of the learning is consistent with it occurring in higher visual centers.

A person does not need to be aware that he or she is learning for it to occur. Consider an experiment in which subjects were first presented with coherent motion stimuli—we will call these invisible practice stimuli—whose coherence was so low that motion was not visible (Wanatabe et al, 2001). The subjects were subsequently tested with stimuli of a higher coherence for various directions of movement. Interestingly, performance at detecting motion was best for the direction of the invisible practice stimuli. Moreover, it was found that as the frequency of exposure to the invisible practice stimuli increased, the performance improved. These results apparently confirm the long-held proposition that exposure to subliminal stimuli (i.e., stimuli that do not reach awareness) can influence behavior.

A *Word of Caution*

Our understanding of cortical physiology is limited by the available technology. As technology becomes more sophisticated, our comprehension of cortical physiology becomes more informed.

For decades, insights regarding cortical function were driven by experiments in which activity was recorded from single neurons. Such experiments continue to enrich our understanding of cortical physiology. These experiments are, however, limited because they do not tell us how information is integrated across populations of cortical neurons.

Consider the processing of color information in striate cortex. Some report that color opponent neurons are not commonly encountered when recording from single neurons in this area—a somewhat controversial finding—leading to the suggestion that it does not play a major role in processing color information (Lennie et al, 1990).[4]

A different picture emerges when striate cortex is studied using fMRI, which shows the activity of a large area of cortex containing many neurons. Such studies reveal that striate cortex (as a whole) manifests significant color opponency (Kleinschmidt et al, 1996; Engel et al, 1997). Consequently, it is important to examine not only the activity of individual neurons, but also the activity of neural networks spanning many neurons.

The controversy regarding the number of color selective neurons in striate cortex, along with the finding of color opponency using fMRI, suggest caution in finalizing our thinking with regard to processing of information within this structure. As technology advances, previously held theories will be modified and replaced by new theories. Although the past decades have seen great leaps in our understanding of cortical functioning, we still have much to learn about this most complex of organs. Further progress is likely to coincide with advances in technology.

Summary

Given the enormous quantity of visual information that is processed by the cortex, it is not surprising that this organ manifests a significant degree of specialization. Cortical areas within the ventral processing stream, including V4 and IT, apparently play a large role in object recognition, and can be thought of as constituting a "what" system. Areas that constitute the dorsal stream, including MT, appear to be important for motion analysis and spatial localization, and can be thought of as being part of a "where" system. Integration of information from the two systems may be coordinated by prefrontal cortex.

The activity of neurons in higher visual centers corresponds more closely with our perceptions than does the activity of neurons in striate cortex. Certain higher-level neurons that manifest changes in sensitivity depending on attentional status may play a role in perceptual learning.

---

4. The number of color selective cells in striate cortex is controversial. See Johnson et al (2001) for a different view.

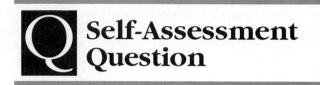

Self-Assessment Question

1. Subsequent to viewing a grating tilted to the left, human subjects note that a vertical grating appears tilted to the right. This is referred to as the tilt-after-effect. Devise a psychophysical experiment that enables you to address the following hypothesis: the tilt-aftereffect is mediated by binocular cortical neurons.

16

Gross Electrical Potentials

Gross electrical potentials are the summed electrical activity of a large number of neurons. Because these potentials can be recorded by noninvasive methods, they can be of clinical value. The electrooculogram (EOG), electroretinogram (ERG), and visually evoked potential (VEP) are discussed in this chapter.

ELECTROOCULOGRAM

As illustrated in Fig. 16–1, the front of the eye has a positive charge relative to the back. This standing (or resting) potential is the basis of the EOG.[1] It is the largest of the gross potentials, on the order of 6 mV (Arden and Barrada, 1962).

Clinical Measurement

To determine the EOG, electrodes that feed into a chart recorder are attached to the inner and outer canthi, as illustrated in Fig. 16–2. The patient is instructed to alternately view fixation points such that the eyes move from extreme left to extreme right gaze. An example of an EOG trace is given in Fig. 16–1.

---

1. For the purpose of understanding the EOG, think of the eye as a battery.

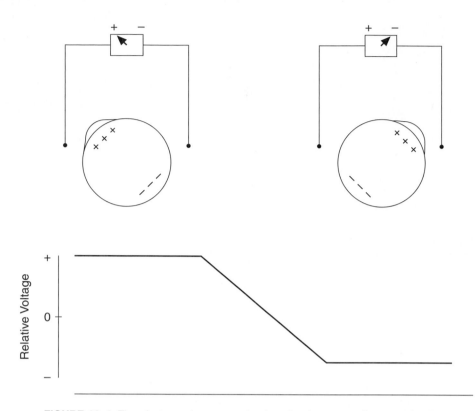

FIGURE 16–1. The electrooculogram can be thought of as a standing potential. The measured polarity of the response changes as the gaze is shifted. This is indicated by the voltmeters in the top diagram and the schematic trace on the bottom.

The EOG is substantially larger under light-adapted than dark-adapted conditions (Arden et al, 1962). It reaches its minimum value **(dark trough)** after about 8 minutes of dark adaptation, whereas the maximum value **(light rise)** is obtained following approximately 10 to 15 minutes of light adaptation (Fig. 16–3) (Berson, 1992).

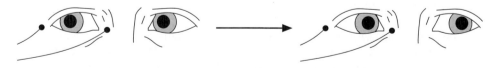

FIGURE 16–2. The electrooculogram is measured with electrodes attached to the inner and outer canthi. The patient shifts his or her gaze from extreme rightward to extreme leftward to cause the change in polarity displayed in Figure 16–1.

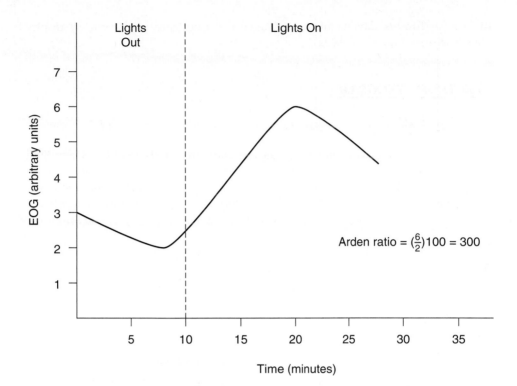

FIGURE 16–3. The electrooculogram reaches a minimum (dark trough) after about 8 minutes of dark adaptation and a maximum (light rise) following approximately 10 to 15 minutes of light adaptation. The Arden ratio is the ratio of the light rise to the dark trough. This diagram is a schematic.

For clinical purposes, it is useful to determine the ratio of the light rise to the dark trough (Arden et al, 1962). This ratio, when expressed as a percentage, is referred to as the **Arden ratio.** Values lower than about 165 to 180 percent are considered abnormal.

Origins and Clinical Applications

The origin of the dark-adapted EOG is most likely the retinal pigment epithelium (RPE) (Brown and Wiesel, 1961). The increased value of the EOG under light-adapted conditions (the light rise) appears to be due primarily to rod activity, although cones play a role in its genesis (Gouras and Carr, 1965).

Although the EOG is occasionally used for the diagnosis of outer retinal disease, it has been largely supplanted by the electroretinogram (ERG). It is, however, useful in the diagnosis of the following four conditions that may not affect the ERG, but often result in a reduced Arden ratio: butterfly-shaped dystrophy of the fovea, fundus flavimaculatus, advanced drusen, and vitelliform dystrophy (Best's disease) (Berson, 1992).

ELECTRORETINOGRAM

Full-Field ERG

The full-field ERG, also referred to as the standard or flash ERG, is a retinal potential elicited by a brief flash of light that evenly illuminates the entire retina. A typical full-field ERG is illustrated in Fig. 16–4A. This potential, unlike the EOG, is not continuously present; it must be elicited by a visual stimulus. The ERG is smaller than the EOG, and is on the order of 1 mV.

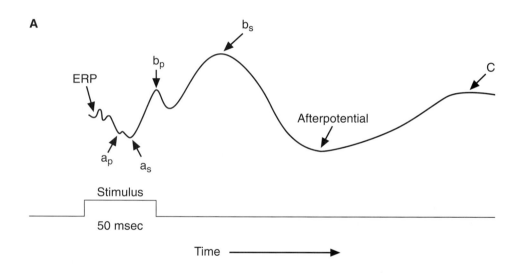

WAVE	PRESUMED ORIGINS
ERP	Outer segments of photoreceptors, primarily cones
a-wave	Photoreceptors
b-wave	Muller/bipolar cells
c-wave	RPE?

FIGURE 16–4. A. Schematic of a full-field flash electroretinogram. Note that the a- and b-waves are each composed of scotopic (a_s, b_s) and photopic (a_p, b_p) components. B. Presumed origins of the various waves that constitute the full-field flash electroretinogram (Armington, 1974; Dowling, 1987; Berson, 1992).

The full-field ERG is composed of a number of different waves (Einthoven and Jolly, 1908). The first is biphasic, referred to as the **early receptor potential (ERP).**[2] It is followed by the negative **a-wave** and the positive **b-wave**, which is the largest ERG component. Next are the **afterpotential** and the **c-wave.**

The full-field ERG is derived primarily from the outer retina (Armington, 1974). The presumed origins of the component waves are given in Fig. 16–4B.

Because the ERG in Fig. 16–4A was produced with stimulus conditions that elicit activity in both rods and cones, the a- and b-wave each consist of a scotopic (a_s, b_s) and photopic component (a_p, b_p). By the proper choice of stimulus conditions, either component can be made to dominate the ERG (Fig. 16–5A). A scotopic-dominated ERG is obtained by stimulating a dark-adapted retina with a dim, short-wavelength light (e.g., 505 nm). To obtain a photopic-dominated ERG, a light-adapted patient is exposed to a relatively bright middle-wavelength stimulus (e.g., 555 nm). In the clinic, a photopic-dominated ERG is often obtained with a stimulus presented at a temporal rate (~30 Hz) that is too high to be resolved by the scotopic system, yet resolvable by the photopic system (Armington, 1974) (Fig. 16–5B).[3]

Note that the scotopic ERG in Fig. 16–5A is both larger and slower than the photopic ERG. This can also be seen by observing the scotopic and photopic contributions in Fig. 16–4A.

Focal Electroretinogram

The ERG represents the summed activity of the retinal tissue that is stimulated by the flash of light (Armington, 1974). Because the stimulus for a full-field ERG illuminates the entire retina, this ERG represents the summed activity of the retina. Full-field flash ERGs are useful clinically for diagnosing widely disseminated choroidal-retinal disease such as retinitis pigmentosa (RP).

Focal lesions, which have relatively little effect on the standard ERG, can be evaluated with so-called focal ERGs, where the light flash is confined to the affected area. Because only the stimulated tissue contributes to the focal ERG, damage to this tissue is noticeable. Figure 16–6 shows schematic full-field and focal flicker ERGs for a patient with a macular lesion. Note that the focal ERG is greatly reduced, whereas the full-field ERG is unaffected.

Multifocal ERG

The multifocal ERG (mfERG), a relatively new technique, enables ERGs to be recorded for many different retinal locations in a brief period of time (about 4

---

2. Elicitation of the ERP requires a much brighter stimulus than necessary to elicit the ERG. Some do not consider the ERP to be part of the ERG.
3. Postreceptoral processes play a significant role in the genesis of the flicker ERG (Kondo and Sieving, 2001).

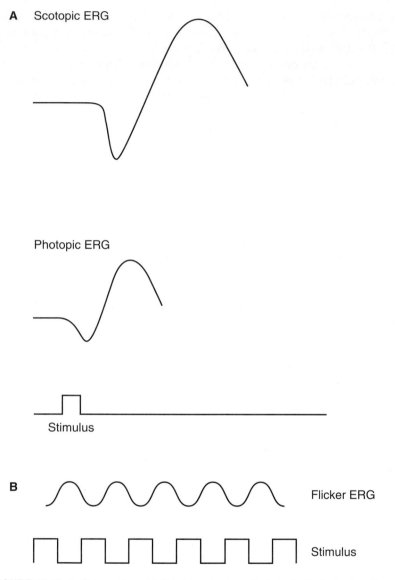

A   Scotopic ERG

Photopic ERG

Stimulus

B   Flicker ERG

Stimulus

FIGURE 16–5. A. Schematics of full-field scotopic and photopic flash electroretinograms (ERGs). Note that the scotopic ERG is larger in amplitude and slower than the photopic ERG. **B.** A flicker ERG can be produced with a high temporal frequency (~30 Hz) square-wave stimulus.

minutes) (Sutter and Tran, 1992). The patient is presented with a stimulus array consisting of about 240 hexagons, half of which are illuminated at any one instance. Each hexagon is modulated independently according to a binary sequence (Fig. 16–7). ERGs for various retinal loci are determined with an algorithm that links recorded electrical activity to the location of a specific hexagon.

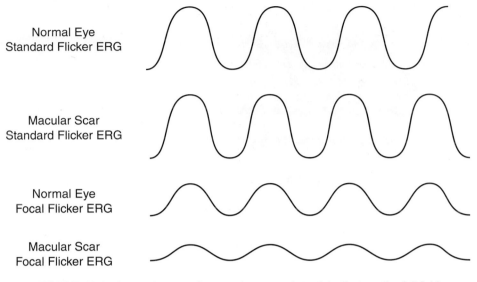

Normal Eye
Standard Flicker ERG

Macular Scar
Standard Flicker ERG

Normal Eye
Focal Flicker ERG

Macular Scar
Focal Flicker ERG

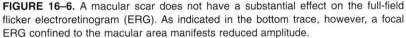

FIGURE 16–6. A macular scar does not have a substantial effect on the full-field flicker electroretinogram (ERG). As indicated in the bottom trace, however, a focal ERG confined to the macular area manifests reduced amplitude.

Although the mfERG potentials have a form that is similar to the full-field flash ERG, they do not have the same origins (Hood et al, 2002).

An important advantage of the mfERG is that it permits the near-simultaneous evaluation of multiple focal regions of the retina. Figure 16–7B presents a mfERG for a 29-year-old patient with suspected central serous retinopathy who presented with a small scotoma located between the fixation point and blind spot. A full-field ERG is normal, yet the mfERG reveals a region between fixation and the blind spot where the ERG waves are abnormal. The mfERG is useful not only in the diagnosis of localized retinal abnormalities, but it might allow the earlier diagnosis of more generalized retinal disease, such as retinitis pigmentosa and glaucoma (Bearse et al, 1996; Hood et al, 1997).

Pattern Electroretinogram

The pattern electroretinogram (PERG) is obtained with a temporally modulated stimulus whose average spatial luminance remains constant (Johnson et al, 1966). Either a grating or checkerboard pattern is typically used (Fig. 16–8A and B). The pattern is phase-shifted by 180 degrees at a moderate temporal rate so that the resultant PERG is elicited by contrast modulation rather than a change in overall luminance.[4]

---

4. In essence, the positions of the white and black components of the pattern are continuously exchanged (counterphase modulation).

A

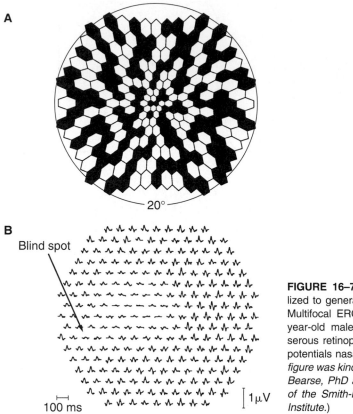

—20°—

B

Blind spot

100 ms   1μV

FIGURE 16–7. **A.** Stimulus array utilized to generate a multifocal ERG. **B.** Multifocal ERG for the left eye of 29 year-old male with suspected central serous retinopathy. Note the abnormal potentials nasal to the blind spot. (*This figure was kindly provided by Marcus A. Bearse, PhD and Erich E. Sutter, PhD of the Smith-Kettlewell Eye Research Institute.*)

An idealized PERG is given in Fig. 16–8C. It is similar in form to a standard flicker ERG, but apparently has different retinal origins. Whereas the outer retina generates the flicker and flash ERGs, the PERG is thought to have origins in the inner retina. In particular, retinal ganglion cells may play a large role in the genesis of the PERG.

A disadvantage of a flashed stimulus is that it produces retinal light scatter. Even if a focal flash is confined to the nonresponsive optic nerve head, an ERG is recorded because light scatters when it is incident upon this structure, stimulating responsive retinal areas. A *focal* PERG minimizes this disadvantage because it is not elicited by an overall increase in luminance, but by an exchange of contrast. For this reason, focal retinal lesions are sometimes examined using a focal PERG.

Clinical Measurement and Applications

The ERG is recorded with an rigid contact lens that contains an electrode connected to an amplifier. For a full-field ERG, the stimulus is typically presented

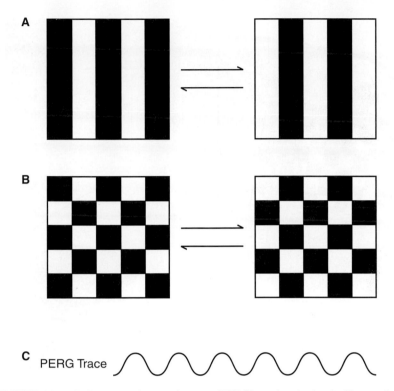

FIGURE 16–8. A. A pattern electroretinogram (PERG) can be obtained with a grating that undergoes a 180-degree phase shift. **B.** A checkerboard pattern that undergoes a 180-degree phase shift also elicits a PERG. **C.** A PERG is a modulated response that follows the phase shifts of the stimulus.

using a **ganzfeld dome,** a sphere that evenly illuminates the patient's retina. The stimuli for a multifocal ERG or PERG can be presented on a computer screen (Fig. 16–9).

The full-field ERG (flash or flicker) is used frequently in the diagnosis of outer retinal disease, such as rod–cone degenerations. It is particularly useful in the diagnosis of retinitis pigmentosa (RP), an inherited retinal degeneration that affects the metabolism of rod and cone outer segments. Rod function is apparently compromised first, with patients often demonstrating night blindness in the early stages of the disease. Subsequently, the disease can affect photopic vision. Visual fields may show a ring scotoma, which can progress, resulting in blindness.

The fundoscopic characteristics typical of RP include superficial bone spicule pigmentation, narrowed arterioles, and optic atrophy (Fig. 16–10). Fundoscopic appearance alone, however, may not be sufficient for a diagnosis since other conditions show similar presentations. Electrodiagnostic testing is often required to make an accurate diagnosis.

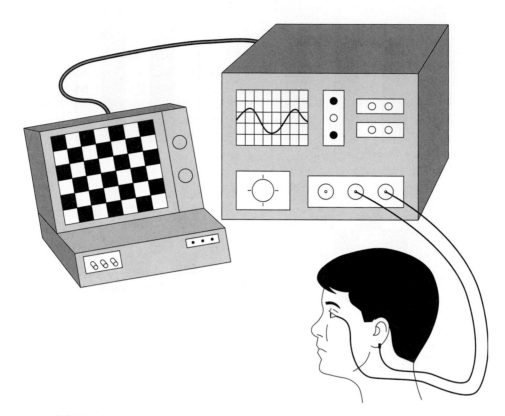

FIGURE 16–9. The PERG is measured with a corneal contact lens electrode that feeds into an amplifier. The stimulus is a checkerboard that undergoes a 180-degree phase shift. The same stimulus can be used to elicit a steady-state visually evoked potential.

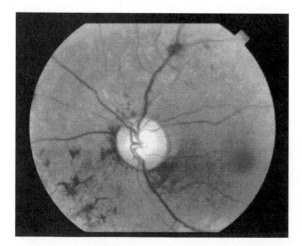

FIGURE 16–10. Fundus photograph showing bone-spicule pigmentation characteristic of retinitis pigmentosa. The pigmentation is most noticeable in the inferior nasal quadrant. Also note the narrowing of arterioles. (*Photograph is courtesy of Dr. Mitchell Dul.*)

Figure 16–11 shows schematic ERGs typical of the early stages of RP. Note that both the photopic and scotopic ERGs are reduced in amplitude. Also of diagnostic value is the time from the stimulus onset to the peak of the response, the so-called **implicit time.** RP, which is progressive, manifests a delayed implicit time. Certain retinal conditions that mimic RP (sector RP, stationary night blindness) may manifest reduced amplitudes but show normal implicit times (Berson, 1992). These conditions are typically nonprogressive.

Whereas the full-field ERG is useful in the diagnosis of outer retinal disease, the PERG may be helpful in the assessment of inner retinal function (Maffei and Fiorentini, 1981). PERGs can be abnormal in early glaucoma, a disease that affects ganglion cell function (Trick, 1985).

VISUALLY EVOKED POTENTIALS

Visually evoked potentials (VEPs), also referred to as evoked potentials (EPs), visually evoked cortical potentials (VECPs), or visually evoked responses (VERs), are very small cortical potentials elicited by visual stimuli. They are on the order of 5 µV, embedded in the randomly fluctuating electroencephalogram (EEG), which has an amplitude of about 60 µV. Because VEPs must be detected against the background noise of the EEG, they are recorded with an averaging computer. Electrodes are positioned on the scalp.

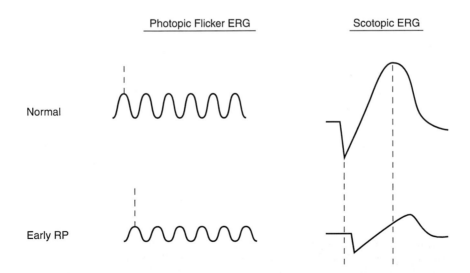

FIGURE 16–11. Schematic photopic flicker and scotopic electroretinograms for a healthy eye and an eye with early retinitis pigmentosa. Note the delayed implicit times in early retinitis pigmentosa.

Transient Visually Evoked Potentials

Transient VEPs are elicited by a flashed stimulus—either patterned or nonpatterned—that is presented multiple times. The computer stores and sums the responses to each individual flash, producing a VEP that is a complex waveform composed of numerous component waves (Fig. 16–12A) (Regan, 1989). It is thought that these individual waves (wavelets) represent the activity of different regions of the brain, primarily cortical areas.

Steady-State Visually Evoked Potentials

A steady-state VEP is obtained with a patterned or nonpatterned stimulus that is presented at a moderate temporal frequency. The stimulus conditions are similar to those used to obtain either a flicker or PERG. The resultant potential is less complex in form than the transient VEP (see Fig. 16-12B).

Multifocal Visually Evoked Potentials

The stimulus arrangement used to elicit a mfERG can be used to elicit a multifocal visually evoked potential (mfVEP) (Baseler et al, 1994). Similar to a mfERG,

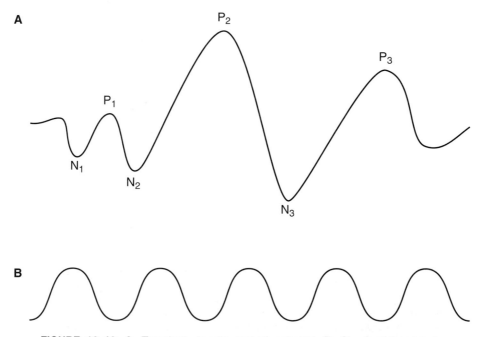

FIGURE 16–12. **A.** Transient visually evoked potential. **B.** Steady-state visually evoked potential. Both traces are schematics.

the mfVEP shows VEPs for many different retinal loci. Interestingly, the mfVEP elicited by a given stimulus location is enhanced when the subject attends to this location (Seiple et al, 2002).

Effect of Contrast on the Amplitude of Visually Evoked Potentials

A high-contrast patterned stimulus elicits a larger amplitude VEP than a low-contrast stimulus (Campbell and Maffei, 1970). This correlation of VEP amplitude with stimulus contrast has been used to assess contrast sensitivity.

Figure 16–13 shows a plot of VEP amplitude as a function of grating contrast for a given spatial frequency. By obtaining VEPs for a sample of moderate- and high-contrast stimuli, it is possible to extrapolate to a zero-amplitude response. The grating contrast that is predicted to elicit this zero-amplitude response typically corresponds well with the psychophysically measured threshold contrast. Consequently, VEPs allow an objective determination of threshold contrast. Likewise, visual acuity can be estimated by presenting high-contrast stimuli of increasing spatial frequency and extrapolating to the zero-amplitude response.

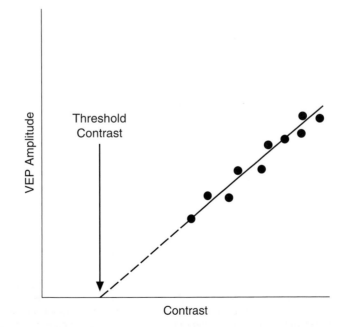

FIGURE 16–13. The amplitude of a visually evoked potential, for a given spatial frequency, is proportional to the stimulus contrast. Threshold contrast is obtained by extrapolation (dashed line) from data obtained at higher contrast levels (circles) (Campbell and Maffei, 1970).

The preceding information has implications for the assessment of visual function in nonresponsive patients. The contrast sensitivity and visual acuity of malingerers, hysterics, the mentally retarded, infants, and other nonresponsive or noncooperative patients can be objectively assessed using VEPs. It should be noted, however, that VEPs produce higher estimates of visual acuity in infants than do behavioral procedures such as forced-choice preferential looking (Norcia et al, 1986; Teller and Movshon, 1986). This is discussed in Chapter 17.

Importance of the Fovea in Visually Evoked Potentials

The majority of the striate cortex is devoted to analyzing foveal vision. Because of this **cortical magnification of foveal vision,** the transient and steady-state VEPs are largely foveal phenomena. Approximately two thirds of the VEP is due to foveal and macular input (Riggs and Wooten, 1972; Berson, 1992).

The importance of the fovea in generating the VEP is illustrated in Fig. 16–14, which shows idealized PERGs and VEPs expected for three different stimuli: a stimulus that covers both the foveal and parafoveal area, a stimulus that covers

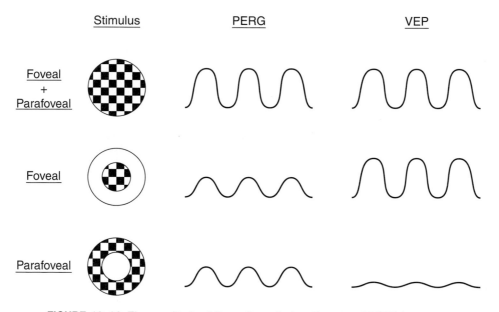

FIGURE 16–14. The amplitude of the pattern electroretinogram (PERG) is proportional to the surface area of the retina stimulated. Reducing the stimulus size in half, as is done in the bottom two PERG traces, reduces the PERG amplitude in half. It does not make any difference that one stimulus is foveal and the other is parafoveal. For the visually evoked potential (VEP), however, the surface area of the retina stimulated is not the critical issue. The VEP is a foveal response; consequently, a parafoveal stimulus does not elicit a significant response.

only the fovea, and a stimulus that covers only the parafoveal region. The bottom two stimuli represent the same area, and each is half the area of the top stimulus.

Note that the PERG amplitude is reduced by half for both the foveal and parafoveal stimuli. This is because the PERG amplitude is primarily dependent on the surface area of retina stimulated. Reducing the stimulated retinal area by half reduces the PERG amplitude by half. A stimulus that stimulates the fovea does not result in a disproportionately large PERG.

The results for the VEP are very different. The foveal stimulus produces a strong VEP, whereas the parafoveal stimulus elicits a weak response, demonstrating the importance of the fovea in generating the VEP.

For the reasons discussed here, it is critical to ensure that patients are fixating the stimulus during a VEP measurement. Malingerers have been known to avert their gaze from the stimulus, thereby reducing the amplitude of the VEP.

Clinical Considerations

Visually evoked potentials provide an objective method to assess contrast sensitivity and visual acuity. Although the results obtained with VEPs are well correlated with psychophysical data, there are occasions when VEPs do not tell the entire story. For example, VEPs overestimate infant acuity (Teller and Movshon, 1986). In addition, certain lesions in higher cortex could presumably have profound effects on vision and little effect on VEPs because they may occur in regions that do not significantly contribute to the VEP (Bodis-Wollner et al, 1977). It is also important to keep in mind that the VEP tests primarily central vision; it allows little assessment of noncentral visual function.

Although VEPs can be useful for establishing the existence of a visual deficit, they do not localize the causative lesion. VEPs may manifest reduced amplitudes in macular, optic nerve, and cortical lesions. Any lesion of the visual pathway that affects central vision may result in an abnormal VEP.

Visually evoked potentials may be used in conjunction with other gross potentials, such as PERGs, to localize a disease process within the visual pathways (Table 16–1). For example, if the VEP is reduced and the PERG is normal, the problem is postretinal. If both the VEP and PERG are reduced, the lesion is retinal.

Normal ERGs are found in amblyopia, whereas VEPs are reduced in magnitude (Sokol, 1990). This is consistent with the notion that amblyopia represents a disorder of cortical development rather than a retinal abnormality (see Chap. 17).

Visually evoked potentials have been used to assist in the diagnosis of multiple sclerosis, a demyelinating disease that can cause optic neuritis. During bouts of optic neuritis, the myelin sheath and axons of the optic nerve are damaged, resulting in reduced saltatory conduction velocity along the optic nerve. Because this condition is typically unilateral, it may result in increased VEP latency for the affected eye relative to the unaffected eye (Halliday et al, 1972). The increased latency may persist after the optic neuritis has resolved.

TABLE 16–1 EXPECTED STATUS OF GROSS ELECTRICAL POTENTIALS IN VARIOUS DISEASE CONDITIONS

Condition	EOG (Arden Ratio)	Standard ERG	Focal PERG	VEP
Macular lesion	Normal	Normal	Abnormal	Abnormal
Retinitis pigmentosa	Abnormal	Abnormal	Abnormal	Abnormal[a]
Optic nerve disease (e.g., glaucoma)	Normal	Normal	Abnormal	Abnormal[a]
Amblyopia	Normal	Normal	Normal	Abnormal
Hysteria, malingering	Normal	Normal	Normal	Normal

[a]The VEP may be normal in the early stages of RP and glaucoma.

Analogous to the use of the mfERG to diagnose localized retinal lesions, the mfVEP can reveal localized damage to the optic nerve. In glaucoma and optic neuritis, mfVEP responses from the affected area of the optic nerve may be abnormal, whereas responses from other regions of the nerve are normal (Hood et al, 2000; Hasegawa and Abe, 2001).

SUMMARY

Gross electrical potentials represent the summed activity of large numbers of neurons. These potentials are obtained using noninvasive techniques. The appropriate use of these potentials, often in combination with each other, is an important clinical tool for diagnosing certain diseases and disorders of the visual system.

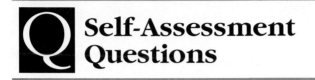
Self-Assessment Questions

1. Malingerers fabricate symptoms to obtain a positive medical diagnosis (i.e., they fake a visual disorder). Most often, these patients claim a reduction in visual acuity. Which electrodiagnostic test would be most useful in making a diagnosis of malingering? Explain.

2. Discuss a potential pitfall of using electrodiagnostic tests to make a diagnosis of malingering. (*Hint:* Could a patient with severely reduced vision show normal electrodiagnostic test results?)

3. Why must the patient look at the stimulus to obtain a normal evoked potential?

4. The pattern electroretinogram (PERG) and steady-state visually evoked potential (VEP) are obtained with the same stimulus. (This stimulus typically is a checkerboard pattern that undergoes a phase shift.) In amblyopia the PERG is normal, whereas the VEP is abnormal. Explain.

Development and Maturation of Vision

The human visual system is not fully developed at birth; rather, it matures over the first several years of life. To do so, it must be exposed to a normal visual environment. Disruption of this environment can have profound consequences for the attainment of normal levels of visual function.

We have, in recent decades, gained important insights regarding the mechanisms of visual development. Procedures that allow the clinical assessment of infant vision have been devised. As a result, eye care clinicians are better equipped to diagnose disorders that impact visual development and to institute treatment when indicated.

We start this chapter by discussing the maturation of the visual system. Both normal and abnormal development are addressed. The final part of the chapter reviews the affect that normal aging has on visual processes.

DEPRIVATION STUDIES

Most neurons in the visual cortex are binocular, receiving input from both eyes (see Chap. 14). However, most neurons do not receive equal input from the two eyes: one eye tends to dominate a given cortical cell. This can be illustrated with

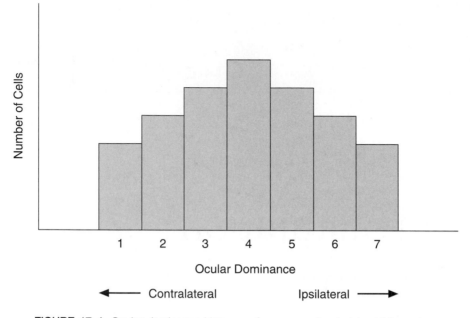

Number of Cells

Ocular Dominance

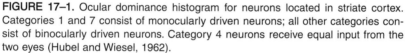

◀——— Contralateral   Ipsilateral ———▶

FIGURE 17–1. Ocular dominance histogram for neurons located in striate cortex. Categories 1 and 7 consist of monocularly driven neurons; all other categories consist of binocularly driven neurons. Category 4 neurons receive equal input from the two eyes (Hubel and Wiesel, 1962).

an **ocular dominance histogram** that is constructed based on recordings from individual neurons in one hemisphere of the adult striate cortex (Fig. 17–1) (Hubel and Wiesel, 1962).[1] Cells in categories 1 and 7 are monocular; category 1 cells receive input from only the contralateral eye, whereas category 7 cells receive input from only the ipsilateral eye. Neurons in category 4 are binocular and receive equal input from both eyes. Cells in the remaining categories are also binocular, but dominated by one of the eyes. Neurons in categories 2 and 3 are dominated by the contralateral eye, and those in categories 5 and 6 are dominated by the ipsilateral eye.

David Hubel and Torston Wiesel, who would later receive the Nobel Prize for their pioneering work on visual development and cortical processing, asked the following question: what is the effect of **visual deprivation** on the development of ocular dominance? To answer this question, they sutured one of a kitten's eyelids closed at birth, and then recorded from striate cortex after the animal had fully matured (Hubel and Wiesel, 1965b). Striate cortex of this monocularly deprived animal is very different from that of a normal animal (Fig. 17–2). Virtually all cells are monocular and responsive only to the nondeprived eye.

---

1. Experiments have been performed in a number of animal models, including cat and monkey.

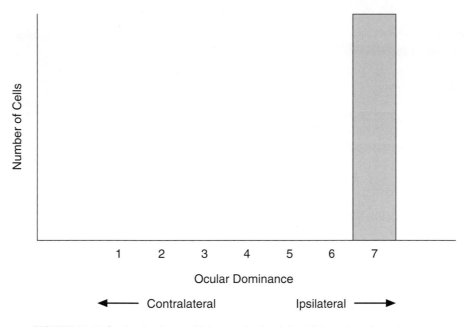

FIGURE 17–2. Ocular dominance histogram for the right striate cortex of a mature cat whose left eye was sutured closed at birth. Note that the nondeprived right eye drives all neurons (Wiesel and Hubel, 1963).

This result leads to an important conclusion. For striate cortex to develop a normal complement of binocular cells, it is necessary for both eyes to provide input during development. The closure of an immature animal's eye results in an absence of cortical cells responsive to this deprived eye. If no cortical cells are responsive to stimulation of an eye, we must conclude that the eye provides no useful vision. It is essentially blind (Harwerth et al, 1987). Moreover, because binocular cells are absent, there is no basis for stereopsis.

What is the result of a similar experiment conducted on a mature cat? When the eye of a 7-year-old cat is closed for 1 year, monocular deprivation has no effect. There is a normal complement of cortical neurons. Although the visual system is plastic (malleable) early in life, it becomes hard-wired (inflexible) later in life (Blakemore and Van Sluyters, 1974). The period during which the visual system can be influenced by environmental manipulation is referred to as the **critical**, or **sensitive**, **period.**

What is the duration of the critical period? If the right eye of a kitten is closed for the first 5 weeks of life and the cortex is examined at the end of these 5 weeks, it is found that cells are responsive only to stimulation of the nondeprived left eye. Now, suppose that the right eye is sutured closed for the first 5 weeks of life, but during the 5 subsequent weeks the right eye is open and the left eye closed (Fig. 17–3). Stimulation of which eye is expected to activate cortical neurons? Because

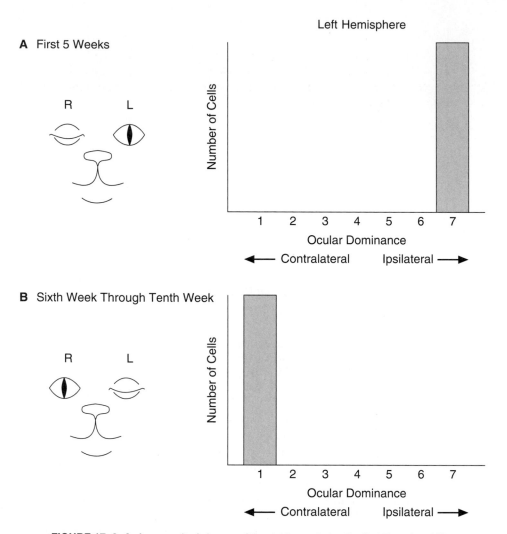

FIGURE 17–3. A. As a result of closure of the right eye during the first 5 weeks of life, most striate cortical cells of this adult cat are driven by the nondeprived left eye. **B.** Closure of the right eye for the first 5 weeks of life followed by monocular closure of the left eye for the next 5 weeks results in most cortical cells being driven by the right eye. This result is obtained because the switch from right eye deprivation to left eye deprivation occurred during the critical period.

the switch occurred early in life, during the critical period, most cortical cells are responsive to stimulation of the right eye.

For the cat, the critical period ends after about 3 months of age (Olson and Freeman, 1980). Consequently, if the suture in the previous experiment had been switched from the right to the left eye at the age of 6 months, cortical cells would still respond primarily to stimulation of the left eye.

The human visual system matures at a much slower pace than does that of the cat and is most sensitive to environmental manipulation during the first 2 years of life. The human critical period is over by about 7 to 9 years of age (Vaegan and Taylor, 1980).

Hubel and Wiesel's work suggests that during the critical period, the two eyes compete with each other to dominate cortical neurons (Hubel, 1988). If both eyes have equal retinal images, then most of the cortical neurons become binocular. However, when one eye is deprived during the critical period, it is at a disadvantage in this binocular competition. The other eye wins out in the competition for cortical neurons, and as a consequence, dominates these neurons.

The underlying assumption for this model is that synaptic connectivity in the cortex is strengthened by neural activity, and that lack of neural activity results in the weakening of these connections.[2] Because a geniculate neuron with input from the nondeprived eye will stimulate a cortical cell more than a geniculate cell from the deprived eye, there is a strengthening of synapses for the nondeprived eye relative to the deprived eye (Fig. 17–4). The synaptic arrangements become permanent as the animal matures, resulting in the critical period.[3]

Monocular deprivation during the critical period results in abnormal striate cortical architecture. Normally, the alternating ocular dominance columns have approximately equal width (see Fig. 14–12). When an eye is deprived, however, the columns receiving input from the nondeprived eye are widened at the expense of those associated with the deprived eye (Hubel et al, 1977).

It appears that ocular dominance columns are initially organized prior to and independent of visual experience (Crowley and Katz, 2000). Removal of an eye prior to the initial development of these columns does not prevent their normal development.[4] Once this basic cortical architecture has been laid down, however, environmental manipulations can be disruptive (i.e., monocular deprivation during the critical period can lead to asymmetrical ocular dominance columns).

How plastic is the cortex during the critical period? Sharma et al (2000) addressed this important question by redirecting retinal ganglion cells to the auditory thalamus in the newly born ferret. Neurons in this structure send projections

---

2. This is referred to as the Hebb synapse model.

3. Single unit recordings in cat extrastriate cortex indicate that monocular deprivation has a more pronounced effect on the ventral pathway than the dorsal pathway (Schroder et al, 2002).

4. This work was performed with ferrets, whose geniculocortical projections form postnatally (unlike cats, whose geniculocortical projections are present at birth).

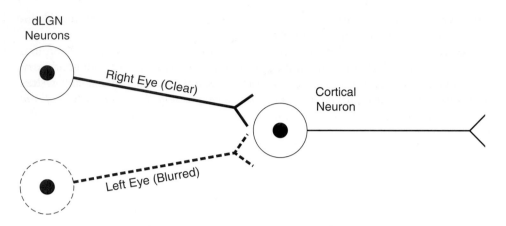

FIGURE 17–4. A relatively high level of neural activity strengthens the connection between the eye that has a clear image and a cortical cell. The relative lack of neural activity produces a weakening of the connection between the eye with a poor image and the same cortical neuron.

to primary auditory cortex. When the auditory cortex was examined following maturation of the animal, the investigators found orientation columns similar to those normally found in striate cortex. Moreover, behavioral experiments demonstrated that these animals were responsive to visual stimuli (von Melchner et al, 2000). In essence, the ferrets were using auditory cortex to see. This finding shows that cortical development is profoundly influenced by the nature of its input.

There is evidence that cortical reorganization, analogous to that in the ferret, may also occur in humans. Imaging studies of individuals blind from an early age reveal striate cortex activity during the use of Braille (Sadato, 1996). Moreover, transcranial magnetic stimulation of the occipital cortex disrupts tactile discrimination in such individuals, but not in normal-sighted individuals (Cohen et al, 1997). These findings suggest that striate cortex, which is normally devoted exclusively to visual processing, may process tactile information in people who become blind early in life.[5]

AMBLYOPIA

For reasons we have discussed previously, monocularly deprived animals may display very poor vision in the deprived eye. Reduction in vision secondary to

---

5. Congenitally blind individuals are better at localizing sounds than sighted people, presumably due to increased cortical area devoted to auditory input (Lessard et al, 1998; Roder et al, 1999).

monocular deprivation during the critical period is referred to as amblyopia (Ciuffreda et al, 1991). It is important to keep in mind that amblyopia results from abnormal cortical development, not an abnormality of the eye itself.

Amblyopia is commonly encountered in clinical practice. It can be secondary to the amblyogenic conditions of monocular occlusion, anisometropia, or strabismus. *A diagnosis of amblyopia should only be made if there is a history of one of these factors.*[6]

Occlusion Amblyopia

Occlusion amblyopia results when an eye is occluded during the critical period. A monocular congenital cataract, monocular lid ptosis (the eyelid covers the pupil, either completely or partially), or other monocular blockage of vision can cause the occlusion. This form of amblyopia can occur iatrogenically, secondary to monocular patching used in the treatment of a disease or injury.[7]

To minimize permanent visual loss, it is necessary to remove the occlusion. In general, the sooner it is removed, the better the visual outcome. Infants with congenital cataracts and ptosis should receive prompt treatment.

Anisometropic Amblyopia

Anisometropia is a condition where the two eyes have unequal refractive errors (Levi and Harwerth, 1977; Bradley and Freeman, 1981). Amblyopia can develop when, during the critical period, one eye has a blurred retinal image at all distances and the fellow eye has a clear retinal image at some distances. This most commonly occurs when one eye manifests a hyperopic refraction and the fellow eye is less hyperopic (compound hyperopic anisometropia), plano (simple hyperopic anisometropia), or myopic (antimetropia).

Consider the following (hypothetical) case of an 8-year-old child who received his first prescription at the age of 7 years:

OD   +6.00DS   20/400
OS   +1.00DS   20/20

---

6. There have been cases where amblyopia has been diagnosed incorrectly, in the absence of an amblyogenic condition. If the reduction in acuity that led to the incorrect diagnosis is due to a progressive disease process, there may be further loss of vision. In such a case, the doctor may be liable for malpractice.

7. Caution should be exercised if monocular patching is indicated for treatment of a disease or injury during the critical period.

Without an optical correction, this patient accommodates 1 diopter to focus the left eye for distance. Because the innervation to accommodation is bilateral and equal, the right eye is always 5 diopters out of focus. Assuming the anisometropia was present during the critical period, the right eye was at a disadvantage in the competition for cortical neurons, and consequently, developed amblyopia.[8] Moreover, because of a paucity of binocular cortical neurons, this patient has greatly reduced stereopsis. Much of the patient's visual loss may have been prevented if he had received an appropriate prescription for spectacles during the critical period.

It is important to note that not all anisometropes develop amblyopia. Consider the following (hypothetical) case of an 8-year-old child who received her first prescription at the age of 7 years[9]:

OD	−3.00DS	20/20
OS	−1.00DS	20/20

Even if this uncorrected refractive error was present during the critical period, each eye had a clear retinal image at certain distances. The right eye was in focus at 33 cm, and the left eye was in focus at 100 cm. Consequently, neither eye developed amblyopia.

Although this patient manifests normal monocular acuities, she will most likely demonstrate reduced stereopsis. Because the retinal images of the two eyes were never simultaneously in focus at any viewing distance, the patient presumably developed relatively few binocular cortical neurons (i.e., most striate cells are expected to fall into ocular dominance categories 1 and 7) (Holopigian et al, 1986; Movshon et al, 1987). This putative reduction in the number of binocular neurons is expected to result in poor stereopsis.

To prevent vision loss due to anisometropic amblyopia, the first eye examination should occur early in life, preferably during the critical period. Using objective tests, such as retinoscopy, a skilled clinician can diagnose anisometropia in a very young child. Consideration should be given to correcting substantial amounts of compound and simple hyperopic anisometropia and antimetropia.

Strabismic Amblyopia

Constant unilateral strabismus (an eye turn), present during the critical period, may lead to amblyopia in the deviated eye. Figure 17–5B shows a case of constant left esotropia. The right eye views the target of regard while the left eye is deviated inward. As a consequence of this deviation, the object of regard, a

---

8. As the amount of image degradation during the critical period increases, the depth of the resultant anisometropic amblyopia also increases (Smith et al, 2000)

9. Anisometropia in which both eyes are myopic is referred to as compound myopic anisometropia.

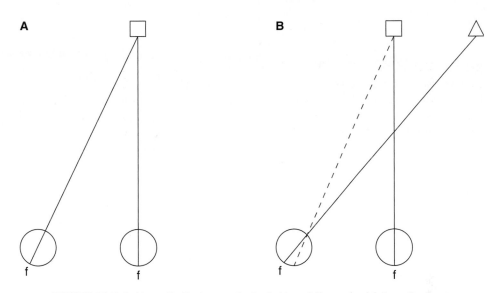

FIGURE 17–5. A. Normally, the image of a fixated target (the square) falls on the fovea of each eye. **B.** In this case of constant left eye esotropia, the fixated square falls on a nonfoveal region of the deviating eye, and the triangle falls on the fovea. This would lead to diplopia in the absence of a sensory adaptation, such as suppression.

square, does not fall on the left fovea. Instead, it is exposed to another image (a triangle). In the absence of a sensory adaptation, the patient will experience diplopia (both a triangle and a square will be seen in the same location because both images fall upon a fovea). To avoid diplopia, the deviating eye may be suppressed, which presumably leads to amblyopia.

Amblyopia develops in constant unilateral deviations, as frequently occur in esotropia, but not in alternating or nonconstant deviations, as is often the case in exotropia (Fig. 17–6A). Because alternating strabismics view objects with each eye, amblyopia does not develop.

Although alternating strabismics may have normal visual acuity in each eye, these patients frequently have little or no stereoscopic vision (Birch and Stager, 1985). During the critical period, cortical neurons do not receive similar images from each eye simultaneously, presumably resulting in a paucity of binocular cells capable of mediating stereopsis. This is similar to the previously discussed example of compound myopic anisometropia.

The scarcity of binocular cells in alternating strabismus can be demonstrated in animal models by experimentally inducing this condition, during the critical period, with surgery or prisms (Hubel and Wiesel, 1965b; Crawford and von Noorden, 1980). Cells in the striate cortex of such an animal are almost exclusively monocular (see Fig. 17–6B).

In adult human strabismics, the relative paucity of binocular cells is indicated by an impaired interocular transfer of the tilt aftereffect (Banks et al, 1975).

A

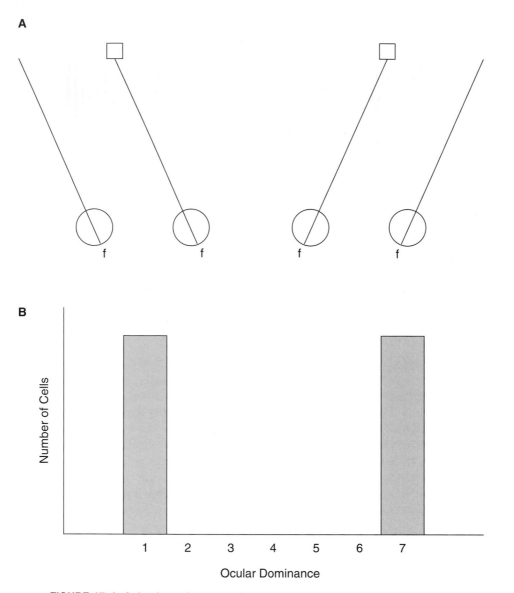

B

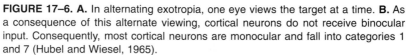

FIGURE 17–6. A. In alternating exotropia, one eye views the target at a time. **B.** As a consequence of this alternate viewing, cortical neurons do not receive binocular input. Consequently, most cortical neurons are monocular and fall into categories 1 and 7 (Hubel and Wiesel, 1965).

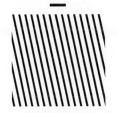 

FIGURE 17–7. To demonstrate interocular transfer of the tilt aftereffect, view the tilted grating for 1 minute with your left eye. Next, view the vertical grating with your right eye. An appearance of the vertical grating tilting to the right is evidence of interocular transfer of the aftereffect. (Because the interocular transfer effect is very subtle, you may not be able to experience it with the stimuli in this diagram. Most observers, however, are able to experience a *monocular* tilt after effect. Cover one eye and move your eye across the length of the horizontal bar for one minute. Next, view the dot with the same eye and note that the vertical lines appear tilted. This is an aftereffect rather than an afterimage because your eye was not stationary during adaptation to the tilted grating.)

Figure 17–7 shows the stimuli used for this psychophysical experiment. Monocularly, the observer views the tilted grating for several minutes. He or she subsequently views the vertical grating with the fellow eye (monocularly). Normal nonstrabismic patients report that the vertical grating appears tilted in a direction opposite to that of the original grating.

Interocular transfer of the tilt aftereffect is mediated by binocular cortical neurons. If few or no such neurons are present, then the phenomenon does not occur. This is the case for patients who develop strabismus early during the critical period—interocular transfer is virtually absent. If, however, the strabismus develops later in the critical period, some residual transfer may be noted.

Treatment of Amblyopia

If the nonamblyopic eye is patched during the critical period, the amblyopic eye may recover vision.[10] Patching outside of the critical period is less effective.

Traditional practice has been to patch the nonamblyopic eye during much of the child's waking hours. Because such patching forces the child to view with the amblyopic eye, patient compliance can be poor. Recent research, however, shows that short periods of patching are as effective as longer periods for the treatment of moderate amblyopia in children (Repka et al, 2003). This finding is expected to lead to better tolerated treatment regimens.

---

10. The treatment of amblyopia involves the "penalization" of the non-amblyopic eye. This can be accomplished with any of number of strategies, including patching or the use of a cycloplegic to induce blur.

MERIDIONAL AMBLYOPIA

In Chapter 14, we learned that most striate cortical neurons are orientation selective. It has been suggested that the development of orientation sensitivity may be influenced by visual experience, just as the development of ocular dominance is influenced by visual experience.

To test this hypothesis, kittens have been raised in visual environments consisting of stripes of only one orientation, such as a room in which the only visible elements are vertical stripes. After the animals mature, recordings are made from single neurons in striate cortex.

If the orientation of the visual world plays a role in visual development, it is expected that a kitten raised in, for example, a vertical environment will display a disproportionate number of cortical cells selective for vertical stimuli. Although the experimental results are somewhat controversial, it appears that the orientation of the visual environment plays a role in visual development (Blakemore and Cooper, 1970; Stryker and Sherk, 1975; Stryker et al, 1978). Animals raised in an environment consisting of only one orientation have a disproportionately large number of cortical cells sensitive to this orientation, and they have disproportionately few neurons sensitive to other orientations.

What are the clinical implications of these findings? When a mature patient is diagnosed with a substantial amount of astigmatism, it is possible that this astigmatism was present during the critical period (Mohindra et al, 1978). Consequently, the patient's visual system may have developed with one meridian more in focus than others. On the basis of the experimental results discussed earlier, the expectation is that the patient's vision will be best for this meridian and less developed for others.

Consider the following (hypothetical) case of a 14-year-old child who has never been examined previously:

OD   pl   −4.00 × 180   20/25
OS   pl   −4.00 × 180   20/25

This type of refractive error, uncorrected, results in focused vertical gratings and defocused horizontal gratings. If visual resolution is determined for this patient when fully corrected, it may be found that the resolution is better for vertical than for horizontal gratings.[11] This patient manifests **meridional amblyopia** (Mitchell et al, 1973).

Meridional amblyopia occurs when a child progresses through the critical period with one visual meridian focused and the other out of focus. The focused meridian presumably wins in the competition for cortical cells, dominates more cortical cells, and manifests better visual resolution. The blurred meridian loses

---

11. Assume that the astigmatism was present during the critical period.

TABLE 17–1 REFRACTIVE ERRORS EARLY IN LIFE

Age (mo)	Average Spherical Equivalent (D)	Percent With > 1D Astigmatism
1	+2.20	4
1.5	+2.08	6
2.5	+2.44	19
4	+2.03	21
6	+1.79	16
9	+1.32	16
12	+1.57	11
18	+1.23	9
24	+1.19	6
30	+1.25	9
36	+1.00	5
48	+1.13	4

Data from Mayer et al (2001).

this competition, drives disproportionately few cortical cells, and manifests relatively poor resolution.

Meridional amblyopia is seen commonly in clinical practice. Patients with high degrees of astigmatism, when first corrected, often have slightly reduced visual acuity. (Over time, the acuity of these patients tends to reach normal levels.) Certain optotypes are especially difficult for these patients to resolve, dependent on the meridian affected. For instance, compound myopic, with-the-rule astigmatism causes horizontal gratings to be out of focus on the retina. Consequently, patients with meridional amblyopia secondary to this refractive error may find it difficult to resolve optotypes such as **E** or **F,** which have substantial horizontal components.[12]

Infants often have astigmatism (Table 17–1). One study showed that half of neonates manifest astigmatism of between 0.75 and 2.00 D (Howland et al, 1983). The axis may depend on the infant's race. Caucasian neonates are likely to show against-the-rule astigmatism, while Chinese neonates are more likely to have with-the-rule (Thorn et al, 1987). The amount of the astigmatism generally decreases over the first 5 to 6 years of life (Gwiazda et al, 1984).

It is unlikely that the low to moderate amounts of astigmatism that are common in neonates lead to meridional amblyopia (Gwiazda et al, 1985). Consequently, it is generally not advisable to optically correct low to moderate amounts of astigmatism in infants. The correction of astigmatism in young,

---

12. There is no clear threshold astigmatic value for the development of meridional amblyopia. In general, the smaller the amount of astigmatism and the earlier that it is corrected, the less likely the development of meridional amblyopia. Since, as previously mentioned, visual acuity tends to recover after the astigmatism is corrected, caution should be exercised in making the diagnosis of meridional amblyopia in patients with corrected astigmatism. Other possible causes for reduced visual acuity (e.g., disease) must be ruled out.

school-age children (4 to 7 years of age) is controversial. It is possible that such a correction could interfere with the normal ocular growth that leads to reductions in astigmatism (emmetropization). However, significant amounts of astigmatism, especially against-the-rule astigmatism, may produce asthenopia (eye strain), which could discourage a child from reading. Based on these various considerations, it is probably best to consider prescribing lenses for young, school-age children if the astigmatism shows no signs of abating and is at least 2.00 D.

PERCEPTUAL CONSEQUENCES OF BILATERAL VISUAL DEPRIVATION

As discussed previously, early monocular visual deprivation leads to profound changes in striate cortex physiology, with resultant amblyopia and loss of stereopsis. What is the effect of bilateral visual deprivation that occurs early in life and continues until maturity? What would a person whose otherwise healthy eyes were occluded from birth see when the occlusion was removed as an adult? There are a few such cases reported in the literature.

Consider the case of S.B., who developed corneal opacities early in life and had vision surgically restored with a corneal transplant at the age of 52 (Gregory, 1974). (Because the opacities did not entirely occlude S.B.'s vision, he had rudimentary vision.) Following the corneal transplant, this patient learned simple visual tasks, such as recognizing letters; however, his vision was profoundly disturbed. Consider the following quote from Gregory (1974):

> He would look at a lamp post, walk round it, stand studying it from a different aspect, and wonder why it looked different and yet the same. . . . He found traffic frightening, and would not attempt to cross even a comparatively small street by himself (p. 111).

This patient had not learned to see an object as being the same regardless of the perspective from which it is viewed, and had difficulty interpreting motion and depth. This case is interesting because it demonstrates the effects that deprivation early in life can have on higher-level visual functions (e.g., form recognition, motion perception) that presumably involve higher cortical areas (see Chap. 15).[13]

DEVELOPMENT OF REFRACTIVE ERRORS

Myopia: Nature versus Nurture

The etiology of myopia has been the subject of intense speculation and investigation for at least a century. For many years, there has been a vigorous debate

---

13. Patients born with dense bilateral cataracts that are removed within the first 187 days of life appear to have permanently reduced ability to discriminate among similar faces, a task that also apparently involves higher coritical areas (LeGrand et al, 2001).

between the advocates of two seemingly opposing theories. The advocates of the nature theory contend that myopia is an inherited condition. Supporters of the nurture theory believe that environmental factors (e.g., prolonged near work) cause myopia. Recent research suggests that both nature and nurture play a role in the development of myopia.

Strong support for a hereditary origin of myopia comes from studies on identical (monozygotic) twins. Such twins, when mature, tend to manifest highly correlated refractive errors (Teikari et al, 1988; Hammond et al, 2001). Other evidence for the heritability of myopia includes the finding that myopic parents are more likely to have myopic children than are parents who are not myopic (Gwiazda et al, 1993).

Most growth of the eyeball occurs during the first 6 years of life. However, myopia is relatively uncommon when children enter school (2 percent of 6-year-old children are myopic), but increases in prevalence throughout the school years (15 percent of 15-year-old children are myopic) (Mutti et al, 1996). This observation has lead to the suspicion that environmental factors, such as prolonged near work, may cause myopia (Saw et al, 2002).

Although prolonged near work appears to be associated with myopia, such correlation does not prove that the near work causes myopia. (Children grow taller during their school years, but attending school does not cause children to grow.) Much of contemporary research in myopia has been aimed at determining if near work causes myopia in certain individuals or is merely associated with the development of myopia.

Support for an environmental role in the development of myopia received much impetus from the finding that suturing an animal's eyelid closed at birth, or optically blurring the retinal image early in life, leads to the development of axial myopia (Wiesel and Raviola, 1977; Raviola and Wiesel, 1978; Siegwart and Norton, 1993). These results not only demonstrate that environmental factors may play a role in the development of myopia, but also suggest that a focused retinal image may be required for normal ocular growth leading to emmetropia.

Additional support for the role of environmental factors comes from experiments in which infant monkeys were raised wearing either minus lenses or plus lenses over one of their eyes (Hung et al, 1995). An eye raised with a minus lens may compensate for this defocus by maturing to a longer axial length than it would have otherwise. Consequently, when the minus lens is removed, the mature eye is myopic. Likewise, an eye that wears a plus lens during development matures to a shorter axial length than it would have otherwise, and is hyperopic when the lens is removed.[14] This and similar experiments demonstrate that the development of emmetropia (emmetropization) is an active process (Wildsoet and Wallman, 1995).

A fairly unambiguous conclusion is that a clear retinal image promotes emmetropization. It has been posited that myopia develops in certain children

---

14. By removing the blurring lens for a little as 1 hour per day, the development of refractive errors secondary to optical defocus can be prevented (Smith et al, 2002).

who do not fully accommodate to near objects, and thereby suffer chronic near blur (Gwiazda et al, 1993). According to this theory, the eye's axial length increases in an attempt to obtain a focused image, causing myopia. It has long been suspected that plus lenses at near, in the form of bifocals or progressive lenses, may lead to a clearer retinal image and forestall the development of myopia (Wallman and McFadden 1995). Recent research, however, seems to indicate that such lenses may have only a minimal impact on the development of myopia (Gwiazda et al, 2003).

Development of Refractive Errors in Humans

It is important to know the course of development of refractive errors from birth through maturity so that the clinician can be aware of what is normal when he or she examines a child. Unfortunately, studies have led to inconsistent results due to the various techniques used to determine the refractive error (i.e., cycloplegia versus noncycloplegia, retinoscopy versus photorefraction). In general, these studies reveal that typical healthy humans are born with or develop a slight amount of hyperopia (less than 2.50 D) during the first year of life (Slataper, 1950; Dobson et al, 1981; Mohindra and Held, 1981). This degree of hyperopia tends to decrease throughout childhood and should not normally be corrected (see Table 17-1) (Howland and Sayles, 1987; Mayer et al, 2001).

The correction of refractive errors in infants and toddlers is controversial because lenses could potentially interfere with emmetropization. For instance, the prescription of minus lenses for myopia could conceivably lead to near defocus, thereby promoting the development of additional amounts of myopia (Hung et al, 1995). There is evidence, however, that the spectacle correction of clinically significant amounts of hyperopia in infants does not interfere with emmetropization (Atkinson et al, 2000).[15] Given the current state of knowledge, lenses should be prescribed for infants and toddlers only after careful consideration of both the benefits that may accrue from the correction (e.g., clear vision, reduced asthenopia, prevention of amblyopia) and the potential interference with the emmetropization process that may result.

DEVELOPMENT OF GRATING ACUITY

The resolution acuity of a 1-month-old infant, as measured behaviorally with spatial gratings, is on the order of 20/600. Adult levels are reached by about 3 to 5 years of age (Teller, 1997). Grating acuity in infants (and other nonverbal patients) has been assessed using several different procedures that do not require the patient to respond verbally. These procedures are discussed next.

---

15. In Atkinson et al (2000), infants with a correction equal or greater than +3.50D in at least one meridian were classified as having significant hyperopia.

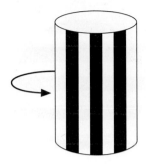

FIGURE 17–8. A drum with stripes is rotated to elicit an optokinetic nystagmus response.

Optokinetic Nystagmus

A moving grating produces a (involuntary) nystagmus, referred to as optokinetic nystagmus (OKN), which consists of a slow following movement (smooth pursuit) followed by fast compensatory eye movement (saccade). A rotating drum that displays a grating can be positioned along the patient's visual axis to produce OKN (Fig. 17–8).

Optokinetic nystagmus is presumably dependent on the ability to resolve the grating. If the grating cannot be resolved, the OKN response may not be elicited. OKN has been used to assess visual capabilities in uncooperative patients including infants, malingerers, hysterics, and the mentally retarded.

Some caution is necessary when interpreting OKN results. It is not established that OKN relies on the same pathways as conscious visual perception (Van Sluyters et al, 1990). Therefore, it is conceivable that a patient could have impaired vision, yet show a normal OKN response.

Preferential Looking

When given a choice between a patterned and nonpatterned stimulus, infants prefer to view the patterned stimulus (Fig. 17–9A). This behavior is referred to as **preferential looking (PL)** (Teller, 1979; Teller and Movshon, 1986).

Preferential looking can be used to determine an infant's grating acuity. The infant typically sits on a parent's lap and views stimuli, as illustrated in Fig. 17–9B. Both the patterned and nonpatterned stimuli have the same average luminance, eliminating luminance as a cue. The examiner is located behind the stimulus display and views the infant's eyes through a peephole. By observing the infant's direction of gaze, the examiner guesses which side the pattern is on. The positions of the patterned and nonpatterned stimuli are randomly interchanged; therefore, the examiner does not know which side the pattern is on and must rely on observation of the child's gaze to determine its location. If the examiner is required to guess which side the pattern is on, the procedure is referred to as **forced-choice preferential looking (FPL).**

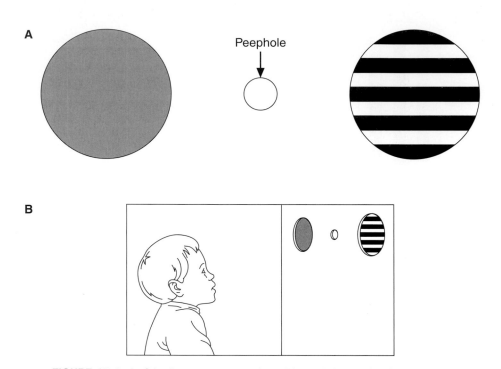

FIGURE 17–9. A. Stimulus arrangement viewed by an infant during forced choice preferential viewing. The examiner observes the infant's eyes through the peephole and guesses which side of the panel contains the grating. (The other side of the panel consists of uniform gray equal in luminance to the grating.) **B.** An infant participating in preferential viewing. The examiner is located behind the stimulus display and views the child's eyes through the peephole.

Several trials are conducted at each of a large number of spatial frequencies, and the results plotted in the form of a psychometric function, similar to that given in Fig. 17–10. The percentage correct for the highest spatial frequencies is 50 percent, which represents chance performance for a two-alternative forced choice (2AFC) procedure (i.e., the infant cannot resolve the spatial frequency gratings). As the spatial frequency decreases, the percentage correct increases. As discussed in Chapter 11, threshold is represented by the point midway between chance performance and 100 percent performance. For a 2AFC procedure, this is 75 percent correct. The spatial frequency that elicits 75 percent correct performance represents the infant's grating acuity.

Although the information provided by FPL is valuable for research purposes, the procedure is time consuming. An alternative form of preferential looking involves the use of Teller acuity cards (McDonald et al, 1985). These rigid, rectangular, hand-held cards have a peephole in the center, with a grating to one side of this peephole. The other side of the card contains no pattern, but has the same average luminance. If the infant looks at the grating, it is assumed that he

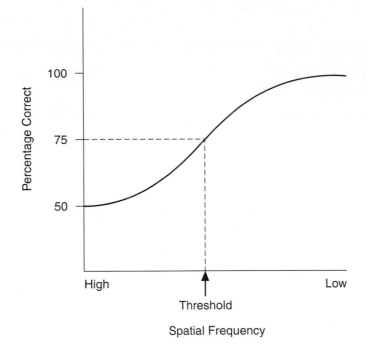

FIGURE 17–10. Psychometric function for a two-alternative forced choice preferential viewing task.

or she can resolve it. Presenting a grating several times is often sufficient to determine if it can be resolved. (The location of the grating can be switched by flipping the card over.) To measure an infant's acuity, the clinician presents gratings of increasing frequency until the infant does not consistently tend to the location of the grating.[16] While the results with Teller acuity cards may be similar to those obtained with the more stringent FPL method, relatively low test-retest reliability limits their effectiveness in diagnosing subtle reductions in acuity that may be associated with clinically significant amblyopia (Dobson, 1993; Teller 1997).

As indicated in Table 17–2 and Fig. 17–11, studies with Teller acuity cards reveal that healthy 1-month-old infants have acuities of about 20/600 (1 cycle/degree) (Mayer et al, 1995). Resolution acuity improves rapidly during the first year of life, with 1-year-old children manifesting acuities of about 20/100 (6 cycles/degree). This is followed by a slower improvement in acuity: adult levels of 20/20 acuity are not reached until 3 to 5 years of age, a finding that is consistent with common clinical experience. Immaturities in the retina, particularly the foveal cones, apparently account for the poor acuity of infants during the first year of life (Abramov et al, 1982; Brown et al, 1987; Banks et al, 1988).

16. Teller acuity cards have also been used to ascertain visual acuity in nonresponsive nursing home residents (Friedman et al, 2002).

TABLE 17–2. MONOCULAR VISUAL ACUITY EARLY IN LIFE

Age (mo)	Average Visual Acuity
1	20/638
1.5	20/540
2.5	20/278
4	20/224
6	20/106
9	20/88
12	20/93
18	20/70
24	20/63
30	20/52
36	20/28
48	20/24

Data from Mayer et al (1995). For binocular acuities see Salomão and Ventura (1995).

Visually Evoked Potentials

Visually evoked potentials (VEPs) give results that are at variance with those obtained with FPL (Norcia and Tyler, 1985; Teller and Movshon, 1986). Whereas FPL suggests that adult levels of resolution acuity are reached between 3 and 5

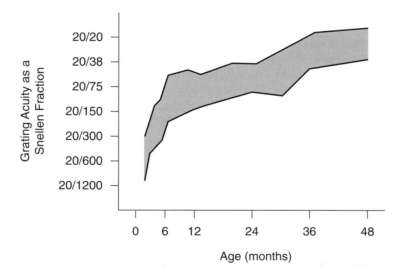

FIGURE 17–11. Monocular visual acuity as a function of age as determined with Teller Acuity Cards. The shaded area shows the 95 percent prediction limits (Mayer et al, 1995).

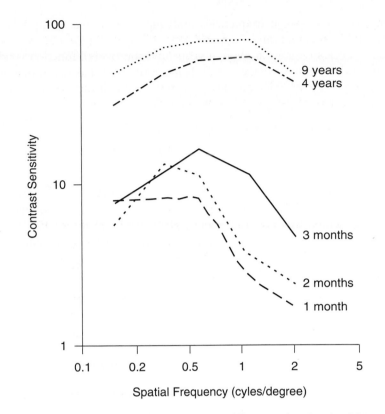

FIGURE 17–12. The contrast sensitivity function shifts upward and to the right as an infant matures, reaching adult form and location at about 9 years of age (Banks and Salapatek, 1978; Adams and Courage, 2002).

years of age, VEPs show adult levels at 6 to 8 months.[17] The different results obtained with FPL and VEPs may be related to the greater cognitive demands associated with FPL (Dobson and Teller, 1978).

DEVELOPMENT OF OTHER VISUAL ATTRIBUTES

Contrast Sensitivity

Figure 17–12 illustrates contrast sensitivity functions (CSFs) at various ages. Note that the CSF for 1-month old infants does not have a band-pass form, suggesting that the lateral interconnections within the retina, which are responsible for lateral inhibition, have not yet fully developed. As infants mature, the CSF assumes a band-pass form and shifts to the right and upward, indicating increased contrast

---

17. Infant visual acuity has been measured with the VEP techniques discussed in Chapter 16 as well as the sweep VEP, where various spatial frequencies are presented in rapid succession (Norcia and Tyler, 1985).

sensitivity for most spatial frequencies and improved visual acuity (Banks and Salapatek, 1978; Movshon and Kiorpes, 1988). The peak of the CSF is at the adult location (~4 cycles/degree) at about 4 years, and the overall function is adult-like by 9 years (Adams and Courage, 2002). Limitations in spatial vision that are present during the first year of life are due primarily to immaturities of the retina rather than the central visual pathways (i.e., the cortex) (Hawken et al, 1997).

Vernier Acuity

Preferential looking reveals that vernier acuity, a form of hyperacuity, matures rapidly during the first year or so of life (similar to grating acuity). It then develops more slowly, reaching adult levels at slightly older ages (~6–8 years of age) than grating acuity (Manny and Klein, 1984; 1985; Kiorpes, 1992). Because vernier acuity is thought to depend on cortical processing, it is not surprising that it reaches adult levels later in life, paralleling the slow maturation of the cortex (Ciuffreda et al, 1991; Levi, 1992).

Stereopsis

Preferential looking can be used to determine if infants respond to stimuli that produce retinal disparity (see Chap. 10). Although few infants manifest stereopsis prior to 3 months of age, it has a rapid onset between 3 and 6 months (Birch et al, 1982; Teller, 1982). Stereoacuity matures rapidly thereafter, often reaching 1 minute of arc by 6 months (Held et al, 1980; Held, 1993).

Temporal Vision: Critical Flicker Fusion Frequency

Whereas spatial vision (i.e., grating and vernier acuity) takes years to reach adult levels, the critical flicker fusion frequency is 40 Hz at 1 month of age and reaches adult levels of about 55 Hz by 3 months (Regal, 1981). The retinal and cortical immaturities that slow the development of grating and vernier acuity apparently have little effect on the maturation of temporal resolution.

Scotopic Sensitivity

The form of the scotopic sensitivity function is adult-like at 1 month of age (Powers et al, 1981). This is not surprising because the shape of the function is determined by the absorption characteristics of rhodopsin and does not depend on postreceptoral processing. The absolute sensitivity of the scotopic system (i.e., the sensitivity for a stimulus of 507 nm presented under conditions that maximize scotopic sensitivity) apparently reaches adult levels by about 6 months of age (Hansen and Fulton, 1993).

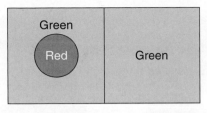

FIGURE 17-13. This stimulus array can be used in a preferential viewing paradigm to assess an infant's ability to discriminate colors. The backgrounds on both the left and right panels are the same color, but not the circle. Infants naturally look at the more interesting panel, which would be the left *if* the infant can discriminate between the colors. If the luminance of the circle can be adjusted so that the infant does not have a preference, he or she does not have wavelength-based discrimination.

Color Vision

Preferential viewing has been used to examine both red–green and blue–yellow color discrimination (Fig. 17–13). Rudimentary red–green discrimination arises during the second month of life (Adams et al, 1990; Allen et al, 1993). Discrimination is worse for smaller stimuli, probably due to poor spatial summation secondary to retinal immaturities (Loop et al, 1979; Packer et al, 1984). Although some investigators find adult-like levels of red–green chromatic discrimination at the end of the first year of life, other researchers provide evidence that chromatic discrimination (both red-green and blue-yellow) improves until adolescence (Morrone et al, 1993; Kelly et al, 1997; Knoblauch et al, 2001). Visually evoked potentials suggest that the photopic spectral sensitivity function is adult-like in young infants (Bieber et al, 1995).

The emergence of blue–yellow color discrimination is less well understood. Certain studies have found crude blue–yellow discrimination in 2-month-old infants, whereas other studies suggest a slower time course for the development of this aspect of color vision (Teller et al, 1978; Varner et al, 1985).

Face Processing

Are infants capable of discriminating one face from another? Consider the stimuli in Fig. 17–14. At 6 months of age, human infants are capable of discriminating between two monkey faces, as well as two human faces (Pascalis et al, 2002). In comparison, older infants (9 months old) and adults are less capable of discriminating between the two monkey faces, revealing that the ability to distinguish among faces becomes more specialized as an infant matures. This suggests that there may be a critical period for the development of face recognition.

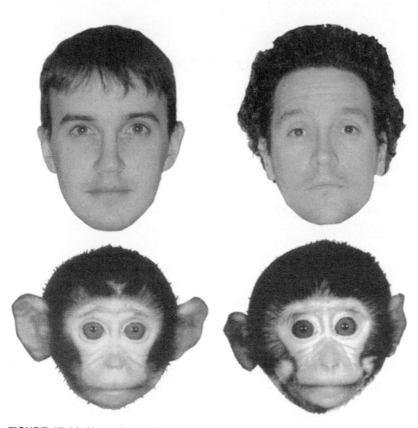

FIGURE 17-14. Not only can 6-month old human infants discriminate between the two human faces, they can also discriminate between the two monkey faces. The ability to distinguish between the monkey faces decreases as the infant ages. (*This figure was kindly provided by Dr. Olivier Pascalis.*)

Summary of Visual Development

Figure 17–15 summarizes the development of various visual attributes in infants and children. Although vision is rudimentary at birth, substantial improvements occur early in life, with certain attributes such as the CFF and the forms of the scotopic and photopic sensitivity functions showing adult-like characteristics within the first 6 months. Other attributes, including stereopsis and color vision, emerge within the first 3 months of life and probably approach adult levels within the first year or so. Grating and vernier acuity improve rapidly during the first year, but then slowly mature until the child is 3 to 5 and 6 to 8 years old, respectively.

The different rates of maturation for the various visual functions are consistent with the notion that each has a different critical period (Harwerth et al, 1987; Levi and Carkeet, 1993). For instance, the critical period for the development of stereopsis may terminate at a younger age than the critical period for the development of vernier acuity.

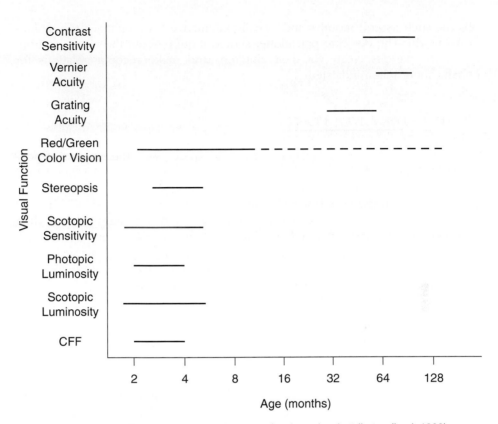

FIGURE 17–15. Time frame for development of various visual attributes (Levi, 1992). The solid lines indicate the period over which adult or near-adult levels of performance are obtained. The dashed line shows that red/green color vision may continue to develop until adolescence.

CLINICAL CONSIDERATIONS

If the developing visual system does not receive normal visual input, it does not develop properly. Conditions such as anisometropia, strabismus, cataracts, and ptosis may produce visual deprivation that can lead to permanent visual loss in the form of amblyopia. Because the visual system becomes hard-wired early in life, it is important that these amblyogenic conditions be diagnosed and treated at the earliest possible time. This necessitates eye examinations early in life.

It is unfortunate that some practitioners continue to inform concerned parents that their children must be of school age before they can be examined. Objective clinical tests can be used to assess the ocular status of nonverbal infants and toddlers. Retinoscopy, the cover and Hirschberg tests, ophthalmoscopy, and other procedures can reveal the presence of conditions that, if treated in a timely manner, are preventable causes of severe visual loss.

Given our current understanding of visual development, it is reasonable to recommend that infants be exposed to a rich visual environment. Visually complex objects, such as crib mobiles and visually interactive toys, enhance the infant's visual world. The eye care practitioner should inquire about the visual environment that parents create for their children, and make recommendations for enhancement when indicated.

VISION IN THE LATER YEARS

The elderly population in America is growing rapidly, with the number of people over 65 years of age increasing by a factor of eleven between 1900 and 1997 and expected to double again by 2030 (Haegerstrom-Portnoy et al, 1999). The rate of growth in the population 85 years and older is even greater. With regard to vision and aging, it has been said that, "things start out badly [infants], then they get better; then, after a long time, they get worse again" (Teller and Movshon, 1986, p. 1483). The changes in visual function that occur with aging can be secondary to ocular disease or can occur in the absence of obvious disease. Some of these are discussed in the following sections.

Contrast Sensitivity

Contrast sensitivity typically remains relatively unchanged until the age of 65 years, declining more rapidly past this age (Haegerstrom-Portnoy et al, 1999). Both senile miosis and nuclear sclerosis probably contribute to reduced contrast sensitivity (Owsley et al, 1983). The aging of neural elements, both retinal and more central, may also play a contributing role.

Are there practical implications of the age-related reduction in contrast sensitivity? For patients who have had undergone cataract removal with subsequent intraocular lens implantation, the rate of automobile accidents is half that of patients who have not undergone the procedure (Owsley et al, 2002). Although this may be related to improvements in contrast sensitivity following the surgery, other factors probably play a role.

Senile Miosis. The pupil becomes smaller and less responsive with age, a condition referred to as senile miosis. A typical 20-year-old has a pupil diameter of about 5.3 mm, whereas a 60-year-old has a pupil diameter of about 3.2 mm (Owsley et al, 1983). Due to the reduction in pupil area, a 60-year-old individual receives one third of the retinal illumination of a 20-year-old. That is, when a 20-year-old looks through a neutral density filter with an optical density of 0.48, the amount of light falling on his or her retina is the same as for a 60-year-old. This reduction in retinal illumination has consequences for visual function, potentially contributing to diminished contrast sensitivity and impaired color discrimination.

An advantage of a small pupil is that it acts as a pinhole, increasing the patient's depth of field (Schwartz, 2002). Therefore, patients with senile miosis often report less reliance on their spectacles, particularly under high illumination that mitigates the loss of light due to reduced pupillary area.

Nuclear Sclerosis. While the crystalline lens of a young adult is colorless, the elderly patient's lens typically appears yellow. The age-related yellowing of the the crystalline lens nucleus, which is readily observed during slit lamp biomicroscopy, is referred to as nuclear sclerosis.

As discussed in Chapter 2, the young crystalline lens absorbs ultraviolet light, which damages it. As the lens ages, this damage accumulates, leading it to absorb increasing amounts of blue light (and appear yellow). The increased lenticular absorption reduces retinal illumination, causing reductions in contrast sensitivity and color discrimination (Weale, 1992).

It is likely that the same (or a similar) process that leads to nuclear sclerosis also leads to senile nuclear cataracts. These cataracts occur at younger ages in populations with substantial exposure to ultraviolet radiation. For this reason, and because ultraviolet radiation may accelerate the development of certain retinal diseases (e.g., age-related macular degeneration), it is important to recommend that patients of all ages wear lenses with ultraviolet filters when outdoors (Weale, 1983).

Resolution Acuity

High levels of visual acuity are usually maintained until at least 65 to 70 years of age (Haegerstom-Portnoy et al, 1999). Thereafter, the data are ambiguous, with some studies showing a gradual decline at older ages, and other studies indicating a more precipitous decline (Slataper, 1950; Kahn et al, 1977). Recent results are summarized in Fig. 17–16. The same factors that contribute to the reduction in contrast sensitivity also play a role in the age-related reduction in visual acuity.

Although visual acuity as normally measured in the clinic—high-contrast acuity—is relatively unaffected through the eighth decade, this is not true for less-than-optimal lighting conditions (see Fig. 17-16). Visual acuity measured under conditions of reduced contrast, reduced illumination, or added glare shows marked reductions in the elderly, especially in the very old (Haegerstrom-Portnoy et al, 1999). The time it takes for visual acuity to recover following exposure to a bright light (**disability glare recovery)** also increases with age (Fig. 17–17).

Visual Fields and Increment Sensitivity

The increment thresholds that are used to measure visual fields are typically determined at light levels where Weber's law is followed (see Chap. 3). Because senile miosis and nuclear sclerosis reduce the retinal illumination produced by the increment and background by the same amount, the Weber fraction ($\Delta I/I_B$) remains unchanged.

Useful Field of View

Elderly people are more likely to be involved in automobile accidents than younger people (Ball and Owsley, 1991). Why is this the case? Age-related

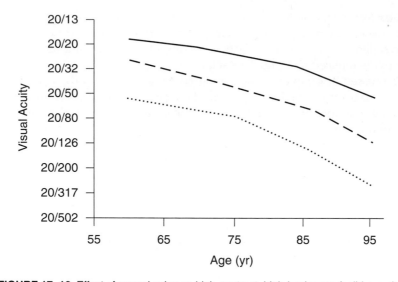

FIGURE 17–16. Effect of normal aging on high-contrast, high-luminance (solid curve), low-contrast, high-luminance (dashed curve), and low-contrast, low luminance visual acuity (dotted curve) (*Data from Haegerstrom-Portnoy et al, 1999*).

declines in visual acuity and other traditional measures of visual function (e.g., contrast sensitivity) may not fully explain this finding and might not be effective for predicting which elderly drivers are at risk for involvement in an automobile accident (Shinar and Schieber, 1991). It has been suggested that an attention-based measure of visual function—the *useful field of view (UFV)*—may be useful for making such predictions (Ball et al, 1993).

In traditional visual field testing, increment thresholds are determined across the visual field (see Chap. 3). This test is exceedingly important for the diagnosis of many ocular and neurological conditions. However, traditional visual fields do not characterize the usefulness of the patient's field of vision. That is, a patient may have a normal visual field, yet not be able to effectively process information presented within this field of vision.

The UFV test requires the patient to divide his or her attention between two stimuli. The task is to *identify* a centrally (foveally) fixated target, while also identifying or detecting a target presented in the peripheral visual field.

Although the standard visual field remains relatively unchanged with increasing age, the UFV decreases, particularly beyond the age of 50 years (Fig. 17–18) (Haegerstrom-Portnoy et al, 1999). There are data suggesting that the size (extent) of the UFV can predict which elderly drivers are more likely to be involved in automobile accidents, with patients manifesting a small UFV more likely to be involved (Ball et al, 1993). This illustrates how clinical psychophysical testing may be used to predict visual function in the patient's natural environment.

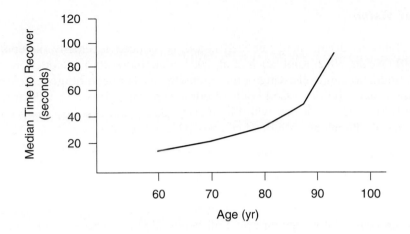

FIGURE 17-17. The amount of time it takes for visual acuity to recover following exposure to a bright light source increases with age beyond about 60 years (*Haegerstrom-Portnoy et al, 1999*).

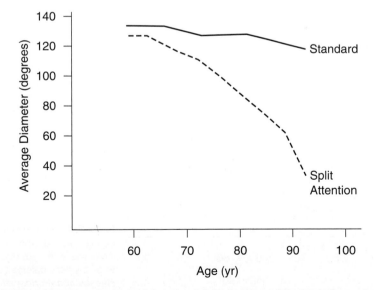

FIGURE 17-18. The diameter of the visual field remains relatively unchanged with age when measured by standard methods, but decreases when divided (split) attention is required *(Data from Haegerstom-Portnoy et al, 1999)*.

Color Vision

The ability to discriminate between colors is reduced in elderly patients (Fig. 17–19) (Weale, 1992; Knoblauch et al, 2001; Shinomori, 2001). Reduction in retinal illumination and yellowing of the crystalline lens are contributory factors. For the most part, the decreased color discrimination manifests as a shift toward a tritan (blue–yellow) defect, with blue-yellow discriminations becoming increasingly more difficult as an individual ages (Hagerstrom-Portnoy et al, 1999).

Temporal and Motion Aspects of Vision

Although not exhaustively studied, it appears that sensitivity to temporal modulation decreases in the ageing eye at all temporal frequencies (Mayer at al, 1988; Casson et al, 1993). There are concomitant reductions in temporal resolution, as measured by the CFF (Lachenmayr et al, 1994). The ability to detect motion, as measured by minimum displacement thresholds, has also been demonstrated to diminish with age (Wood and Bullimore, 1995). Data showing reductions in preferred speed for neurons in the aged rat cortex suggest a neural origin for the changes in motion perception (Spear et al, 1994; Mendelson and Wells, 2002).

Stereopsis

The elderly manifest decreased stereopsis (Fig. 17–20). Stereoacuity thresholds typically become increasingly elevated beyond the age of 50 years (Wright and Wormald, 1992; Haegerstrom et al, 1999).

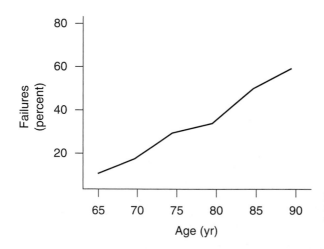

FIGURE 17-19. The percentage of people failing the D-15 test increases with age, due primarily to blue-yellow defects (*Data from Haegerstrom-Portnoy et al, 1999*).

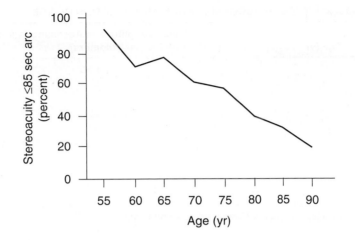

FIGURE 17-20. The percentage of people with steroacuity thresholds equal or better than 85 seconds decreases with age (*Data from Haegerstrom-Portnoy et al, 1999*).

Presbyopia

The ability to accommodate decreases with age (Table 17–3) (Donders, 1864). When this reduction in accommodation produces symptoms such as blur and eyestrain when reading, it is referred to as presbyopia. Symptoms are usually first noticed when patients are in their mid-40s. Presbyopia is one of the primary reasons patients seek eye care.

Although somewhat controversial, it appears that one factor in the development of presbyopia is decreased elasticity of the lens capsule (Weale, 1992). When the ciliary muscle constricts, it releases tension on the lens zonules and capsule, allowing the lens to bulge anteriorly (see Fig. 2–2). The decreasing elasticity of the aging lens capsule presumably interferes with this process. Presbyopia can be treated with convex (plus) lenses that compensate for the loss of near dioptric power.

Astigmatism

The aging crystalline lens shows increasing dioptric power in the horizontal meridian relative to the vertical meridian. Clinically, this manifests as a gradual shift from with-the-rule to against-the-rule astigmatism as the eye ages (Morgan and Rosenbloom, 1993).

TABLE 17–3 AMPLITUDE OF ACCOMMODATION AS A FUNCTION OF AGE

Age (y)	Typical Amplitude of Accommodation (diopters)
10	12.50
20	9.75
30	7.25
40	4.00
50	2.50
60	1.25
70	0.50
75	0.00

Extrapolated from the data of Donders (1864) and Duane (1912) This table is From Schwartz, *Geometrical and Visual Optics: A Clinical Introduction* (2002).

Summary of Vision in the Later Years: Clinical Considerations

As the population ages, eye care practitioners will see increasing numbers of elderly patients. These patients should be educated with regard to expected changes in their visual capabilities and the manner in which these changes can affect their daily activities. Eye care practitioners should make practical recommendations that enable patients to enhance their visual environment.

One factor all too often overlooked by patients and doctors alike is the proper use of light. In this chapter, we stressed that reduction in retinal illumination is an important factor in reducing visual function in elderly patients. It cannot be overemphasized that elderly patients need sufficient light to maximize their visual capabilities. Patients should be questioned with respect to the lighting conditions they use for various tasks. On the basis of the patient's visual status, work, and hobbies, specific practical recommendations should be made.

Q Self-Assessment Questions

1. An infant has a high spatial frequency cutoff of 4 cycles/degree. Express the visual acuity as a Snellen function.

2. At the age of 20 years, a patient's pupillary diameter is 7 mm. At age 70 years, this same patient's pupillary diameter is 2 mm. **A.** Calculate the percentage reduction in the amount of light reaching the patient's retina. **B.** What is the optical density of a neutral density filter, which when placed in front of the 20-year-old eye, will reduce the light level to that experienced by the 70-year-old eye?

3. A 4-year-old child who has never worn spectacles has the following refraction and corrected acuities:

OD	plano	20/20
OS	+3.00 DS	20/200

   A. Given that all other ocular findings are unremarkable, what is your diagnosis? **B.** Would you expect this patient's stereoacuity to be normal? **C.** Provide a treatment plan for the patient.

4. A 30-year-old patient presents with a dense cataract in the left eye. The patient claims that this cataract has been present for the past 15 years. Following cataract extraction, the best-corrected acuity in the left eye is 20/1000. Assuming that the left eye is otherwise healthy and has never suffered trauma, and that there are no neurological issues or postsurgical complications, provide an explanation for this reduction in acuity.

5. A 10-year-old child undergoes strabismus surgery to correct a congenital constant right eye esotropia. The child has received no previous treatment and the presurgical acuity in the deviated eye is 20/1000. **A.** Do you expect the child to regain normal or near-normal acuity in the right eye following surgery? **B.** What degree of stereopsis is expected following the surgery?

A Answers to Self-Assessment Questions

1. A. Photophobia, squinting, poor daytime vision, reduced visual acuity ($\approx$ 20/200), nystagmus, poor fixation.
   B. Long-pass sunglasses (red) are helpful because long wavelength light is least effective at bleaching rhodopsin.

2. Locate these wavelengths on the photopic and scotopic spectral sensitivity functions. The 507- and 555-nm stimuli are equally bright under photopic conditions only when the 507-nm stimulus has more energy. (This is because the photopic system is less sensitive to 507 nm than to 555 nm.) If the intensities of these two equally bright stimuli are decreased by equal amounts, the 507-nm stimulus continues to contain more energy. Under scotopic conditions, the 507-nm stimulus appears brighter because it has more energy and because the scotopic system is more sensitive to 507 nm than to 555 nm.

3. The scotopic visual system is most sensitive to 507 nm because this wavelength is most effective at bleaching rhodopsin.

4. A. Red, because threshold detection of 610 nm, after 20 minutes of dark adaptation, is mediated by the cones.
   B. The 465-nm stimulus has no color after 20 minutes of dark adaptation because it is detected by the scotopic system.

5. A. About 4 log units (photochromatic interval).
   B. About 0.5 log unit (photochromatic interval).

6. A. After 1.5 minutes, 50 percent of the photopigment has regenerated and 50 percent remains bleached. Over the next 1.5 minutes, 50 percent of the remaining photopigment recovers. Consequently, the total amount of cone photopigment that recovers after 3 minutes is 50 percent plus 25 percent, or 75 percent.
   B. The rod–cone break occurs at about 35 minutes. The half-life for rhodopsin regeneration is 5 minutes. Therefore, after 5 minutes, 50 percent has regenerated. And after 10 minutes, 75 percent has regenerated. Carrying out this calculation to 35 minutes shows that at this time 99.22 percent of the rhodopsin has regenerated.

7. A. Although the cones are more sensitive after 11 minutes of dark adaptation, the rods are capable of detecting the stimulus if it is sufficiently intense. According to Fig. 3–9B, the stimulus would need to be on the order of 6 relative log units to be detected by the rods. (Note that after 5 minutes of dark adaptation, the rods could not detect the stimulus because their threshold approaches infinity.)
   B. The cones plateau at about 3.75 relative log units. They maintain this same threshold at 20 minutes (and beyond).
   C. The difference between the cone and rod plateaus is about 3 log units.

8. A. The 507-nm patch is brighter because it results in more quantal absorptions by rhodopsin.
   B. Both patches have the same brightness because they bleach the same number of rhodopsin molecules.

CHAPTER 4.
PHOTOMETRY

1. Formula:

(number of watts) (visual efficiency) (680 lumens/watt) = number of lumens

Solve for number of watts:

$$(\text{number of watts}) \ (0.62) \ (680 \text{ lumens/W}) = 1000 \text{ lumens}$$
$$\text{number of watts} = 2.37 \text{ W}$$

A

2. Use the formula from Problem 4–1 to calculate the number of lumens for each wavelength. Abney's law allows the addition of these amounts to determine the total number of lumens.

500 nm: (10 W) (0.35) (680 lumens/W) = 2380 lumens
550 nm: (5 W) (1.00) (680 lumens/W) = 3400 lumens
650 nm: (20 W) (0.10) (680 lumens/W) = 1360 lumens
Total = 7140 lumens

3. Observe $V'(\lambda)$. There are 680 scotopic lumens/W at 555 nm. The number of scotopic lumens per watt at other wavelengths is determined by a proportionality factor.

500 nm: (10 W) (1.0/0.4) (680 scotopic lumens/W) = 17,000 scotopic lumens
550 nm: (5 W) (0.50/0.40) (680 scotopic lumens/W) = 4250 scotopic lumens
650 nm: (20 W) (0) (680 scotopic lumens/W) = 0 scotopic lumens
Total = 21,250 scotopic lumens

4. Seventy foot-candles fall on a probe that measures 3 × 3 cm. The area of this probe is 0.0097 ft^2. Therefore,

$$(70 \text{ lumens/ft}^2) (0.0097 \text{ ft}^2) = 0.67 \text{ lumens.}$$

5. Place a filter with the transmission characteristics of the $V(\lambda)$ function in front of the probe. The device would then need to be calibrated.

6. $E = I/d^2$

$E = 100 \text{ lumens}/(2\text{ft})^2 = 25 \text{ lumen/ft}^2$ or 25 foot-candles

Convert to lux:

$$(25 \text{ foot-candles}) (10 \text{ lux/foot-candle}) = 250 \text{ lux}$$

7.

$$E_1 = E_2$$
$$I_1/d_1^2 = I_2/d_2^2$$
$$50 \text{ cd}/(1 \text{ ft})^2 = X/(3 \text{ ft})^2$$

$$X = 450 \text{ cd}$$

A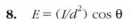

8. $E = (I/d^2) \cos \theta$

As lux is metric, convert distance to meters:

$$2 \text{ ft} = 0.6096 \text{ m}$$

Substitute:

$$100 = I/(0.6096)^2 (\cos 60)$$
$$I = 74.32 \text{ cd}$$

9.
$$OD = \log (1/T)$$
$$OD = \log (1/0.25)$$
$$OD = 0.60$$

10. Combined OD = 0.50 + 1.0 = 1.5

$$OD = \log(1/T)$$
$$1.5 = \log(1/T)$$
$$10^{1.5} = 1/T$$
$$31.62 = 1/T$$
$$T = 0.032$$
$$\text{Percent transmitted} = (100)(0.032) = 3.2\%$$
$$\text{Percent absorbed} = 100 - 3.2 = 96.8\%$$

11.
$$L = rE$$
$$50 = 0.7E$$
$$E = 71.43 \text{ foot-candles}$$

12. $(25 \text{ cd}) (4\pi \text{ lumens/cd}) = 314 \text{ lumens}$

13. $L = rE$
Convert 100 lumens/m² to foot-candles:

$$(100 \text{ lumens/m}^2) \left(\frac{1 \text{ foot-candle}}{10 \text{ lumens/m}^2} \right) = 10 \text{ foot-candles}$$

$$L = rE$$
$$5 = r(10)$$
$$r = 0.5$$

A

CHAPTER 5.
COLOR VISION

1. The observer will behave as a monochromat because he or she continues to have only one photopigment. (If, however, the observer compares vision with the red sunglasses to vision without the red sunglasses, he or she will behave as a dichromat.)

2. A. About 500 nm.
   B. About 0.64.
   C. A nonspectral purple.

3. A. About 595 nm.
   B. About 0.50.
   C. About 480 nm.

4. Illuminant D_{65}, because it has a higher color temperature, appears more blue than illuminant A. That is, relative to illuminant D_{65}, illuminant A appears reddish yellow. This is consistent with the location of illuminant D_{65} in the "blue corner" of the CIE diagram; illuminant A is located relatively closer to the red–yellow region of this diagram.

5. A. Trichromacy of vision.
   B. Paints, when mixed together, produce a subtractive color mixture. This subtractive mixture is less bright than any of the original paints. Consequently, mixing of paints produces a dim color. This can be alleviated by brightly illuminating the picture. Alternatively, access to more than three primaries allows the artist to optimize brightness, as well as to match hues.

6. A red filter (or almost any colored filter) would be useful. The metameric match, which the camouflaged clothing produces with the background, holds up only under normal viewing conditions. When viewed with a colored filter, which results in a subtractive color mixture, the metameric match no longer holds.

A ⸻

7. The invariant hues presumably represent those wavelengths that perfectly balance one of the opponent color channels. For example, 578 nm perfectly balances the red–green channel and stimulates only the yellow channel. As the stimulus intensity increases, the red–green channel remains "neutralized," and there is no change in hue.

CHAPTER 6.
ANOMALIES OF COLOR VISION

1. A. Typically, yes.
   B. The number on the plate is not seen by a color-defective patient because it is a metameric match with the background. The red filter forms a subtractive mixture with the plate and eliminates the metamerism, enabling the color-defective patient to see the number. Another way to think of this is that a combined filter and retinal photopigment absorption spectrum is displaced from that of the photopigment alone. Consequently, the original metameric match no longer holds.

2. A. No.
   B. Top mixture field appears red and the bottom test field appears black.
   C. The red filter transmits only the longer wavelengths that emerge from the anomaloscope (subtractive mixture). Consequently, for the top mixture field, only red is transmitted. For the bottom test field, little or no light is transmitted.

3. A. Yes.
   B. Both the mixture and test field appear green.
   C. Exposure of the eye to a red light produces a disproportionate bleaching of erythrolabe. The result is that subsequently viewed objects appear relatively more green. This is true for the mixture and test fields that initially appeared yellow. They remain metamers, but now appear green.

4. A. 670 nm is matched by a very dim yellow test field, whereas 546 nm is matched by a relatively bright test field.
   B. The scotopic spectral sensitivity curve peaks at 510 nm; consequently, 546 nm is brighter than 670 nm.

A

CHAPTER 7.
SPATIAL VISION

1. A. The visual acuity is 20/15. First, calculate the minimum angle of resolution (MAR):

$$15/20 = 0.75'\text{ arc}$$

Therefore, the size of the threshold detail is 0.75′ arc. This means each bar of the grating subtends 0.75′ arc (see Fig. 7–19). If each bar subtends 0.75′ arc, then a cycle of a grating (a dark and bright bar together) subtends 1.50′ arc. Convert this to cycles/degree:

$$\left(\frac{1\text{ cycle}}{1.5'\text{ arc}}\right)\left(\frac{60'\text{ arc}}{1\text{ degree}}\right) = 40\text{ cycles/degree}$$

  B. 7.5 cycles/degree.
  C. 4.0 cycles/degree.

2. A. The contrast sensitivity function cutoff is 5 cycles/degree. If the grating has 5 cycles in one degree, then each cycle must subtend one fifth of a degree. Each cycle of a grating consists of both a bright and dark bar. The bars themselves represent the detail of the grating (see Fig. 7–19). Therefore, the detail is one half of one cycle of the grating, or (1/2)(1/5 degree) = 1/10 degree. This is the MAR in degrees. We must convert this MAR to minutes of arc:

$$\left(\frac{1}{10}\text{ degree}\right)\left(\frac{60'\text{ arc}}{1\text{ degree}}\right) = 6'\text{ arc}$$

The MAR is 6′ arc. Because the acuity measurement is at 20 feet, the Snellen fraction is 20/120 (120/20 = 6′ arc). An alternative solution involves recalling that a 20/20 acuity corresponds to 30 cycles/degree. Five cycles/degree represents a MAR six times as large (30/5 = 6) as does an acuity of 20/20. Therefore, the Snellen fraction corresponding to 5 cycles/degree is 20/120.
  B. 20/30.
  C. 20/10.

3. The visual acuity is 20/100.

A. By definition, the threshold letter subtends 5′ arc overall at 100 feet. The tangent relationship is used to calculate the letter's physical size. First, convert 5′ arc to degrees:

$$(5'\ arc) \left(\frac{1\ degree}{60'\ arc} \right) = 0.0833\ degree$$

Next, convert 100 ft to millimeters:

$$(100\ ft) \left(\frac{12\ in}{1\ ft} \right) \left(\frac{25.4\ mm}{1\ in} \right) = 30{,}480\ mm$$

Tangent relationship:

$$\tan (0.0833\ degree) = \frac{overall\ letter\ size}{30{,}480\ mm}$$

$$overall\ letter\ size = 44.31\ mm$$

B. The detail of the letter is one fifth this overall size or

$$(1/5)(44.31\ mm) = 8.86\ mm$$

4. For 20/80, the MAR is 4′ arc (i.e., 80/20 = 4). To maintain a MAR of 4′ arc, the fraction would need to be 10/40.

5. A. The patient's high-frequency cutoff is 30 cycles/degree. This measurement represents a MAR of 1′ arc. This MAR does not change with distance. The size of the stimulus (grating bars or acuity letters) required to produce this MAR will change, but the MAR remains constant. Consequently, the patient's high-frequency cutoff will be 30 cycles/degree at both 20 and 10 ft.

B. As there is 30 cycles/degree, each cycle must subtend 1/30th of a degree. A single bar is one half of a cycle (see Fig. 7–19). Therefore, each bar subtends (1/2)(1/30 degree) = 1/60 degree. We can use the tangent relationship to calculate the size of a bar. First, we must convert the distance to millimeters:

$$(20\ ft) \left(\frac{12\ in}{1\ ft} \right) \left(\frac{25.4\ mm}{1\ in} \right) = 6096\ mm$$

Tangent relationship:

A

$$\tan\left(\frac{1}{60}\right) = \frac{\text{bar width}}{6096 \text{ mm}}$$

$$\text{bar width} = 1.77 \text{ mm}$$

C. The angle is the same as in B, but the distance is now 10 ft. Convert 10 feet to millimeters and substitute as follows:

$$\tan\left(\frac{1}{60}\right) = \frac{\text{bar width}}{3048 \text{ mm}}$$

$$\text{bar width} = 0.89 \text{ mm}$$

This means that to obtain 30 cycles/degree, the bars used at 10 feet are one half the size as those used at 20 feet. The key is to recognize that the angle of resolution remains constant.

6. A. The measured acuity is expected to be less than 20/20.
B. The overhead lights decrease the contrast of the optotypes on the projected chart, resulting in a reduction in visual acuity.

CHAPTER 8.
TEMPORAL ASPECTS OF VISION

1. 20 Hz = 20 cycles/s. Each cycle is 1/20th of a second or 0.05 second. One half of a cycle is the on-phase; its duration is (1/2)(0.05) = 0.025 second. Convert to milliseconds:

$$(0.025 \text{ s}) (1000 \text{ ms/s}) = 25 \text{ milliseconds}$$

2. A total cycle is 40 milliseconds, or 1 cycle/40 ms. Convert to hertz:

$$(1 \text{ cycle/40 ms}) (1000 \text{ ms/s}) = 25 \text{ cycles/s or 25 Hz}$$

3. The percentage modulation, $(A/I_{ave})(100)$, remains constant at low frequencies as I_{ave} is increased. Because the amplitude (A) remains a constant fraction of the background illumination (I_{ave}), Weber's law is followed (see Chap. 11)

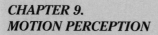

CHAPTER 9.
MOTION PERCEPTION

1. Cortical activity can be measured in alert human subjects with functional magnetic resonance imaging (fMRI) or positron emission tomography (PET). As described in Chapter 15, the subject views a moving object while cortical activity is measured. The level of cortical activity is then measured when the same object is stationary. The difference in activity between the moving and stationary conditions is presumably greatest in those cortical areas that are involved in motion perception.

CHAPTER 10.
DEPTH PERCEPTION

1. Because monovision contact lenses interfere with stereopsis, we need to consider the importance of stereopsis for flying an airplane. Many of a pilot's visual tasks are performed at far distances. At these far distances, stereopsis is of little or no value because objects would need to be separated by great linear distances to produce a threshold disparity. For comparatively close tasks, such as a visual landing, stereopsis may play a role.

CHAPTER 11.
PSYCHOPHYSICAL METHODOLOGY

1. A Perfect performance = 100%.
   Chance performance = 33%.
   B. Perfect performance = 100%.
   Chance performance = 20%.

2. Forced choice methodology is preferable because different criteria may be used for the detection of stable and flickering gratings.

CHAPTER 12.
FUNCTIONAL RETINAL PHYSIOLOGY

1. Gratings are optimal stimuli for ganglion cells, which have evolved to detect contrast. The various spatial frequencies may be coded by ganglion cells with various receptive field dimensions. That is, low spatial frequencies may be coded by peripheral ganglion cells with large receptive fields, and high frequencies may be coded by foveal ganglion cells with small receptive fields.

2. The receptive fields of foveal ganglion cells are smaller than those of peripheral ganglion cells. These smaller foveal receptive fields manifest less spatial summation, but higher spatial resolution, than the larger peripheral receptive fields.

3. The antagonistic surround of ganglion cells is less apparent under dark adaptation. This allows greater spatial summation with a resultant increase in sensitivity (and reduction in resolution) (Barlow et al, 1957).

CHAPTER 13.
PARALLEL PROCESSING

1. Cats respond to movement but may ignore stationary objects. This presumably reflects a highly developed "where" system and a less well developed "what" system.

2. The color detection function is expected to manifest reduced sensitivity relative to the flicker detection function.

3. Visual acuity targets are high spatial frequency targets. If glaucoma initally affects the magno pathway, which codes low spatial frequencies, it is unlikely to result in reduced visual acuity. (As it progresses, glaucoma results in reduced acuity due to damage to the parvo system.)

4. This procedure assumes that magno neurons code luminance and that all magno neurons have the same spectral sensitivity. The first assumption is controversial. The second assumption is not correct; not all magno neurons demonstrate the same spectral sensitivity (Cavanagh, 1991).

CHAPTER 14.
STRIATE CORTEX

1. Injection of a radioactive tracer into the optic nerve of one eye at various stages of development would provide such information.

2. *Left cell:* A red light falling on the cell's receptive field center, surrounded by a green annulus on the surround, would elicit maximum excitation. *Right cell:* A green light falling on the cell's receptive field center, surrounded by a red annulus falling on the surround, would elict maximum excitation.

3. See Chapters 12, 13, and 14.

CHAPTER 15.
INFORMATION STREAMS AND EXTRASTRIATE PROCESSING

1. If the tilt aftereffect is mediated by binocular cortical neurons, it should be transferrable from one eye to the other eye. That is, if a subject stares at lines tilted slightly counterclockwise with his or her left eye, vertical lines subsequently viewed with the right eye should appear tilted clockwise. If an effect does not show interocular transfer, it is probably mediated by monocular neurons located lower in the visual system (e.g., dLGN). (As discussed in Chapter 17, the tilt aftereffect does show interocular transfer.)

A

CHAPTER 16.
GROSS ELECTRICAL POTENTIALS

1. Visually evoked potential (VEP). If the VEP is normal, the visual pathways are intact up through at least primary visual cortex.

2. A patient with a lesion in the higher visual centers could manifest a normal electrooculogram, electroretinogram, and visually evoked potential because these tests sample the visual system at lower levels.

3. The evoked potential is primarily a foveal response. Aversion of gaze will result in a reduced potential.

4. The pattern electroretinogram (PERG) test retinal function, whereas the VEP tests cortical function. Amblyopia affects the cortex, not the retina. Consequently, the VEP is abnormal, and the PERG is normal.

CHAPTER 17.
DEVELOPMENT AND MATURATION OF VISION

1. Each cycle = 1/4 degree
Each half-cycle = 0.5/4 degree
Convert to minutes of arc:

$$\left(\frac{0.5}{4} \text{ degree}\right)\left(\frac{60' \text{ arc}}{\text{degree}}\right) = 7.5'$$

Convert to a Snellen fraction:

$$\text{visual acuity} = 20/150$$

(See Chap. 7 for a detailed discussion of these calculations.)

A

2. A. Twenty-year-old patient:

$$r = 3.5 \text{ mm}$$
$$A_1 = \pi r^2$$
$$A_1 = \pi (3.5)^2$$
$$A_1 = 12.15\pi$$

Seventy-year-old patient:

$$r = 1 \text{ mm}$$
$$A_2 = \pi r^2$$
$$A_2 = \pi (1)^2$$
$$A_2 = \pi$$

Percentage reduction:

$$(A_1 - A_2)/A_1 = (12.25\ \pi - \pi)/12.25\pi = 92\%$$

B. $OD = \log(1/T)$

$T = \pi/12.25\pi$

$T = 0.0816$

$OD = \log(1/T)$

$OD = 1.09$

3. A. Anisometropic amblyopia of the left eye.
  B. No. The expected reduction in binocular cortical neurons results in reduced stereoacuity.
  C. i. Fully correct the refractive error.
   ii. Encourage use of left eye by part-time patching of the right eye.
   iii. Prescribe orthoptics which require the simultaneous use of both eyes.
   iv. Carefully monitor the patient's progress.

4. As there are no indications of disease or injury, the left eye may be amblyopic. However, a cataract that develops at 15 years of age does not produce amblyopia. Perhaps the cataract was present earlier in life, during the critical period, but was cosmetically noticeable at age 15.

5. A. No. The child is past the critical period.
  B. Very poor stereopsis. No binocular cortical cells have developed.

P Practice Examination 1

This examination consists of 57 items. For each item, select the single best answer.

1. What percentage of the eye's refractive power is provided by the cornea?
    a. 25 percent
    b. 33 percent
    c. 50 percent
    d. 67 percent

2. The nonphotosensitive pigment that covers the surface of the macula lutea shows maximal absorption for
    a. blue light
    b. green light
    c. yellow light
    d. red light

3. The thickness of the retina is about
    a. 0.02 mm
    b. 0.20 mm
    c. 2.00 mm
    d. 20.00 mm

4. UV C is absorbed primarily by the
    a. cornea
    b. crystalline lens
    c. RPE

P

5. A rod monochromat views the following four patches of monochromatic light: 440 nm, 510 nm, 555 nm, and 565 nm. Each patch produces 20 quantal absorptions. Which is brightest?

      a. 440 nm

      b. 510 nm

      c. 555 nm

      d. 565 nm

      e. all of the above are equally bright

6. Threshold contrast, under photopic conditions, is closest to

      a. 1.000

      b. 0.100

      c. 0.010

      d. 0.001

7. The rod-cone break of the dark adaptation curve will be most prominent when the stimulus is

      a. foveal and green

      b. foveal and orange

      c. nonfoveal and green

      d. nonfoveal and orange

8. Consider the region of the light adaptation curve that follows Weber's law. As the background intensity decreases, contrast sensitivity

      a. decreases

      b. increases

      c. remains constant

9. Assume that the absorption of 10 quanta of 510 nm by rhodopsin results in vision. If the wavelength was 450 nm, how many quanta would need to be absorbed to produce vision?

      a. 10 quanta

      b. < 10 quanta

      c. > 10 quanta

P ――――――――――――――――――――――――

10. One patient has a pupil diameter of 8 mm and another has a pupil diameter of 4 mm. How much more light reaches the retina of the eye with the larger pupil (compared to the eye with the smaller pupil)?

    a. 2X

    b. 4X

    c. 6X

    d. 8X

11. Appropriate units for luminous power, illuminance, and luminance are, respectively

    a. candelas, candelas/m^2, lumens/m^2

    b. candelas, foot-candelas, foot-lamberts

    c. candelas, foot-lamberts, foot-candles

    d. lumens, foot-lamberts, foot-candles

    e. lumens, foot-candles, foot-lamberts

12. You are asked to measure the lighting conditions in a classroom to determine if they are adequate. The lighting conditions should be specified in which of the following units?

    a. lumens/m^2

    b. candelas/m^2

    c. lumens

    d. candelas

13. When measured at an angle of 30 degrees to its surface, a matte surface with a reflectance factor of 0.70 has a luminance of 50 foot lamberts. What is the luminance when measured perpendicular to the surface?

    a. 25 foot-lamberts

    b. 43 foot-lamberts

    c. 50 foot-lamberts

    d. 75 foot-lamberts

P ━━━━━━━━━━━━━━━━━━━━━━━━━━━━━━━━━

14. A subject views two patches of light. One patch consists of an additive mixture of 475 and 510 nm, and the other patch consists of an additive mixture of 490 and 520 nm. By adjusting the intensities of each of the wavelengths that constitute these patches, the subject is able to perfectly match the two patches. The subject:

    a. must be a monochromat

    b. must be a dichromat

    c. must be a trichromat

    d. could be either a dichromat or trichromat

    e. could be either a monochromat, dichromat, or trichromat

15. An isoluminant grating consists of red and green bars. Compared to the red bars, the green bars have:

    a. greater radiance

    b. less radiance

    c. greater luminance

    d. less luminance

16. Which of the following is not a perceptual attribute of color?

    a. hue

    b. colormetric purity

    c. saturation

17. The colorimetric purity of a monochromatic patch of 440 nm is closest to

    a. 1.00

    b. 0.75

    c. 0.50

    d. 0.25

    e. 0.00

P

18. The following five pairs of wavelengths are viewed by a trichromat. Which pair contains wavelengths that appear most similar to each other?

     a. 485 nm, 490 nm

     b. 490 nm, 495 nm

     c. 585 nm, 590 nm

     d. 590 nm, 595 nm

     e. 640 nm, 645 nm

19. A sample has chromaticity coordinates of $y = 0.6$ and $z = 0.1$. What is the dominant wavelength of this sample?

     a. 470

     b. 490

     c. 510

     d. 550

     e. 590

20. What is the dominant wavelength of a mixture that consists of 33 percent of 490 nm and 66 percent of 580 nm?

     a. 480 nm

     b. 500 nm

     c. 510 nm

     d. 520 nm

     e. 560 nm

21. A yellow background is used when performing short-wavelength automated perimetry because this background

     a. increases the absolute sensitivity of the S-cones

     b. suppresses the S-cones

     c. suppresses the M-and L-cones

22. According to Kollner's rule, age-related macular degeneration is most likely to result in which type of color vision defect?

     a. deutan

     b. protan

     c. tritan

P ───────────────────────────

23. A deuteranomalous trichromat adjusts the Nagel anomaloscope so that the mixture and test fields match each other. He subsequently stares at a large green light and then views his original match. He will report that:

    a. the two fields are no longer matched to each other for hue

    b. the two fields are no longer matched to each other for brightness

    c. the two fields remain perfectly matched to each other

24. Screening for red/green defects in children is important because such a defect could

    a. affect later career choices

    b. develop into a monochromacy

    c. develop into tritanomaly

    d. be reversed with available treatments

25. Which of the following pairs of colors is least likely to be confused by a deutan?

    a. purple and green

    b. purple and blue

    c. red and yellow

    d. red and blue

26. A protanomalous trichromat makes a match on the Nagel anomaloscope. When viewed by a normal trichromat, the mixture field appears:

    a. green

    b. red

    c. achromatic

27. The bright bar of a sine wave grating has a luminance of 90 foot-lamberts, and the dark bar has a luminance of 30 foot-lamberts. The contrast of the grating is

    a. 0.25

    b. 0.33

    c. 0.50

    d. 0.75

    e. 1.00

P ────────────────────────────────

28. All of the gratings listed below have equally low contrast. Which is most visible?
    a. 10 cycle/deg sine wave grating
    b. 20 cycle/deg sine wave grating
    c. 30 cycle/deg sine wave grating
    d. 40 cycle/deg sine wave grating

29. Prior adaptation to a sine wave grating of 5 c/d will result in a subsequent reduction of a sensitivity at
    a. 5 c/d
    b. 10 c/d
    c. 15 c/d
    d. "a" and "b" are both correct
    e. "a" and "c" are both correct
    f. "b" and "c" are both correct

30. Which of the following acuities is most related to increment threshold?
    a. resolution
    b. recognition
    c. minimum detectable
    d. vernier

31. What prevents our visual world from disappearing when we fixate an object?
    a. lateral inhibition
    b. optical defocus
    c. spatial antagonism
    d. small, involuntary eye movements

32. The CFFs for a given percentage modulation are 2.5 and 50 Hz. A stimulus of 55 Hz, presented at this given percentage modulation, is seen as
    a. steady
    b. flickering
    c. either steady or flickering

P ━━━━━━━━━━━━━━━━━━━━━━━━━━━━━━━━━━

33. Which of the following is a pictorial cue to depth?

    a.   accommodation

    b.   convergence

    c.   motion parallax

    d.   texture

34. During monocular ophthalmoscopy, you notice a small brown spot. When using the iris as a reference, motion parallax shows with-motion. The brown spot is most likely located on the

    a.   cornea

    b.   iris

    c.   posterior surface of the lens

35. Compared to a lax criterion, a strict criterion results in (relatively)

    a.   few false positives and many hits

    b.   few false positives and few hits

    c.   many false positives and many hits

    d.   many false positives and few hits

36. When determining a threshold, which psychophysical method minimizes the importance of a subject's criterion?

    a.   staircase

    b.   adjustment

    c.   forced choice

    d.   constant stimuli

    e.   descending limits

37. In frequency doubling, what appears to double?

    a.   the spatial frequency of the stimulus

    b.   the temporal frequency of the stimulus

    c.   both "a" and "b"

P ─────────────────────────

38. The depolarization that occurs under the myelin sheath of a ganglion cell axon is

     a. an action potential

     b. electrotonic spread

     c. "a" and "b" are both correct

39. Which of the following would elicit the largest response in an off-center ganglion cell?

     a. light covering the cell's entire receptive field

     b. darkness covering the cell's entire receptive field

     c. spot of darkness covering only the center of the cell's receptive field

40. Isoluminant gratings, when used in experiments involving human subjects, are thought to be detected by

     a. magno cells

     b. parvo cells

     c. parasol cells

41. With regard to magno cells of the dLGN, which is false?

     a. easily saturate

     b. sensitive to high spatial frequencies

     c. transient neural response

     d. synapse in layer $4C\alpha$ of the cortex

42. Parvo cells constitute what percentage of the nonfoveal ganglion cells?

     a. 10

     b. 30

     c. 40

     d. 90

43. The interblob region of striate cortex receives its primary input from layer
    a. 4B
    b. $4C\alpha$
    c. $4C\beta$

44. The more superficial layers of striate cortex project to
    a. brain stem
    b. higher cortical area
    c. midbrain
    d. both "a" and "c" are correct

45. Double color opponent neurons are located in the
    a. retina
    b. dLGN
    c. striate cortex blobs
    d. V5

46. The inability to recognize faces is referred to as
    a. achromatopsia
    b. alexia
    c. dyslexia
    d. prosopagnosia

47. Which of the following does NOT describe the visual pathway that processes motion?
    a. temporal processing stream
    b. dorsal processing stream
    c. parietal pathway
    d. "where" pathway

P ⸺⸺⸺⸺⸺⸺⸺⸺⸺⸺⸺⸺⸺⸺⸺

48. Which of the following is (are) expected to be abnormal following an episode of optic neuritis?
    a. EOG
    b. standard ERG
    c. VEP
    d. "a" and "b"
    e. "b" and "c"

49. Which of the following is (are) are often abnormal in retinitis pigmentosa?
    a. ERG amplitude
    b. ERG implicit time
    c. both "a" and "b"

50. Which of the following is (are) normal in amblyopia?
    a. EOG
    b. PERG
    c. VEP
    d. "a" and "b"
    e. "a" and "c"

51. The standing potential of the eye is at its maximum:
    a. immediately after the lights are turned off
    b. immediately after the lights are turned on
    c. after 15 minutes of dark adaptation
    d. after 15 minutes of light adaptation

52. Which of the following potentials is least affected by a macular lesion?
    a. full-field ERG
    b. flash VEP
    c. steady state VEP

P ————————————————————————————

53. The prevalence of astigmatism among 5-year-old children compared to 1-year-old children is

    a. the same

    b. less

    c. greater

54. A patient progresses through her critical period with the following refractive error

        OD   - 2.50 DS
        OS   plano

When examined at 12 years of age, this patient will most likely manifest

    a. right eye amblyopia

    b. left eye amblyopia

    c. reduced stereopsis

    d. "a" and "b"

    e. "a" and "c"

    f. "b" and "c"

55. Preferential looking suggests that visual acuity reaches adult levels of maturity at which age?

    a. 0 to 12 months

    b. 13 to 35 months

    c. 36 to 60 months

    d. 61 to 72 months

56. Alternating strabismus, induced by surgery during the critical period of a cat, causes

    a. most of the striate cortical cells to be monocular

    b. most of the striate cortical cells to be binocular

    c. blindness of one of the eyes

    d. "a" and "c"

    e. "b" and "c"

P ━━━━━━━━━━━━━━━━━━━━━━━━━━

57. An otherwise normal adult cat has its right eyelid sutured closed for 1 year. At the end of this year it, is expected that the cat will show

      a.   amblyopia of the right eye

      b.   amblyopia of the left eye

      c.   reduced stereopsis

      d.   no deficits in vision

P Practice Examination 2

This examination consists of 54 items. For each item, select the single best answer.

1. The aqueous humor is located within the
     a. anterior chambers
     b. posterior chamber
     c. vitreous chamber
     d. both "a" and "c" are correct

2. The range for UV A radiation is
     a. 200–280 nm
     b. 280–320 nm
     c. 320–400 nm
     d. 800–2500 nm
     e. 2,500–50,000 nm
     f. 50,000–10^6 nm

3. Which of the following layers of the right dLGN receives input from the right eye?
     a. 1
     b. 2
     c. 4
     d. 6

4. Your patient, a rod monochromat, has asked for advice regarding tinted lenses. You should advise a darkly tinted lens of which color?
     a. red
     b. yellow
     c. green
     d. blue

P

5. What percentage of cone photopigment has regenerated 3.0 minutes following a 100 percent bleaching?

    a. 12.5

    b. 25.0

    c. 50.0

    d. 75.0

    e. 87.5

6. Under scotopic conditions, a blue and yellow flower appear equally bright. Under photopic conditions, which flower will most likely appear brighter?

    a. the blue flower

    b. the yellow flower

    c. the blue and yellow flowers appear equally bright

7. When foveally fixated, a small target (0.5 deg) of which of the following wavelengths will be least visible?

    a. 430 nm

    b. 535 nm

    c. 565 nm

8. A patient has a condition that results in the total elimination of his SWS cones without affecting any other retinal structure. The patient's expected visual acuity is

    a. 20/20

    b. 20/50

    c. 20/100

    d. 20/150

    e. 20/200

9. A patient has degenerative disease that has destroyed her cones. The expected visual acuity for this patient is closest to

    a. 20/20

    b. 20/40

    c. 20/200

    d. 20/1000

P ━━━━━━━━━━━━━━━━━━━━━━━━━━━━━━━━

10. One candela is equal to

     a. 1 lumen per m^2

     b. 1 lumen per steradian

     c. 1 lumen per ft^2

11. A source with which of the following color temperatures will appear most red?

     a. 2000°K

     b. 3000°K

     c. 5000°K

     d. 10,000°K

12. A neutral density filter transmits 35 percent of the light that is incident upon it. The optical density of the filter is closest to

     a. 0.19

     b. 0.46

     c. 0.54

     d. 0.81

13. A mixture of equal amounts of 490 and 560 nm has a dominant wavelength of

     a. 480 nm

     b. 510 nm

     c. 540 nm

     d. 570 nm

14. The excitation purity of a mixture that consists of 75 percent of 500 nm and 25 percent of 550 nm is closest to?

     a. 0.15

     b. 0.25

     c. 0.50

     d. 0.75

     e. 1.00

15. The complement of 580 nm is
    a. 400 nm
    b. 480 nm
    c. 520 nm
    d. 510 nm
    e. 520 nm

16. A patient with which of the following color vision deficiencies is most likely to have a recent history of color naming errors?
    a. deutan
    b. protan
    c. tritan

17. Which of the following pairs of wavelengths appear most similar to a protanope?
    a. 495 nm, 500 nm
    b. 500 nm, 505 nm
    c. 520 nm, 525 nm
    d. 540 nm, 545 nm

18. As the mixture field of the Nagel anomaloscope is adjusted
    a. luminance remains constant
    b. radiance remains constant
    c. both luminance and radiance remain constant

19. A patient is a deuteranomalous trichromat. Our best guess as to the location of the peak of his/her M-cone absorption spectra is
    a. 525 nm
    b. 530 nm
    c. 550 nm
    d. 565 nm
    e. 575 nm

P ————————————————————————————————

20. A women's mother is a deutan and her father and husband have normal color vision. What percentage of her sons are expected to have a color anomaly?

   a. 0 percent

   b. 25 percent

   c. 50 percent

   d. 75 percent

   e. 100 percent

21. The foveola of a red-green dichromat contains how many types of photopigments?

   a. one

   b. two

   c. three

   d. four

22. At a distance of 20 feet, a patient has a CSF that peaks at 4 cycles per degree. When measured at 40 feet, this patient's CSF is expected to peak at

   a. 2 c/d

   b. 4 c/d

   c. 6 c/d

   d. 8 c/d

23. A patient has a Snellen acuity of 10/20. The expected high spatial frequency cut-off is how many cycles per degree?

   a. 5

   b. 10

   c. 15

   d. 20

   e. 25

   f. 30

24. Which of the following is the correct name for an eye chart that consists of letters of constant size and diminishing contrast?

    a. Bailey–Lovie

    b. Bailey–Robson

    c. Pelli–Lovie

    d. Pelli–Robson

25. At a distance of 100 ft, a patient can barely resolve a sine wave grating. The dark bar of this grating has a width of 75.00 mm. What is the expected acuity of this patient when measured at 20 feet?

    a. 20/85

    b. 20/128

    c. 20/150

    d. 20/169

    e. 20/338

26. The disappearance of stabilized retinal images is caused by

    a. lateral inhibition

    b. optical defocus

    c. the Nyguist theorem

    d. involuntary eye movements

27. Under scotopic conditions, the CFF is closest to

    a. 20 Hz

    b. 30 Hz

    c. 40 Hz

    d. 50 Hz

    e. 60 Hz

28. Monovision contact lenses typically cause

    a. stereopsis to improve

    b. stereopsis to become worse

    c. no change in stereopsis

P

29. Which of the following is not a monocular depth cue?
    a. motion parallax
    b. accommodation
    c. convergence
    d. linear perspective

30. Which of the following cues to depth is much more useful at near distances than at farther distances?
    a. interposition
    b. retinal disparity
    c. linear perspective
    d. motion parallax

31. A yes–no experiment consists of 100 trials. The stimulus is present on 80 of the trials. The subject reports seeing the stimulus on 70 trials, and there are 55 hits. How many false alarms are there?
    a. 5
    b. 15
    c. 25
    d. 55

32. Which of the following experiments is expected to result in the least steep (i.e., shallowest) psychometric function?
    a. 2 AFC
    b. 4 AFC
    c. 6 AFC
    d. 8 AFC

33. Which method of determining thresholds is commonly used during auto-mated visual field testing?
    a. adjustment
    b. constant stimuli
    c. forced choice
    d. staircase

P

34. The inert portion of rhodopsin is the
    a. chromophore
    b. opsin
    c. transducin

35. Immediately prior to exposure to a light, the resting potential of a rod is closest to
    a. −30 mV
    b. −50 mV
    c. −70 mV
    d. −90 mV

36. With regard to a conventional flat synapse made by a bipolar cell, which is true?
    a. it is located in the inner plexiform layer
    b. the bipolar cell is on-center
    c. the neurotransmitter is glutamate
    d. both" a" and "b" are true
    e. both "a" and "c "are true
    f. both "b" and "c" are true

37. Intracellular techniques are necessary for recording the activity of
    a. simple cells
    b. bipolar cells
    c. ganglion cells

38. A monkey with a lesion in layers 3, 4, 5, and 6 of its dLGNs will manifest reductions in
    a. contrast sensitivity for low spatial frequencies
    b. high frequency temporal resolution
    c. wavelength based discrimination
    d. both "a" and "b" are correct

P ─────────────────────────────────────

39. Which of the following are part of the magno pathway?
    a. pale stripes
    b. thick dark stripes
    c. thin dark stripes

40. The neurons located in the most dorsal layer the primate dLGN manifest which of the following properties?
    a. color-opponent
    b. transient
    c. maximum sensitivity to low spatial frequencies
    d. rapidly saturate to increasing contrast
    e. both "a" and "d" are correct
    f. both "c" and "d" are correct
    g. "a", "c," and "d" are all correct

41. The receptive fields of which cells cannot be mapped out with small spots of light?
    a. complex
    b. simple
    c. "a" and "b" are correct

42. Cortical cells that receive input from magno neurons are probably
    a. spatially linear
    b. direction selective
    c. position selective

43. Abnormal connections between cortical modules is thought to be the cause of
    a. blindsight
    b. prosopagnosia
    c. achromatoposia
    d. synaesthesia

P ────────────────────────

44. A hypercolumn contains a complete set of
     a. ocular dominance and orientation columns
     b. thin and thick dark stripes
     c. blobs

45. Inferotemporal cortex appears to be involved in the analysis of
     a. form
     b. motion
     c. color

46. The motion aftereffect is associated with activity in which area of the brain?
     a. LGN
     b. striate cortex
     c. V4
     d. V5

47. Which of the following is an example of bottom-up attention?
     a. looking for a friend in a crowd of people
     b. responding to the slamming of a door
     c. searching for quarters in a drawer of loose change

48. Which of the following waves of the ERG is typically the smallest?
     a. a_p
     b. a_s
     c. b_p
     d. b_s

49. The primary contributors to the dark adapted aspect of the EOG are the
     a. cones
     b. rods
     c. cells of the RPE
     d. Muller cells
     e. bipolar cells

P

50. Suturing an animal's eyelid closed at birth is most likely to result in the eye developing
    a. axial hyperopia
    b. axial myopia
    c. refractive hyperopia
    d. refractive myopia

51. The expected corrected visual acuity for a healthy 50 year old is closest to
    a. 20/20
    b. 20/30
    c. 20/50
    d. 20/70
    e. 20/90

52. The prevalence of hyperopia among 5-year-old children, compared to 1-year-old children, is
    a. the same
    b. less
    c. greater

53. FPL reveals an acuity of 5 c/d. What is the equivalent Snellen fraction?
    a. 20/120
    b. 20/240
    c. 20/480
    d. 20/960
    e. 20/1200

54. Which of the following reaches maturity latest in life?
    a. absolute threshold
    b. dark adaptation
    c. grating acuity
    d. stereopsis

P Practice Examination 3

This examination consists of 51 items. For each item, select the single best answer.

1. The length of an average adult human eye is closest to
    a. 5 mm
    b. 10 mm
    c. 15 mm
    d. 20 mm
    e. 25 mm

2. The nuclei of which of the following cells are located innermost in the retina?
    a. amacrine cells
    b. bipolar cells
    c. horizontal cells

3. UV radiation is not a factor in the development of
    a. glaucoma
    b. age-related macular degeneration
    c. cataracts

4. Under daylight conditions, a red and yellow surface look equally bright. Compared to the yellow surface, the red surface most likely emits
    a. less energy
    b. more energy
    c. equal energy

P ——————————————————————

5. Photopic and scotopic thresholds are most similar to each other for which wavelength?

    a. 400 nm

    b. 420 nm

    c. 507 nm

    d. 555 nm

    e. 650 nm

6. The percentage of rhodopsin that is bleached at rod saturation is closest to

    a. 10

    b. 30

    c. 50

    d. 70

    e. 90

7. The photochromatic interval is expected to be smallest for a

    a. centrally fixated 5.0° orange target

    b. centrally fixated 0.5° orange target

    c. peripherally viewed 5.0° orange target

    d. peripherally viewed 0.5° orange target

8. Sensitivity regulation is most associated with the portion of the light adaptation curve that has a slope of

    a. ∞

    b. 1

    c. 1/2

    d 0

9. A neutral density filter transmits 50 percent of 500 nm light that is incident upon it. If 40 watts of 550 nm are incident on the filter, how many watts are transmitted?

    a. 20

    b. 30

    c. 40

P ————————————————————

    d. 340

    e. 680

    f.   1020

10. The color temperature of an incandescent bulb is 3300°K. This means that

    a. the temperature of the bulb is 3300°K

    b. when the bulb is heated to 3300°K, it matches the spectral distribution of a blackbody radiator

    c. the bulb matches the spectral distribution of a blackbody radiator whose temperature is 3300°K

11. In the minimally distinct border method of photometry, the perception of the border is minimized when the two surfaces are matched for

    a. radiant intensity

    b. radiance

    c. luminous intensity

    d. luminance

12. Which of the following classes of cones contributes least to the photopic spectral sensitivity curve?

    a. L-cones

    b. M-cones

    c. S-cones

13. The excitation purity of a mixture that consists of 33 percent of 490 nm and 66 percent of 580 nm is closest to?

    a. .30

    b. .60

    c. .75

    d. .85

    e. 1.0

P ————————————————————————

14. Which of the following hues cannot be produced by monochromatic light?

    a. blue

    b. green

    c. purple

    d. red

    e. violet

15. A rod monochromat views two patches of light. One patch consists of a single wavelength (540 nm) and the other patch consists of an additive mixture of three wavelengths (425 nm, 475 nm, and 510 nm). If the subject is allowed to independently adjust the intensity of each of the wavelengths, which of the following will occur?

    a. The subject will be able to match the two patches after adjusting the intensity of the wavelengths.

    b. The subject will not be able to match the two patches even after adjusting the intensity of the wavelengths.

    c. The two patches will be matched at all intensity settings.

16. As the intensity of a stimulus of 540 nm is decreased, it appears more

    a. blue

    b. green

    c. yellow

    d. red

17. A monochromat compares his vision when looking through a red filter to his vision without a red filter. Using the red filter in this way, the subject will function as if they have

    a. one photopigment

    b. two photopigments

    c. three photopigments

    d. four photopigments

P ─────────────────────────────

18. A protanope is presented with two patches of light. One patch consists of 570 nm and the other of 610 nm. By proper adjustment of their intensity, this subject can match these two patches so that they appear to have the same

    a. brightness

    b. hue

    c. saturation

    d. "a," "b," and "c" are all correct

19. A protanope matches 670 nm to 590 nm in an anomaloscope. When viewed by a normal subject, the 590 nm will appear

    a. brighter than the 670 nm

    b. dimmer than the 670 nm

    c. the same brightness as the 670 nm

20. The expected visual acuity for an adult deuteranope is closest to

    a. 20/20

    b. 20/40

    c. 20/200

    d. 20/1000

21. A deuteranomalous trichromat observes the match made by a normal observer on a Nagel I anomaloscope. To this deuteranomalous trichromat, the mixture field most likely appears

    a. more green than the test field

    b. more red than the test field

    c. the same hue as the test field

22. Which of the following color vision tests is best suited to test a patient suspected of having outer retinal disease?

    a. red-green plate test

    b. anomaloscope

    c. D-15

P ────────────────────────────────

23. A child with normal visual acuity fails a pseudoisochromatic plate test. The most likely diagnosis is

    a. anomalous trichromacy

    b. dichromacy

    c. monochromacy

    d. trichromacy

24. Each dark stripe on an OKN drum has a width of 1 cm. What is the spatial frequency of the drum when viewed at a distance of 2 meters?

    a. 0.88 c/d

    b. 1.75 c/d

    c. 2.63 c/d

    d. 5.25 c/d

    e. 7.88 c/d

25. The adult hyperacuity threshold is closest to

    a. 0.05 min arc

    b. 0.30 min arc

    c. 0.50 min arc

    d. 1.00 min arc

    e. 1.30 min arc

26. A patient has a high frequency CSF cutoff of 35 c/d. At a distance of 10 feet, what is the width of a single dark bar of the smallest grating the patient can resolve?

    a. 0.19 mm

    b. 0.38 mm

    c. 0.57 mm

    d. 0.76 mm

27. Recognition acuity is a form of

    a. hyperacuity

    b. resolution acuity

    c. minimal detectable acuity

P

28. A monocular individual may use which of the following to determine the depth of an object?

    a. motion parallax

    b. stereopsis

    c. angular declination

    d. both "a" and "c" are correct

29. A subject fixates a target (a square) located at a distance of 175 cm. While fixating this square, the subject is aware of a circle located at a distance of 125 cm. This circle

    a. produces crossed retinal disparity

    b. produces uncrossed retinal disparity

    c. is viewed by the fovea of each eye

30. When measuring visual acuity with a typical Snellen visual acuity test, which psychophysical method is typically utilized?

    a. ascending limits

    b. descending limits

    c. adjustment

    d. constant stimuli

    e. staircase

31. Steven's law is based upon the use of

    a. indirect scaling

    b. magnitude estimation

    c. both "a" and "b" are correct

32. A quantum of light is absorbed by rhodopsin. The event immediately preceding the closing of Na+ pores in the rod outer segment is

    a. cGMP $\rightarrow$ GMP

    b. GMP $\rightarrow$ cGMP

    c. all-trans retinal $\rightarrow$ 11-cis retinal

    d. 11-cis retinal $\rightarrow$ all-trans retinal

P

33. With regard to horizontal cells, which is false?
    a. show spatial antagonism
    b. hyperpolarize in response to light
    c. postsynaptic to photoreceptors
    d. manifest spatial summation

34. Which is not a characteristic of on-center bipolar cells?
    a. spatial antagonism
    b. glutamate causes hyperpolarization
    c. presynaptic to ganglion cells
    d. generate action potentials

35. Which of the following would elicit the smallest response (either excitatory or inhibitory) in an on- center ganglion cell?
    a. spot of light covering the cell's entire receptive field
    b. spot of light covering only the center of the cell's receptive field
    c. spot of darkness covering only the center of the cell's receptive field

36. With regard to the invaginating synapse formed by photoreceptors, horizontal cells, and bipolar cells, which is false?
    a. It is located in the outer layer.
    b. The associated bipolar cell is off-center.
    c. The neurotransmitter is glutamate.

37. Cells in which category are always spatially nonlinear?
    a. M-cells
    b. P-cells
    c. X-cells
    d. Y-cells

38. The neurons that constitute the parvo pathway are
    a. noncolor opponent
    b. easily saturated
    c. sustained

P

39. Which of the following does not characterize the receptive field properties of simple cells?
    a. orientation selectivity
    b. spatially linear
    c. position selective
    d. center-surround organization

40. Disparity detectors are found in the
    a. retina
    b. dLGN
    c. cortex

41. Prosopagnosia is often accompanied by
    a. achromatopsia
    b. akinetopsia
    c. object agnosia

42. Which of the following cortical areas is not part of the ventral processing system?
    a. V4
    b. V5
    c. IT

43. In order to maximize the size of the b_p wave of the ERG, the stimulus should be what wavelength?
    a. 450 nm
    b. 500 nm
    c. 550 nm
    d. 600 nm

44. The EOG has an amplitude closest to
    a. 0.01 mV
    b. 0.1 mV
    c. 10 mV
    d. 100 mV

P ━━━━━━━━━━━━━━━━━━━━━━━━━━

45. VEPs suggest that visual acuity reaches adult levels at what age?
    a.   6 to 8 months
    b.   12 to 24 months
    c.   36 to 48 months
    d.   60 to 72 months

46. Which of the following lists the gross potentials in order of increasing voltage?
    a.   ERG, EOG, VER
    b.   VER, ERG, EOG
    c.   VER, EOG, ERG
    d.   EOG, ERG, VER
    e.   ERG, VER, EOG
    f.   EOG, VER, ERG

47. A patient has the following uncorrected refractive error during his critical period

    OD   pl = -3.50 × 090
    OS   pl = -3.50 × 090

    Which of the following may be most difficult to resolve when wearing the correction?
    a.   a horizontal grating
    b.   an oblique grating
    c.   a vertical grating

48. Strabismic amblyopia is most likely to be found in
    a.   exotropia
    b.   esotropia
    c.   esophoria
    d.   exophoria

P

49. The interocular transfer of the tilt aftereffect will be weakest when constant strabismus first develops at which age?
    a. 1 year
    b. 2 years
    c. 3 years
    d. 4 years

50. Which of the following reaches maturity earliest in life?
    a. red-green color vision
    b. stereopsis
    c. vernier acuity
    d. CFF

51. The expected corrected visual acuity for a healthy 70 year-old is closest to
    a. 20/20
    b. 20/40
    c. 20/60

A Answers to Practice Examinations

A Answers to Practice Examinations

PRACTICE EXAMINATION 1

1. D
2. A
3. B
4. A
5. E
6. C
7. C
8. C
9. A
10. B
11. E
12. A
13. C
14. E
15. B
16. B
17. A
18. E
19. D
20. E
21. C
22. C
23. C
24. A
25. D
26. B
27. C
28. A
29. A
30. C
31. D
32. A
33. D
34. C
35. B
36. C
37. A
38. B
39. C
40. B
41. B
42. D
43. C
44. B
45. C
46. D
47. A
48. C
49. C
50. D
51. D
52. A
53. B
54. C
55. C
56. A
57. D

PRACTICE EXAMINATION 2

1. A
2. C
3. B
4. A
5. D
6. B
7. A
8. A
9. C
10. B
11. A
12. B
13. B
14. D
15. B
16. C
17. D
18. A
19. C
20. C
21. A
22. B
23. C
24. D
25. D
26. A
27. A
28. B
29. C
30. B
31. B
32. A
33. D
34. B
35. B

A

36. C	**3.** A	**29.** A
37. B	**4.** B	**30.** B
38. C	**5.** E	**31.** B
39. B	**6.** A	**32.** A
40. A	**7.** B	**33.** A
41. A	**8.** B	**34.** D
42. B	**9.** A	**35.** A
43. D	**10.** C	**36.** B
44. A	**11.** D	**37.** D
45. A	**12.** C	**38.** C
46. D	**13.** A	**39.** D
47. B	**14.** C	**40.** C
48. A	**15.** A	**41.** A
49. C	**16.** B	**42.** B
50. B	**17.** B	**43.** C
51. A	**18.** D	**44.** C
52. B	**19.** B	**45.** A
53. A	**20.** A	**46.** B
54. C	**21.** B	**47.** C
	22. C	**48.** B
	23. A	**49.** A
ANSWERS TO	**24.** B	**50.** D
PRACTICE	**25.** A	**51.** A
EXAMINATION 3	**26.** D	
	27. B	
1. E	**28.** D	
2. A		

References

Abney WW. *Researches in Color Vision and the Trichromatic Theory*. London: Longmans, Green; 1913.

Abramov I, Gordon J, Hendrickson A, et al. The retina of the newborn human infant. *Science*. 1982;217:265–267.

Adams AJ. Impact of new and emerging instrumentation on optometry. *Optom Vis Sci*. 1993;70:272–278.

Adams AJ, Bodis-Wollner I, Enoch JM, et al. Normal and abnormal mechanisms of vision: Visual disorders and visual deprivation. In: Spillman L, Werner JS, eds. *Visual Perception: The Neurophysiological Foundations*. New York: Academic Press; 1990:381–416.

Adams AJ, Haegerstrom-Portnoy G. Color deficiency. In: Amos JF, ed. *Diagnosis and Management in Vision Care*. Boston: Butterworths; 1987.

Adams AJ, Rodic R, Husted R, Stamper R. Spectral sensitivity and color discrimination changes in glaucoma and glaucoma-suspect patients. *Invest Ophthalmol Vis Sci*. 1982;23:516–524.

Adams RJ, Courage ML. Using a single test to measure human contrast sensitivity from early childhood to maturity. *Vision Res*. 2002;42:1205-1210.

Adams RJ, Maurer D, Cashin HA. The influence of stimulus size on newborn's discrimination of chromatic from achromatic stimuli. *Vision Res*. 1990;30:2023–2030.

Adelson EH, Movshon JA. Phenomenal coherence of moving visual patterns. *Nature*. 1982;300:523– 525.

Aguilar M, Stiles WS. Saturation of the rod mechanism of the retina at high levels of stimulation. *Opt Acta*. 1954;1:59–65.

Albright JD. Direction and orientation selectivity of neurons in visual area MT of the macaque. *J Neurophysiol*. 1984;52:1106–1130.

Allen D, Banks MS, Norcia AM. Does chromatic sensitivity develop more slowly than luminance sensitivity? *Vision Res*. 1993;33:2553–2562.

Alpern M, Moeller J. The red and green cone visual pigments of deuteranomalous trichromacy. *J Physiol*. 1977;266:647–675.

Alpern M, Torii S. The luminosity curve of the protanomalous fovea. *J Gen Physiol*. 1968a;52:717–737.

Alpern M, Torii S. The luminosity curve of the deuteranomalous fovea. *J Gen Physiol*. 1968b;52:738–749.

Alpern M, Wake T. Cone pigment in human deutan colour vision defects. *J Physiol*. 1977;266:595–612.

Apple DJ, Rabb MF. *Ocular Pathology: Clinical Applications and Self Assessment*. St. Louis: Mosby-Year Book; 1991.

Applegate RA, Bonds AB. Induced movement of receptor alignment toward a new pupillary aperture. *Invest Ophthalmol Vis Sci.* 1981;21:869–873.

Arden GB, Barrada A. Analysis of the electrooculograms of a series of normal subjects. *Br J Ophthalmol.* 1962;46:468–481.

Arden GB, Barrada A, Kelsey JH. New clinical test of retinal function based upon the standing potential of the eye. *Br J Ophthalmol.* 1962;46:449–467.

Armington JC. *The Electroretinogram.* New York: Academic Press; 1974.

Atkinson J, Anker S, Bobier W, et al. Normal emmetropization in infants with spectacle correction for hyperopia. *Invest Ophthalmol Vis Sci.* 2000;41:3726-3731.

Bailey IL, Lovie JE. New design principles of visual acuity letter charts. *Am J Optom Physiol Opt.* 1976;53:740–745.

Ball K, Owsley C. Identifying correlates of accident involvement in older drivers. *Hum Factors.* 1991;33:583–595.

Ball K, Owsley C, Sloane ME, et al. Visual attention problems as a predictor of vehicle crashes in older adults. *Invest Ophthalmol Vis Sci.* 1993;34:3110–3123.

Ball KK, Sekuler R. A specific and enduring improvement in visual motion discrimination. *Science.* 1982;218:697–698.

Banks MS, Aslin RN, Letson RD. Sensitive period for the development of human binocular vision. *Science.* 1975;190:675–677.

Banks M, Bennett P. Optical and photoreceptor immaturaties limit the spatial and chromatic vision of human neonates. *J Opt Soc Am A.* 1988;5:2059–2079.

Banks M, Salapatek P. Acuity and contrast sensitivity in 1-, 2-, and 3-month-old human infants. *Invest Ophthalmol Vis Sci.* 1978;17:361–365.

Barlow HB. Retinal noise and absolute threshold. *J Opt Soc Am.* 1956;46:634–639.

Barlow HB. Temporal and spatial summation in human vision at different background intensities. *J Physiol.* 1958;141:337–350.

Barlow HB. Optic nerve impulses and Weber's law. *Cold Spring Harb Symp Quant Biol.* 1965;30:539–546.

Barlow HB, Blakemore C, Pettigrew JP. The neural mechanisms of binocular depth discrimination. *J Physiol.* 1967;193:327–342.

Barlow HB, Fitzhugh R, Kuffler SW. Change in organization in the receptive fields of the cat's retina during dark adaptation. *J Physiol.* 1957;137:338–354.

Barmack NH. Dynamic visual acuity as an index of eye movement control. *Vision Res.* 1970;10:1377–1391.

Barnes S, Werblin F. Gated currents generate single spike activity in amacrine cells of tiger salamander retina. *Proc Natl Acad Sci USA.* 1986;83:1509–1512.

Bartley SH. Subjective brightness in relation to flash rate and the light/dark ratio. *J Exp Psychol.* 1938;23:313–319.

Bartley SH. *Vision: A Study of Its Basis.* New York: Hafner; 1963.

Barton JJS, Sharpe JA, Raymond JE. Directional defects in pursuit and motion perception in humans with unilateral cerebral lesions. *Brain.* 1996;119:1535–1550.

Baseler HA, Sutter EE, Klein SA, Carney T. The topography of visual evoked response properties across the visual field. *Electroenceph Clin Neurophysiol.* 1994;90:65-81.

Baylor DA, Nunn BS, Schnapf JL. The photocurrent, noise and spectral sensitivity of rods of the monkey *Macaca fascicularis. J Physiol.* 1984;357:575–607.

Beard BL, Levi DM, Reich LN. Perceptual learning in parafoveal vision. *Vision Res.* 1995;35:1679–1690.

Bearse MA, Sutter EE, Sim D, et al. Glaucomatous dysfunction revealed in higher order components of the electroretinogram. In: *Vision Science and Its Applications, 1996 OSA Technical Digest Series, Vol. 1,* Washington, D.C.: Optical Society of America; 1996:104–107.

Berson DM, Dunn FA, Takao M. Phototransduction by retinal ganglion cells that set the circadian clock. *Science.* 2002;295: 1070-1073.

Berson EL. Electrical phenomena in the retina. In: Hart MH, ed. *Adler's Physiology of the Eye,* 9th ed. St. Louis: Mosby-Year Book; 1992:641–707.

Bieber M, Volbrecht V, Werner J. Spectral efficiency measured by heterochromatic flicker photometry is similar in human infants and adults. *Vision Res.* 1995;35:1385–1392.

Birch E, Gwiazda J, Held R. Stereoacuity development for crossed and uncrossed disparities in human infants. *Vision Res.* 1982;22:507–513.

Birch EE, Stager DR. Monocular acuity and stereopsis in infantile esotropia. *Invest Ophthalmol Vis Sci.* 1985;26:1624–1630.

Birch J. *Diagnosis of Defective Colour Vision.* Oxford: Oxford University Press; 1993.

Bisiach E, Rusconi ML. Breakdown of perceptual awareness in unilateral neglect. *Cortex.* 1990;26:643–649.

Blakemore C, Campbell FW. On the existence of neurones in the human visual system selectively sensitive to the orientation and size of retinal images. *J Physiol.* 1969;203: 237–260.

Blakemore C, Cooper CF. Development of the brain depends on the visual environment. *Nature.* 1970;228:477–478.

Blakemore CB, Van Sluyters RC. Reversal of the physiological effects of monocular deprivation in kittens: Further evidence for a sensitive period. *J Physiol.* 1974;237:195–216.

Bodis-Wollner I, Atkin A, Rabb E, Wolkstein M. Visual association cortex and vision in man: Pattern-evoked occipital potentials in a blind boy. *Science.* 1977;198:629-630.

Bodis-Wollner I, Camisa JM. Contrast sensitivity measurement in clinical diagnosis. In: Lessel S, Van Dalen JTW, eds. *Neuroophthalmology 1980.* Amsterdam: Excerpta Medica; 1980;1:373–401.

Bosworth CF, Sample PA, Weinreb RN. Motion perception thresholds in areas of glaucomatous visual field loss. *Vision Res.* 1997;37:355–364.

Boycott B, Wassle H. Parallel processing in the mammalian retina. *Invest Ophthalmol Vis Sci.* 1999;40:1313-1327.

Boynton RM. Implications of the minimally distinct border. *J Opt Soc Am.* 1973;63:1037– 1043.

Boynton RM. *Human Color Vision.* New York: Holt, Rinehart, and Winston; 1979.

Bradley A, Freeman RD. Contrast sensitivity in anisometropic amblyopia. *Invest Ophthalmol Vis Sci.* 1981;21:467–476.

Brannan JR, Williams MC. The effects of age and reading ability on flicker threshold. *Clin Vision Sci.* 1988;3:137–142.

Breitmeyer BG. *Visual Masking.* New York: Oxford University Press; 1984.

Breitmeyer BG. Parallel processing in human vision: History, review, and critique. In: Brannon H, ed. *Applications of Parallel Processing in Vision.* Amsterdam: Elsevier; 1992:37–38.

Brenner E, Van Damme WJM. Judging distance from ocular convergence. *Vision Res.* 1998;38:493–498.

Broca A, Sulzer D. La sensation lumineuse en fonction du temps. *J Physiol Pathol Gen.* 1902;4:632–640.

Broca A, Sulzer D. La sensation lumineuse en fonction du temps. *J Physiol Pathol Gen.* 1904;6:55–68.

Brown A, Dobson V, Maier J. Visual acuity of human infants at scotopic, mesopic and photopic luminances. *Vision Res.* 1987;27:1845–1858.

Brown KT, Wiesel JW. Localization of origins of electroretinogram components by intraretinal recording in the intact cat eye. *J Physiol.* 1961;158:257–280.

Bullimore MA, Wood JM, Swenson K. Motion perception in glaucoma. *Invest Ophthalmol Vis Sci.* 1993;34:3526–3533.

Burr DC, Morrone MC, Ross J. Selective suppression of the magnocellular visual pathway during saccadic eye movements. *Nature.* 1994:371:511–513.

Calkins DJ, Sterling P. Evidence that circuits for spatial and color vision segregate at the first retinal synapse. *Neuron.* 1999;24:313-321.

Campbell FW, Maffei L. Electrophysiological evidence for the existence of orientation and size detectors in the human visual system. *J Physiol.* 1970;207:635–652.

Campbell FW, Robson JG. Application of Fourier analysis to the visibility of gratings. *J Physiol.* 1968;197:551–566.

Casson EJ, Johnson CA, Nelson-Quigg JM. Temporal modulation perimetry: The effects of aging and eccentricity on sensitivity in normals. *Invest Ophthalmol Vis Sci.* 1993; 34:3096–3102.

Cavanagh P. Vision at equiluminance. In: Kulikowski JJ, Walsh V, Murray IJ, eds. *Limits of Vision.* Boca Raton, FL: CRC Press; 1991:234–250.

Cavanagh P. When colours move. *Nature.* 1996;379:26.

Cavanagh P, MacLeod DIA, Anstis SM. Equiluminance: Spatial and temporal factors and the contribution of blue-sensitive cones. *J Opt Soc Am [A].* 1987;4:1428–1438.

Chapanis A. Spectral saturation and its relation to color-vision defects. *J Exp Psychol.* 1944;34:24–44.

Ciuffreda KJ, Levi DM, Selenow A. *Amblyopia.* Boston: Butterworth-Heinemann; 1991.

Ciuffreda KJ, Tannen B. *Eye Movement Basics for the Clinician.* St. Louis: Mosby; 1995.

Cohen LG, Celnik P, Pascual-Leone A, et al. Functional relevance of cross-modal plasticity in blind humans. *Nature.* 1997;389:180-183.

Corbetta M, Miezin FM, Dobmeyer S, et al. Attentional modulation of neural processing of shape, color, and velocity in humans. *Science.* 1990;248:1556–1559.

Cornsweet T. *Visual Perception.* New York: Academic Press; 1970.

Crawford MLJ, von Noorden GK. Optically induced concomitant strabismus in monkeys. *Invest Ophthalmol Vis Sci.* 1980;19:1105–1109.

Cropper SJ, Derrington AM. Rapid colour-specific detection of motion in human vision. *Nature.* 1996;379:72–74.

Crowley JC, Katz LC. Early development of ocular dominance columns. *Science.* 2000;290: 1321-1324.

Curcio CA, Allen KA. Topography of ganglion cells in human retina. *J Comp Neurol.* 1990; 300:5–25.

Curcio CA, Allen KA, Sloan KR et al. Distribution and morphology of human cone photoreceptors stained with anti-blue opsin. *J Comp Neur.* 1991;312:610-624.

Curcio CA, Owsley C, Jackson GR. Spare the rods, save the cones in aging and age-related maculopathy. *Invest Ophthalmol Vis Sci.* 2000;41:2015-2018.

Curcio CA, Sloan KR, Kalina RE, Hendrickson AE. Human photoreceptor topography. *J Comp Neurol.* 1990;292:497-523.

Dacey DM, Lee BB. The "blue-on" opponent pathway in primate retina originates from a distinct bistratified ganglion cell type. *Nature.* 1994;367:731-735.

Dacey DM, Lee BB, Stafford DK, et al. Horizontal cells of the primate retina: cone specificity without spectral opponency. *Science.* 1996;271:656-659.

Dacheux RF, Raviola E. Physiology of H1 horizontal cells in the primate retina. *Proc R Soc Lond B.* 1990;239:213-230.

Damasio A, Yamada T, Damasio H, et al. Central achromatopsia: Behavioral anatomic and physiologic aspects. *Neurology.* 1980;30:1064–1071.

deLange H. Research into the dynamic nature of the human fovea cortex systems with intermittent and modulated light: II. Phase shift in brightness and delay in color perception. *J Opt Soc Am.* 1958;48:784–789.

DeMonasterio FM, Gouras P. Functional properties of ganglion cells of the rhesus monkey retina. *J Physiol.* 1975;251:167–195.

Derrington AM, Krauskopf J, Lennie P. Chromatic mechanisms in lateral geniculate nucleus of macaque. *J Physiol.* 1984;357:241–265.

Desimone R, Duncan J. Neural mechanisms of selective visual attention. *Ann Rev Neurosci.* 1995;18:193–222.

DeValois RL, Abramov I, Jacobs GH. Analysis of response patterns of LGN cells. *J Opt Soc Am.* 1966;56:966–977.

DeValois RL, Albrecht DG, Thorell LG. Spatial frequency selectivity of cells in macaque visual cortex. *Vision Res.* 1982;22:545–549.

DeValois RL, Morgan HC, Polson MC, et al. Psychophysical studies on monkey vision. I. Macaque luminosity and color vision tests. *Vision Res.* 1974;14:53–67.

DeVries HL. The quantum character of light and its bearing upon threshold of vision, the differential sensitivity and visual acuity of the eye. *Physica.* 1943;10:553–564.

DeYoe EA, Van Essen DC. Concurrent processing streams in monkey visual cortex. *Trends Neurosci.* 1988;11:219–226.

Dixon MJ, Smilek D, Cudahy C, Merikle PM. Five plus two equals yellow. *Nature.* 2000; 406:365.

Dobson V. Visual acuity testing in infants: From laboratory to clinic. In: Simons K, ed. *Early Visual Development: Normal and Abnormal.* New York: Oxford University Press; 1993:318–334.

Dobson V, Fulton AB, Manning K, et al. Cycloplegic refractions of premature infants. *Am J Ophthalmol.* 1981;91:490–495.

Dobson V, Teller D. Visual acuity in human infants: A review and comparison of behavioral and electrophysiological studies. *Vision Res.* 1978;18:1469–1483.

Donders FC. *On the Anomalies of Accommodation and Refraction of the Eye.* London: New Sydenham Society; 1864.

Dowling JE. *The Retina: An Approachable Part of the Brain.* Cambridge, MA: Harvard University Press; 1987.

Dowling JE, Boycott BB. Organization of the primate retina: electron microscopy. *Proc R Soc Lond Biol Sci.* 1966;166:80–111.

Dreher B, Fukada Y, Rodieck RW. Identification, classification and anatomical segregation of cells with X-like and Y-like properties in the lateral geniculate nucleus of old-world primates. *J Physiol.* 1976;258:433–452.

Einthoven W, Jolly WA. The form and magnitude of the electrical response of the eye to stimulation by light at various intensities. *Q J Exp Physiol.* 1908;1:373–416.

Engel S, Zhang X, Wandell B. Colour tuning in human visual cortex measured with functional magnetic resonance imaging. *Nature.* 1997;388:68–71.

Enoch JM, Birch DG. Inferred positive phototropic activity in human photoreceptors. *Philos Trans R Soc Lond Biol Sci.* 1981;291:293–303.

Enoch JM, Fry GA. Characteristics of a model retinal receptor studied at microwave frequencies. *J Opt Soc Am.* 1958;48:899–911.

Enroth-Cugell C, Robson JG. The contrast sensitivity of retinal ganglion cells of the cat. *J Physiol.* 1966;187:517–552.

Fain GL, Mathews, HR. Calcium and the mechanism of light adaptation in vertebrate photoreceptors. *Vis Neurosci.* 1990;10:981–989.

Famiglietti EV, Kolb H. Structural basis for ON- and OFF-center responses in retinal ganglion cells. *Science.* 1976;194:193–195.

Fechner GT. *Elemente der Psychophysik.* Leipzig: Breitkopf und Hartel; 1860.

Ferry ES. Persistence of vision. *Am J Sci.* 1892;44:192–207.

Fiorentini A, Berardi N. Perceptual learning specific for orientation and spatial frequency. *Nature*. 1980;287:43–44.

Flom MC, Weymouth FW, Kahneman D. Visual resolution and contour interaction. *J Opt Soc Am*. 1963;53:1026–1032.

Friedman D, Munoz B, Massof RW, et al. Grating visual acuity using the preferential-looking method in elderly nursing home residents. *Invest Ophthalmol Vis Sci*. 2002;43:2572-2578.

Fuster JM, Jervey JP. Inferotemporal neurons distinguish and retain behaviorally relevant features of visual stimuli. *Science*. 1981;212:952–955.

Gale CR, Hall NF, Phillips DIW, Martyn CN. Lutein and zeaxanthin status and risk of age-related macular degeneration. *Invest Ophthalmol Vis Sci*. 2003;44:2461-2465.

Gallant JL, Braun J, Van Essen DC. Selectivity for polar, hyperbolic, and cartesian gratings in macaque visual cortex. *Science*. 1993;259:100–103.

Gegenfurtner KR, Mayser H, Sharpe LT. Seeing movement in the dark. *Nature*. 1999;398-399.

Gilbert CD. Laminar differences in receptive field properties of cells in cat primary visual cortex. *J Physiol*. 1977;268:391–421.

Goebel R, Muckli L, Zanella FE,, et el. Sustained extrastriate cortical activation without visual awareness revealed by fMRI studies of hemianopic patients. *Vision Res*. 2001;41:1459-1474.

Goldstone RL. Perceptual Learning. *Annu Rev Psychol*. 1998;49:585-612.

Gouras P. Identification of cone mechanisms in monkey ganglion cells. *J Physiol*. 1968;199:533-547.

Gouras P, Carr RE. Cone activity in the light-induced DC response of monkey retina. *Invest Ophthalmol*. 1965;4:318–321.

Gouras P, Du J, Yamamoto S, Kjeldbye H. Anatomy and physiology of photoreceptor transplants in degenerate C3H mouse retina. *Invest Ophthalmol Vis Sci*. 1993;34:1096.

Granit R, Harper P. Comparative studies on the peripheral and central retina: II. Synaptic reaction in the eye. *Am J Physiol*. 1930;95:211–228.

Grassman H. On the theory of compound colors. *Philos Mag*. 1854;7:254–264.

Graziano MSA. Awareness of space. *Nature*. 2001;411:903-904.

Gregory RL. *Concepts and Mechanisms of Perception*. London: Duckworth; 1974.

Gregory RL. *Eye and Brain*. 3rd ed. New York: McGraw-Hill; 1978.

Grill-Spector K, Kourtzi Z, Kanwisher N. The lateral occipital complex and its role in object recognition. *Vision Res*. 2001;41:1409-1422.

Gross CG. Inferotemporal cortex and vision. *Prog Physiol Psychol*. 1973;5:77–115.

Grossman Ed, Blake R. Brain activity evoked by inverted and imagined biological motion. *Vision Res*. 2001;41:1475-1482.

Gwiazda J, Hyman L, Hussein M, et al. A randomized clinical trial of progressive addition lenses versus single vision lenses on the progression of myopia in children. *Invest Ophthalmol Vis Sci*. 2003;44:1492-1500.

Gwiazda J, Mohindra I, Brill S, Held R. Infant astigmatism and meridional amblyopia. *Vision Res*. 1985;25:1269–1276.

Gwiazda J, Scheiman M, Mohindra I, Held R. Astigmatism in infants: Changes in axis and amount from birth to six years. *Invest Ophthalmol Vis Sci*. 1984;25:88–92.

Gwiazda J, Thorn F, Bauer J, et al. Emmetropization and the progression of manifest refraction in children followed from infancy to puberty. *Clin Vision Sci*. 1993;8:337–344.

Haegerstrom-Portnoy G. The vision of rod monochromats. *Optom Vis Sci*. 1991;68(12s): 21.

Haegerstrom-Portnoy G, Schneck ME, Brabyn JA. Seeing into old age: vision beyond acuity. *Optom Vis Sci*. 1999;76:141-158.

Halliday AM, McDonald WI, Mushin J. Delayed visual responses in optic neuritis. *Lancet*. 1972;1:982–985.

Hammond CJ, Snieder H, Gilbert CE, Spector TD. Genes and environment in refractive error: twin eye study. *Invest Opthalmol Vis Sci.* 2001; 42:1232-1236.

Hansen RM, Fulton AB. Development of scotopic retinal sensitivity. In: Simons K, ed. *Early Visual Development: Normal and Abnormal.* New York: Oxford Press; 1993:130–142.

Harwerth RS, Smith EL, Duncan GC, et al. Multiple sensitive periods in the development of the primate visual system. *Science.* 1987;232:235–238.

Hasegawa S, Abe H. Mapping of glaucomatous visual field defects by multifocal VEPs. *Invest Ophthalmol Vis Sci.* 2001;42:3341-3348.

Hattar s. Liao H-W, Takao M, et al. Melopsin-containing retinal ganglion cells: architecture, projections, and intrinsic photosensitivity. *Science.* 2002;295:1065-1069

Hawken MJ, Blakemore C, Morley JW. Development of contrast sensitivity and temporal-frequency selectivity in primate lateral geniculate nucleus. *Exp Brain Res.* 1997;114:86–98.

Heath GG. Color vision. In: Wick R, Hirsch MJ, eds. *Children's Vision.* Philadelphia: Chilton; 1963.

Hecht S. Rods, cones and the chemical basis of vision. *Physiol Rev.* 1937;17:239–290.

Hecht S, Haig L, Chase AM. The influence of light adaptation on subsequent dark adaptation of the eye. *J Gen Physiol.* 1937;20:831–850.

Hecht S, Shlaer S, Pirenne MH. Energy, quanta, and vision. *J Gen Physiol.* 1942; 25:819–840.

Heijl A, Leske MC, Bengtsson B, et al. Reduction of intraocular pressure and glaucoma progression: results from the Early Manifest Glaucoma Trial. *Arch Ophthalmol.* 2002;120:1268-1279.

Held R. What can rates of development tell us about underlying mechanisms? In: Granrud C, ed. *Visual Perception and Cognition in Infancy.* Hillsdale: Erlbaum; 1993:75–89.

Held R, Birch EE, Gwiazda J. Stereoacuity of human infants. *Proc Natl Acad Sci USA.* 1980;77:5572–5574.

Hendry SHC, Yoshioka T. A neurochemically distinct third channel in the macaque dorsal lateral geniculate nucleus. *Science.* 1994;264:575-577.

Hering E. *Outlines of a Theory of Light Sense* (translated by Hurvich LM, Jameson D). Cambridge, MA: Harvard University Press; 1964 (originally published 1920).

Hess RF, Carney LG. Vision through an abnormal cornea. *Invest Ophthalmol Vis Sci.* 1979;18:470–483.

Hess RF, Woo G. Vision through cataracts. *Invest Ophthalmol Vis Sci.* 1978;17:428–435.

Higgins KE, Moskowitz–Cook A, Knoblauch K. Color vision testing: An alternative "source" of illuminant C. In: Verriest G, ed. *Modern Problems in Ophthalmology.* Basel: Karger; 1978;19:113–121.

Hill GT, Raymond JE. Deficits of motion transparency perception in adult developmental dyslexics with normal unidirectional motion senstivity. *Vision Res.* 2002;42:1195-1203.

Hitchcock PF, Hickey TL. Ocular dominance columns: Evidence for their presence in humans. *Brain Res.* 1980;182:176–179.

Hoffman KP, Stone J. Conduction velocity of afferents to cat visual cortex: A correlation with cortical receptive field properties. *Brain Res.* 1971;32:460–466.

Holopigian K, Blake R, Greenwald MJ. Selective losses in binocular vision in anisometropic amblyopes. *Vision Res.* 1986;26:621–630.

Hood DC, Frishman LJ, Saszik S, Viwanathan S. Retinal origins of the primate multifocal ERG: Implications for the human response. *Invest Ophthalmol Vis Sci.* 2002;43:1673-1685.

Hood DC, Holopigian K, Greenstein V, et al. A comparison of visual field loss to multifocal ERG changes in patients with RP. In: *Vision Science and Its Applications, 1997 OSA Technical Digest Series, Vol. 1,* Washington, D.C.: Optical Society of America; 1997:272–275.

Howland HC, Braddick O, Atkinson J, Howland B. Optics of photorefraction: Orthogonal and isotropic methods. *J Opt Soc Am*. 1983; 73:1701–1708.

Howland HC, Sayles N. A photorefractive characterization of focusing ability of infants and young children. *Invest Ophthalmol Vis Sci*. 1987;28:1005–1015.

Hsia Y, Graham CH. Spectral luminosity curves for protanopic, deuteranopic and normal subjects. *Proc Natl Acad Sci USA*. 1957;43:1011–1019.

Hubel DH. *Eye, Brain, and Vision*. New York: Scientific American Library; 1988.

Hubel DH, Wiesel TN. Receptive fields of single neurons in the cat's striate cortex. *J Physiol*. 1959;148:574–591.

Hubel DH, Wiesel TN. Receptive fields, binocular interaction and functional architecture in the cat's visual cortex. *J Physiol*. 1962;160:106–154.

Hubel DH, Wiesel TN. Receptive fields and functional architecture in two non-striate visual areas (18 and 19) of the cat. *J Physiol*. 1965a;28:229–289.

Hubel DH, Wiesel TN. Binocular interaction in striate cortex of kittens reared with artificial squint. *J Neurophysiol*. 1965b;28:1041–1059.

Hubel DH, Wiesel TN. Receptive fields and functional architecture of monkey striate cortex. *J Physiol*. 1968;195:215–243.

Hubel DH, Wiesel TN. Sequence regularity and geometry of orientation columns in the monkey striate cortex. *J Comp Neurol*. 1974;158:267–294.

Hubel DH, Wiesel TN. Functional architecture of macaque monkey visual cortex. *Proc R Soc Lond Biol Sci*. 1977;198:1–59.

Hubel DH, Wiesel TN, LeVay S. Plasticity of ocular dominance columns in monkey striate cortex. *Philos Trans R Soc Lond*. 1977;278:377–409.

Hubel DH, Wiesel TN, Stryker MP. Anatomical demonstration of orientation columns in macaque monkey. *J Comp Neur*. 1978;177:361–380.

Hung L-F, Crawford MLJ, Smith EL. Spectacle lenses alter eye growth and the refractive status of young monkeys. *Nature Med*. 1995;1:761–765.

Hurvich LM. *Color Vision*. Sunderland, MA: Sinauer Associates; 1981.

Hurvich LM, Jameson D. Some quantitative aspects of an opponent-colors theory. II. Brightness, saturation, and hue in normals and dichromatic vision. *J Opt Soc Am*. 1955;45:602-616.

Ingling CR, Martinez-Uriegas E. Simple opponent receptive fields are asymmetrical: G-cone centers predominate. *J Opt Soc Am*. 1983;73:1527–1532.

Ishai A, Sagi D. Common mechanisms of visual imagery and perception. *Science*. 1995; 268:1772–1774.

Ittleson WH, Kilpatrick FP. Experiments in perception. *Sci Am*. 1951;185:50–55.

Johnson CA. Early losses of visual function in glaucoma. *Am J Optom Physiol Opt*. 1995; 72:359–370.

Johnson CA, Casson EJ, Adams AJ, et al. Progression of glaucomatous visual field loss over five years: A comparison of white-on-white and blue-on-yellow perimetry. *Invest Ophthalmol Vis Sci*. 1992;33:1384.

Johnson EN, Hawken MJ, Shapley R. The spatial transformation of color in the primary visual cortex of the macaque monkey. *Nat Neurosci*. 2001;4:409–416.

Johnson EP, Riggs LA, Schick AML. Photopic retinal potentials evoked by phased alterations of a barred pattern. In: Burian HM, Jacobson JH, ed. *Clinical Electroretinography, Proceedings of the Third International Symposium*. Oxford: Pergamon; 1966:75–91.

Judd DB. *Color in Business, Science, and Industry*. New York: Wiley; 1952.

Judd DB, Wyszecki G. *Color in Business, Science, and Industry*. New York: Wiley; 1963.

Kahn HA, Leibowitz HM, Ganley JP, et al. The Framingham Eye Study. I. Outline and major prevalence findings. *Am J Epidemiol.* 1977;106:17-32.

Kaiser PK, Comerford JP, Bodinger DM. Saturation of spectral lights. *J Opt Soc Am.* 1976;66:818–826.

Kalmus H. The familial distribution of congenital tritanopia with some remarks on some similar conditions. *Ann Hum Genet.* 1955;20:39–56.

Kaufman L, Rock I. The moon illusion. I. *Science.* 1962;136:953–961.

Kelly DH. Visual responses to time-dependent stimuli. 1. Amplitude sensitivity measures. *J Opt Soc Am.* 1961;51:422–429.

Kelly DH. Spatiotemporal variation of chromatic and achromatic contrast thresholds. *J Opt Soc Am.* 1983;73:742–750.

Kelly JP, Borchert K, Teller DY. The development of chromatic and achromatic contrast sensitivity in infancy as tested with the sweep VEP. *Vision Res.* 1997;37:2057–2072.

King-Smith PE, Carden D. Luminance and opponent-color contributions to visual detection and adaptation and to temporal and spatial integration. *J Opt Soc Am.* 1976;66: 709–717.

Kiorpes L. Development of vernier acuity and grating acuity in normally reared monkeys. *Vis Neurosci.* 1992;9:243–251.

Kleinschmidt A, Lee BB, Requardt M, Frahm J. Functional mapping of color processing by magnetic resonance imaging of responses to selective P- and M-pathway stimulation. *Exp Brain Res.* 1996;110:279-288.

Knau H, Kremers, J, Schmidt H-J et al. M-cone opsin gene number does not corrlelate with variation in L/M-cone sensitivity. *Vision Res.* 2002;42:1888-1896.

Knoblauch K, Vital-Durand F, Barbur JL. Variation of chromatic sensitivity across the life span. *Vision Res.* 2001:41:23-36.

Knowles A. The biochemical aspects of vision. In: Barlow HB, Mollon JD, eds. *The Senses.* Cambridge: Cambridge University Press; 1982;82–101.

Kolb H, DeKorver L. Midget ganglion cells of the parafovea of the human retina: a study by electron microscopy and serial-section reconstructions. *J Comp Neurol.* 1991;303:617-636.

Köllner H. *Die Störungen des Farbensinnes. ihre klinische Bedeutung und ihre Diagnose.* Berlin: Karger; 1912.

Kondo M, Sieving PA. Primate photopic sine-wave flicker ERG: vector modeling analysis of component origins using glutamate analogs. *Invest Ophthalmol Vis Sci.* 2001;42:305-312.

Korte A. Kinematoskopische Untersuchungen. *Z Psychol.* 1915;72:193–206.

Kosslyn SM, Oschner KN. In search of occipital activation during visual mental imagery. *Trends Neurosci.* 1994;17:290–292.

Krauskopf J, Mollon JD. The independence of the temporal integration properties of individual chromatic mechanisms in the human eye. *J Physiol.* 1971;219:611–623.

Kuffler SW. Discharge patterns and functional organization of mammalian retina. *J Neurophysiol.* 1953;16:37–68.

Lachenmayr BJ, Kojetinsky S, Ostermaier N, et al. The different effects of aging on normal sensitivity in flicker and light-sense perimetry. *Invest Ophthal Vis Sci.* 1994;35: 2741–2748.

Lamb T. Transduction in vertebrate photoreceptors: The roles of cyclic GMP and calcium. *Trends Neurosci.* 1986;May:224–228.

Land EH. The retinex. *Sci Am.* 1964;52:247–264.

Lee BB, Martin PR, Valberg A. The physiological basis of heterochromatic flicker photometry demonstrated in the ganglion cells of the macaque retina. *J Physiol.* 1988;404: 323–347.

Lee BB, Pokorny J, Smith VC, et al. Luminance and chromatic modulation sensitivity of macaque ganglion cells and human observers. *J Opt Soc Am* [A]. 1990;7:2223– 2236.

Lee BB, Sun H. The physiological origin of chromatic response components in signals of the magnocellular pathway of the macaque. *Invest Ophthalmol Vis Sci.* 2003;44:E-Abstract 3191.

Le Grand R, Mondloch CJ, Maurer D, Brent HP. Early visual experience and face processing. *Nature.* 2001;410:890.

LeGrand Y. *Light Color and Vision.* London: Chapman and Hall; 1968.

Lennie P. Recent developments in the physiology of color vision. *Trends Neurosci.* 1984;7:243–248.

Lennie P, Krauskopf J, Sclar G. Chromatic mechanisms in striate cortex of macaque. *J Neurosci.* 1990a;2:649–669.

Lennie P, Trevarthen C, Van Essen D, Wässle H. Parallel processing of visual information. In: Spillman L, Werner JS, eds. *Visual Perception: The Neurophysiological Foundations.* New York: Academic Press; 1990b:103–128.

Leopold DA, Logothetis NK. Activity changes in early visual cortex reflect monkeys' percepts during binocular rivlary. *Nature.* 1996;379:549–553.

Lerman S. *Radiant Energy and the Eye.* New York: MacMillan; 1980.

Lessard N, Pare M, Lepore F, Lassonde M. Early-blind human subjects localize sound sources better than sighted subjects. *Nature.* 1998;395;278-280.

Lettvin JY, Maturana HR, McCulloch WS, Pitts WH. What the frog's eye tells the frog's brain. *Proc Inst Radio Eng.* 1959;47:1940–1951.

Levi DM. Amblyopia: A developmental disorder of spatial vision. *Optom Vis Sci.* 1992;69 (12s):123.

Levi DM, Carkeet A. Amblyopia: A consequence of abnormal visual development. In: Simons K, ed. *Early Visual Development: Normal and Abnormal.* New York: Oxford Press; 1993:391–408.

Levi DM, Harwerth RS. Spatiotemporal interactions in anisometropic and strabismic amblyopia. *Invest Ophthalmol Vis Sci.* 1977;16:90–95.

Levi DM, Klein SA, Aitsebaomo AP. Vernier acuity, crowding, and cortical magnification. *Vision Res.* 1985;25:963–977.

Levi DM, Polat U, Ying-Sheng H. Improvement in vernier acuity in adults with amblyopia. *Invest Ophthal Vis Sci.* 1997;38:1493–1510.

Levine MW, Shefner JM. *Fundamentals of Sensation and Perception.* 2nd ed. Pacific Grove, CA: Brooks/Cole; 1991.

Lindberg KA, Fisher SK. An ultrastructural study of inter-plexiform cell synapses in human retina. *J Comp Neurol.* 1986;243:561–576.

Livingstone MS, Hubel DH. Psychophysical evidence for separate channels for the perception of form, color, movement, and depth. *J Neurosci.* 1987;7:3466–3468.

Livingstone MS, Hubel DH. Segregation of form, color, movement, and depth: Anatomy, physiology, and perception. *Science.* 1988;240:740–749.

Livingstone MS, Rosen GD, Drislane FW, Galaburda AM. Physiological and anatomical evidence for a magnocellular defect in developmental dyslexia. *Proc Natl Acad Sci USA.* 1991;88:7943–7947.

Logothetis NK. Physiological studies of motion inputs. In: Smith AT, Snowden RJ, eds. *Visual Detection of Motion.* New York: Academic Press; 1994:177–216.

Logothetis NK, Schiller PH, Charles ER, Hurlbert AC. Perceptual deficits and the activity of the color-opponent and broad-band pathways at isoluminance. *Science.* 1990;247:214–217.

Loop MS, Bruce LL, Petuchowski, S. Cat color vision: The effect of stimulus size, shape, and viewing distance. *Vision Res.* 19;1979:507-513.

Lovegrove WJ, Garzia RP, Nicholson SB. Experimental evidence for a transient system deficit in specific reading disability. *J Am Optom Assoc*. 61;1990:137–146.

Lund JS, Henry GH, MacQueen CL, Harvey AR. Anatomical organization of the primary visual cortex (area 17) of the cat. A comparison with area 17 of the macaque monkey. *J Comp Neurol*. 1979;184:599–618.

MacAdam DL. *Sources of Color Vision*. Cambridge, MA: The MIT Press; 1970.

Maddess T, Henry GH. Performance of nonlinear visual units in ocular hypertension and glaucoma. *Clin Vision Sci*. 1992;7:371–383.

Maffei L, Fiorentini A. Electroretinographic responses to gratings before and after section of the optic nerve. *Science*. 1981;211:953–955.

Manny RE, Klein SA. The development of vernier acuity in infants. *Curr Eye Res*. 1984;3:453–462.

Manny RE, Klein SA. A three alternative tracking paradigm to measure vernier acuity of older infants. *Vision Res*. 1985;25:1245–1252.

Matin E. Saccadic suppression: A review and analysis. *Psychol Bull*. 1974;81:899–917.

Matin E, Clymer A, Matin L. Metacontrast and saccadic suppression. *Science*. 1972;178:179–182.

Martin P. Colour processing in the primate retina: recent progress. *J Physiol*. 1998;513.3:631-638.

Mattingley JB, Rich AN, Yelland G, Bradshaw JL. Unconscious priming eliminates automatic binding of colour and alphanumeric form in synaesthesia. *Nature*. 2001;410:580-582.

Maunsell JHR. The brain's visual world: Representation of visual targets in cerebral cortex. *Science*. 1995;270:764–769.

Maunsell JHR, Nealey TA, DePriest DD. Magnocellular and parvocellular contributions to responses in the middle temporal visual area (MT) of the macaque monkey. *J Neurosci*. 1990;10:3323–3334.

Maunsell JHR, Newsome WT. Visual processing in monkey extrastriate cortex. *Ann Rev Neurosci*. 1987;10:363–401.

Maunsell JH, Van Essen DC. Functional properties of neurons in the middle temporal area of the macaque monkey. I. Selectivity for stimulus direction, speed, and orientation. *J Neurophysiol*. 1983;49:1127–1147.

Mayer DL, Beiser AS, Warner AF, et al. Monocular acuity norms for the Teller Acuity Cards between ages one month and four years. *Invest Ophthalmol Vis Sci*. 1995;36: 671–685.

Mayer DL, Hansen RM, Moore BD, et al. Cycloplegic refractions in healthy children aged 1 through 48 months. *Arch Ophthalmol*. 2001;119:1625-1628.

Mayer MJ, Kim CBY, Svingos A, Glucs A. Foveal flicker sensitivity in healthy aging eyes: I: Compensating for pupil variation. *J Opt Soc Am A*. 1988;5:2201–2209.

Mayer MJ, Spiegler JJ, Ward B, et al. Mid-frequency loss of foveal flicker sensitivity in early stages of age-related maculopathy. *Invest Ophthalmol Vision Sci*. 1992;33: 3136–3142.

McDonald MA, Dobson V, Sebris SL, et al. The acuity card procedure: A rapid test of infant acuity. *Invest Ophthalmol Vis Sci*. 1985;26:1158–1162.

McKendrick AM, Johnson CA, Anderson AJ, Fortune B. Elevated vernier acuity thresholds in glaucoma. *Invest Ophthalmol Vis Sci*. 2002;43:1393-1399.

Mendelson JR, Wells EF. Age-related changes in the visual cortex. *Vision Res*. 2002;42:695-703.

Merabet L, Desautels A, Minville K, Casanova C. Motion integration in a thalamic visual nucleus. *Vision Res*. 1998;396:265-268.

Merbs SL, Nathans J. Absorption spectra of human cone pigments. *Nature*. 1992;356: 433–435.

Merigan WH. Chromatic and achromatic vision of macaques: Role of the P pathway. *J Neurosci*. 1989;9:776–783.

Merigan WH, Maunsell JHR. Macaque vision after magnocellular lateral geniculate lesions. *Vis Neurosci.* 1990;5:347–352.

Merigan WH, Maunsell JHR. How parallel are the primate pathways? *Ann Rev Neurosci.* 1993;16:369–402.

Miller JW, Ludvigh E. The effect of relative motion on visual acuity. *Surv Ophthalmol.* 1962;7:83–116.

Miller K. Understanding layer 4 of the cortical circuit: a model based on cat V1. *Cerebral Cortex.* 2003;13:73-82.

Millodot M. Image formation in the eye. In: Barlow HB, Mollon JD, eds. *The Senses.* Cambridge: Cambridge University Press; 1982:46–61.

Mishkin M, Ungerleider LG, Macko KA. Object vision and spatial vision: Two cortical pathways. *Trends Neurosci.* 1983;6:414–417.

Mitchell DE, Freeman RD, Millodot M, Haegerstrom G. Meridional amblyopia: Evidence for modification of the human visual system by early visual experience. *Vision Res.* 1973;13:535–558.

Mitchell DE, Reardon J, Muir DW. Interocular transfer of motion aftereffect in normal and stereo blind observers. *Exp Brain Res.* 1975;22:163–173.

Mohindra I, Held R. Refraction in human infants from birth to five years. *Doc Ophthalmol.* 1981;28:19–27.

Mohindra I, Held R, Gwiazda J, Brill S. Astigmatism in human infants. *Science.* 1978;202:329–331.

Moran J, Desimone R. Selective attention gates visual processing in extrastriate cortex. *Science.* 1985;229:782–784.

Morgan MW, Rosenbloom AA. *Vision and Aging.* 2nd ed. Boston: Butterworth-Heinemann; 1993.

Morrone MC, Burr DC, Fiorentini A. Development of infant contrast sensitivity to chromatic stimuli. *Vision Res.* 1993;33:2535–2552.

Motter BC. Neural correlates of attentive selection for color or luminance in extrastriate area V4. *J Neurosci.* 1994;14:2178–2189.

Movshon JA, Adelson EH, Gizzi MS, Newsome WT. The analysis of moving visual patterns. In: Chagas C, Gattass R, Gross C, eds. *Pattern Recognition Mechanisms.* Vatican City: Pontifical Academy of Sciences; 1985:117–151.

Movshon JA, Eggers HM, Gizzi MS, et al. Effects of early unilateral blur on the macaque's visual system: III. Physiological observations. *J Neurosci.* 1987;7:1340–1351.

Movshon JA, Kiorpes L. Analysis of the development of spatial contrast sensitivity in monkey and human infants. *J Opt Soc Am A.* 1988;5:2166–2172.

Mutti DO, Zadnick K, Adams AJ. The nature versus nurture debate goes on. *Invest Ophthalmol Vis Sci.* 1996;37:952–957.

Nakayama K. Biological motion processing: A review. *Vision Res.* 1985;25:625–660.

Nakayama K, Tyler CW. Psychophysical isolation of movement sensitivity by removal of positional cues. *Vision Res.* 1981;21:427–433.

Nathans J. The genes for color vision. *Sci Am.* 1989;260(2):42–49.

Nathans J. The evolution and physiology of human color vision: insights from molecular genetic studies of visual pigments. *Neuron.* 1999;24:299-312.

Nathans J, Piantanida TP, Eddy RL, et al. Molecular genetics of inherited variation in human color vision. *Science.* 1986a;232:203–210.

Nathans J, Thomas D, Hogness DS. Molecular genetics of human color vision: the genes encoding blue, green, and red pigments. *Science.* 1986b;232:193–202.

Neitz J, Jacobs GH. Polymorphism of long-wavelength cone in normal human colour vision. *Nature*. 1986;323:623–625.

Neitz J, Neitz M. Color Vision Defects. In: Wright AF, Barrie, J, eds. *Molecular Genetics of Inherited Eye Disorders*. Harwood Academic Publishers; 1994:217–257.

Neitz J, Neitz M, Kainz PM. Visual pigment gene structure and the severity of color vision defects. *Science*. 1996;274:801–803.

Neitz M, Neitz J. Molecular genetics of color vision and color vision defects. *Arch Ophthalmol*. 2000;118:691-700.

Nelson R, Famiglietta EV, Kolb H. Intracellular staining reveals different levels of stratification for on- and off-center ganglion cells in cat retina. *J Neurophysiol*. 1978;41:472-483.

Newman N. *Neuro-Ophthalmology: A Practical Text*. Norwalk, CT: Appleton & Lange; 1992.

Newsome WT, Paré EB. A selective impairment of motion perception following lesions of middle temporal visual area (MT). *J Neurosci*. 1988;8:2201–2211.

Newsome WT, Wurtz RH. Probing visual cortical function with discrete chemical lesions. *Trends Neurosci*. 1988;11:394–400.

Norcia AM, Tyler CW. Spatial frequency sweep VEP: Visual acuity in the first year of life. *Vision Res*. 1985;25:1399–1408.

Norcia AM, Tyler CW, Allen D. Electrophysiological assessment of contrast sensitivity in human infants. *Am J Optom Physiol Opt*. 1986;63:12–15.

Olson CR, Freeman RD. Profile of the sensitive period for monocular deprivation in kittens. *Exp Brain Res*. 1980;39:17–21.

Osterberg G. Topography of the layer of rods and cones in the human retina. *Acta Ophthalmol Suppl*. 1935;6:1–103.

Ooi TL, Wu B, He ZJ. Distance determined by the angular declination below the horizon. *Nature*. 2001;414:197-200.

Osorio D, Vorobyov M. Colour Vision as an adaptation to frugivory in primates. *Proc R Soc Lond B Biol Sci*. 1996;263:593-599.

Owsley C, McGwin G, Sloane M, et al. Impact of cataract surgery on motor vehicle crash involvement by older adults. *J Am Med Assoc*. 2002;288:841-849.

Owsley C, Sekular R, Siemsen D. Contrast sensitivity throughout adulthood. *Vision Res*. 1983;23:689–699.

Packer O, Hartmann EE, Teller DY. Infant color vision: The effect of field size on Rayleigh discriminations. *Vision Res*. 1984;24:1247–1260.

Pascalis O, de Haan M, Nelson, CA. Is face processing species-specific during the first year of life? *Science*. 2002;296:1321-1323.

Pascual-Leone A, Walsh V. Fast backprojections from the motion to the primary visual area necessary for visual awareness. *Science*. 2001;292:510-512.

Peichl L, Wassle H. Morphological identification of on- and off-centre brisk transient (Y) cells in the cat retina. *Proc R Soc Lond B*. 1981;212:139-156.

Pelli PG, Robson JG, Wilkins AJ. The design of a new letter chart for measuring contrast sensitivity. *Clin Vision Sci*. 1988;2:187–199.

Pirenne MH. *Vision and The Eye*. London: Chapman and Hall; 1967.

Pitt FHG. *Characteristics of Dichromatic Vision with an Appendix on Anomalous Trichromatic Vision*. Great Britain Medical Report Series, no. 200; 1935.

Pitts DG. The human ultraviolet action spectrum. *Am J Optom Arch Am Acad Optom*. 1974;51:946–960.

Pokorny J, Smith VC. Wavelength discrimination in the presence of chromatic fields. *J Opt Soc Am*. 1970;60:562–569.

Pokorny J, Smith VC, Verriest G, Pinckers AJLG. *Congenital and Acquired Color Vision Defects*. New York: Grune and Stratton; 1979.

Polyak SL. *The Retina*. Chicago: University of Chicago Press; 1941.

Popovic Z, Sjostrand J. Resolution, separation of retinal ganglion cells, and cortical magnification in humans. *Vision Res*. 2001;41:1313-1319.

Porter TC. Contributions to the study of flicker, II. *Proc R Soc Lond*. 1902;70A:313–329.

Posner MI. Seeing the mind. *Science*. 1993;262:673–674.

Powers MK, Schneck M, Teller DY. Spectral sensitivity of human infants at absolute visual threshold. *Vision Res*. 1981;21:1005–1016.

Priest IG, Brickwedde FG. The minimum perceptible colorimetric purity as a function of dominant wavelength. *J Opt Soc Am*. 1938;28:133–139.

Provencio I, Rollag MD, Castrucci AM. Photoreceptive net in mammalian retina. *Nature*. 2002;415:493

Pugh EN, Cobbs WH. Visual transduction in vertebrate rods and cones. *Vision Res*. 1986;26:1613–1643.

Purkinje J. *Opera Omnia Beobachtungen und Versuche zur Physiologie der Sinne*. Vol. 1. Prague: JG Calve; 1819.

Quigley HA, Addicks EM, Green WR. Optic nerve damage in human glaucoma. III. Quantitative correlation of nerve fiber loss and visual field defect in glaucoma, ischemic neuropathy, papilledema, and toxic neuropathy. *Arch Ophthalmol*. 1982;100: 135–146.

Quigley HA, Sanchez RM, Dunkelberger GR, et al. Chronic glaucoma selectivity damages large optic nerve fibers. *Invest Ophthalmol Vis Sci*. 1987;28: 913–920.

Ramus F. Talk of two theories. *Nature*. 2001;412:393-395.

Rao SC, Rainer G, Miller EK. Integration of what and where in the primate prefrontal cortex. *Science*. 1997;276:821–824.

Ratliff F, Hartline HK, Miller WH. Spatial and temporal aspects of retinal inhibitory interaction. *J Opt Soc Am*. 1963;53:110–120.

Ratliff F, Riggs LA. Involuntary motions of the eye during monocular fixation. *J Exp Psychol*. 1950;40:687–701.

Raviola E, Wiesel TN. Effect of dark-rearing on experimental myopia in monkeys. *Invest Ophthalmol Vis Sci*. 1978;17:485–488.

Lord Rayleigh. Experiments on colour. *Nature*. 1881;25:64–66.

Rea MS. *Lighting Handbook: Reference and Application*. New York: Illuminating Engineering Society of North America; 1993.

Reeves BC, Wood JM, Hill AR. Vistech VCTS 6500 Charts—within and between session reliability. *Optom Vis Sci*. 1991;68:728–737.

Regal DM. Development of critical flicker fusion frequency in infants. *Vision Res*. 1981; 21:549–555.

Regan D. *Human Brain Electrophysiology: Evoked Potentials and Evoked Magnetic Fields in Science and Medicine*. New York: Elsevier; 1989.

Repka MX, Beck RW, Holmes JM et al. A randomized trial of patching regimens for treatment of moderate amblyopia in children. *Arch Ophthalmol*. 2003;121:603-611.

Riggs LA, Ratliff F, Cornsweet JC, Cornsweet TN. The disappearance of steadily fixated test objects. *J Opt Soc Am*. 1953;43:495–501.

Riggs LA, Wooten BR. Electrical measures and psychophysical data on human vision. In: Jameson D, Hurvich LM, eds. *Handbook of Sensory Physiology*. Vol. VII/4. *Visual Psychophysics*. New York: Springer-Verlag; 1972:690–731.

Rodenstock HB, Swick DA. Color discrimination for the color blind. *Aerospace Med*. 1974;145:1194–1197.

Roder B, Teder-Salejarvi W, Sterr A, et al. Improved auditory spatial tuning in blind humans. *Nature*. 1999;400:162-166.

Rodieck RW. Which cells code for color? In: Valberg A, Lee BB, eds. *From Pigments to Perception: Advances in Understanding Visual Processes*. New York: Plenum; 1991:83–93.

Rodman HR, Albright TD. Single-unit analysis of pattern-motion selective properties in the middle temporal visual area (MT). *Exp Brain Res*. 1989;75:53–64.

Rolls ET, Tovée MJ. Sparseness of the neuronal representation of stimuli in the primate temporal cortex. *J Neurophysiol*. 1995;73:713–726.

Roorda A, Metha AB, Lennie P, Williams DR. Packing arrangement of the three cone classes in primate retina. *Vision Res*. 2001;41:1291-1306.

Roorda A, Williams DR. The arrangement of three cone classes in the living human eye. *Nature*. 1999;397:520-522.

Rose A. The sensitivity performance of the human eye on an absolute scale. *J Opt Soc Am*. 1948;38:196–208.

Rushton WAH. A cone pigment in the protanope. *J Physiol*. 1963a;168:345–359.

Rushton WAH. Cone pigment kinetics in the protanope. *J Physiol*. 1963b;168:374–388.

Rushton WAH. The Ferrier lecture. Visual adaptation. *Proc R Soc Lond Biol Sci*. 1965a;162: 20–46.

Rushton WAH. A foveal pigment in the deuteranope. *J Physiol*. 1965b;176:24–37.

Sadato N, Pascual-Leone A, Grafman J, et al. Activation of the primary visual cortex by Braille reading in blind subjects. *Nature*. 1996;380:526-528.

Salzman CD, Newsome WT. Neural mechanisms for forming a perceptual decision. *Science*. 1994;264:231–237.

Saw S-M, Chua W-H, Hong C-Y, et al. Nearwork in early-onset myopia. *Invest Ophthalmol Vis Sci*. 2002;43:332-339.

Schiller PH. The effects of V4 and middle temporal (MT) area lesions on visual performance in the rhesus monkey. *Vis Neurosci*. 1993;10:717–746.

Schiller PH, Finlay BL, Volman SF. Quantitative studies of single-cell properties in monkey striate cortex. I. Spatiotemporal organization of receptive fields. *J Neurophysiol*. 1976;39:1288–1319.

Schiller PH, Logothetis NK, Charles ER. Functions of the color-opponent and broad-band channels of the visual system. *Nature*. 1990a;343:68–70.

Schiller PH, Logothetis NK, Charles ER. Role of color-opponent and broad-band channels in vision. *Vis Neurosci*. 1990b;5:321–346.

Schiller PH, Malpeli JG. Functional specificity of lateral geniculate laminae of the rhesus monkey. *J Neurophysiol*. 1978;41:788–797.

Schnapf JL, Baylor DA. How photoreceptors respond to light. *Sci Am*. 1987;256(4):40–47.

Schnapf JL, Kraft TW, Baylor DA. Spectral sensitivity of human cone photoreceptors. *Nature*. 1987;325:439–441.

Schneck ME, Haegerstrom-Portnoy G. Color vision defect type and spatial vision in the optic neuritis trial. *Invest Ophthalmol Vis Sci*. 1997;38:2278–2289.

Schroder J-H, Fries P, Roelfsema PR. Ocular dominance in extrastriate cortex of strabismic amblyopic cats. *Vision Res*. 2002;42:29-39.

Schwartz SH. Reaction time distributions and their relationship to the transient/sustained nature of the neural discharge. *Vision Res*. 1992;32:2087–2092.

Schwartz SH. Colour and flicker thresholds for high frequency increments. *Ophthalmic Physiol Opt*. 1993;13:299–302.

Schwartz SH. Spectral sensitivity of dichromats: Role of postreceptoral processes. *Vision Res*. 1994;34:2983–2990.

Schwartz SH. Spectral sensitivity as revealed by isolated step onsets and step offsets. *Ophthalmic Physiol Opt*. 1996;16:58-63.

Schwartz, SH. *Geometrical and Visual Optics: A Clinical Introduction*. New York: McGraw-Hill; 2002.

Schwartz SH, Godwin LD. Masking of the achromatic system: Implications for saccadic suppression. *Vision Res*. 1996;36:1551–1559.

Schwartz SH, Loop, MS. Evidence for transient luminance and quasi-sustained color mechanisms. *Vision Res*. 1982;22:445-447.

Seiple W, Clemens C, Greentein VC, et al. The spatial distribution of selective attention assessed using the multifocal visual evoked potential. *Vision Res*. 2002;42:1513-1521.

Shapley R. Visual sensitivity and parallel retinocortical pathways. *Annu Rev Psychol*. 1990;41:635–658.

Sharma J, Angelucci A, Sur M. Induction of visual orientation modules in auditory cortex. *Nature*. 2000;404:841-847.

Shinar D, Schieber F. Visual requirements for safety and mobility of older drivers. *Hum Factors*. 1991;33:507–519.

Shinomori K, Schefrin BE, Werner JS. Age-related changes in wavelength discrimination. *J Opt Soc Am A*. 2001;310-318.

Sekuler R, Blake, R. *Perception*. New York: McGraw-Hill; 1990.

Siegwart JT, Norton TT. Refractive and ocular changes in tree shrews raised with plus or minus lenses. *Invest Ophthalmol Vis Sci*. 1993;34:1208.

Silverman SE, Trick GL, Hart WM. Motion perception is abnormal in primary open-angle glaucoma and ocular hypertension. *Invest Ophthalmol Vis Sci*. 1990;31:722–729.

Slaghuis WL, Lovegrove WJ. Spatial-frequency-dependent visible persistence and specific reading disability. *Brain Cogn*. 1985;4:219–240.

Slataper FJ. Age norms of refraction and vision. *Arch Ophthalmol*. 1950;43:466–481.

Slaughter MM, Miller RF. The role of glutamate receptors in information processing in the distal retina. In: Gallego A, Gouras P, eds. *Neurocircuitry of the Retina, A Cajal Memorial*. New York: Elsevier; 1985:51–65.

Smallman HS, MacLeod DIA, Doyle P. Realignment of cones after cataract removal. *Nature*. 2001;412:604-605.

Smith EL, Hung L-F, Kee, C-s, Qiao Y. Effects of brief periods of unrestricted vision on the development of form-deprivation myopia in monkeys. *Invest Ophthalmol Vis Sci*. 2002;43:291-299.

Smith EL, Hung L-F, Harwerth RS. The degree of image degredation and the depth of amblyopia. *Invest Ophthalmol Vis Sci*. 2000;41:3775-3781.

Smith VC, Pokorny J. Spectral sensitivity of the foveal cone photopigments between 400 nm and 500 nm. *Vision Res*. 1975;15:161–171.

Smith VC, Pokorny J, Gamlin PD, et al. Functional architecture of the photoreceptive ganglion cell in primate retina: spectral sensitivity and dynamics of the intrinsic response. *Invest Ophthalmol Vis Sci*. 2003;44: E-Abstract 5185.

Sokol S. The visually evoked cortical potential in optic nerve and visual pathway disorders. In: Fishman GA, Sokol S, eds. *Electrophysiologic Testing in Disorders of the Retina, Optic Nerve, and Visual Pathway*. San Francisco: American Academy of Ophthalmology; 1990:105–141.

Sowden PT, Rose D, Davies IRL. Perceptual learning of luminance contrast detection: specific for spatial frequency and retinal location but not orientation. *Vision Res*. 2002;42:1249-1258.

Spear PD, Moore RJ, Kim CBY, et al. Effects of aging on the primate visual system: Spatial and temporal processing by lateral geniculate neurons in young adult and old rhesus monkeys. *J Neurophysiol*. 1994;72:402–420.

Sperling HG, Harwerth RS. Red-green cone interactions in the increment-threshold spectral sensitivity of primates. *Science*. 1971;172:180–184.

Sperling HG, Jolliffe CL. Intensity-time relationships at threshold for spectral stimuli in human vision. *J Opt Soc Am*. 1965;55:191–199.

Steinman BA, Steinman SB, Lehmkuhle S. Visual attention mechanisms show a center-surround organization. *Vision Res*. 1995;35:1859–1869.

Steinman SB, Levi DM, McKee SP. Discrimination of time and velocity in the amblyopic visual system. *Clin Vision Sci*. 1988;2:265–276.

Steinman SB, Steinman BA. Vision and Attention. I: Current models of visual attention. *Optom Vis Sci*. 1998;75:146–155.

Steinman SB, Steinman BA, Garzia RP, *Foundations of Binocular Vision: A Clinical Perspective*. New York: McGraw-Hill; 2000.

Stell WK, Ishida AT, Lightfoot DO. Structural basis for on- and off-center responses in retinal bipolar cells. *Science*. 1977;198:1269–1271.

Stevens SS. On the psychophysical law. *Psychol Rev*. 1957;64:153–181.

Stiles WS. The directional sensitivity of the retina and the spectral sensitivities of the rods and cones. *Proc R Soc Lond Biol Sci*. 1939;127:64–105.

Stiles WS. Further studies of visual mechanisms by the two-colour threshold method. In: *Collequio Sobre Problemas Opticos de la Vision*. Madrid; 1953:63–103.

Stone J, Dreher B, Levanthal A. Hierarchical and parallel mechanisms in the organization of visual cortex. *Brain Res Rev*. 1979;1:345–394.

Stoner GR, Albright TD. The interpretation of visual motion: Evidence for surface segmentation mechanisms. *Vision Res*. 1996;36:1291–1310.

Stryer L. Cyclic GMP cascade of vision. *Annu Rev Neurosci*. 1986;9:87–119.

Stryker MP, Sherk H. Modification of cortical orientation selectivity in the cat by restricted visual experience: A reexamination. *Science*. 1975;190:904–906.

Stryker MP, Sherk H, Levanthal AG, Hirsch HVB. Physiological consequences for the cat's visual cortex of effectively restricting early visual experience with oriented contours. *J Neurophysiol*. 1978;41:896–909.

Sutter E, Tran D. The field topography of ERG components in man-1. The photopic luminance response. *Vision Res*. 1992;32:433–446.

Svaetichin G. Spectral response curves from single cones. *Acta Physiol Scand*. 1956;39 (suppl 134):17–46.

Swanson WH, Ueno T, Smith VC, Pokorny J. Temporal modulation sensitivity and pulse-detection thresholds for chromatic and luminance perturbations. *J Opt Soc Am* [A]. 1987;4:1992–2005.

Swets JA, Tanner WP Jr, Birdsall TG. Decision processes in perception. *Psychol Rev*. 1961; 68:301–340.

Tanaka K, Saito H, Fukada Y, Moriya M. Coding visual images of objects in the inferotemporal cortex of the macaque monkey. *J Neurophysiol*. 1991;66:170–189.

Teikari JM, Kaprio J, Koskenvuo MK, et al. Heritability estimate for refractive errors: A population-based sample of adult twins. *Gen Epidemiol*. 1988;5:171–181.

Teller DY. The forced-choice preferential looking procedure: A psychophysical technique for use with human infants. *Infant Behav Dev*. 1979;2:135–153.

Teller DY. Scotopic vision, color vision, and stereopsis in infants. *Curr Eye Res*. 1982;2: 199–210.

Teller DY. First glances: The vision of infants. *Invest Ophthalmol Vis Sci*. 1997;38: 2183–2203.

Teller DY, Morse R, Borton R, Regal D. Visual acuity for vertical and diagonal gratings in human infants. *Vision Res*. 1974;14:1433–1439.

Teller DY, Movshon JA. Visual development. *Vision Res*. 1986;26:1483–1506.

Teller DY, Peeples DR, Sekel M. Discrimination of chromatic from white light by two-month-old human infants. *Vision Res.* 1978;18:41–48.

Theile A, Henning M, Kubischik M, Hoffmann K-P. Neural mechanisms of saccadic suppression. *Science.* 2002;295;2460-2462.

Thorn F, Held R, Fang L. Orthogonal astigmatic axes in Chinese and Caucasian infants. *Invest Ophthalmol Vis Sci.* 1987;28:191–194.

Tomita T. Electrical activity of vertebrate photoreceptors. *Q Rev Biophys.* 1970;3:179–222.

Tong F, Nakayama K, Vaughan JT, Kanwisher N. Binocular rivalry and visual awareness in human extrastriate cortex. *Neuron.* 1998;21:753-759.

Tootell RBH, Reppas JB, Dale AM, et al. Visual motion aftereffect in human cortical area MT revealed by functional magnetic resonance imaging. *Nature.* 1995;375:139–141.

Tovée MJ. *An Introduction to the Visual System.* Cambridge: Cambridge; 1996.

Tovée MJ, Cohen-Tovée EM. The neural substrates of face processing: A review. *Cogn Neuropsychol.* 1993;10:505–528.

Trick GL. Retinal potentials in patients with primary open angle glaucoma: Physiological evidence for temporal frequency tuning defects. *Invest Ophthalmol Vis Sci.* 1985;26:1750–1758.

Trick GL, Steinman SB, Amyot, M. Motion perception deficits in glaucomatous optic neuropathy. *Vision Res.* 1995;35:2225–2233.

Troxler D. Ueber das verschwinden gegebener Gegenstande innerhalb unseres Gesichtskreises. In: Himly K, Schmidt JA, eds. *Ophthalmische Bibliothek.* Jena: Fromann; 1804;2:51–53.

Ts'o DY, Gilbert CD. The organization of chromatic and spatial interactions in the primate striate cortex. *J Neurosci.* 1988;8:1712–1727.

Ts'o DY, Roe AW, Gilbert CD. A hierarchy of the functional organization for color, form and disparity in primate visual area V2. *Vision Res.* 2001;41:1333-1349.

Tyler CW. Specific defects of flicker sensitivity in glaucoma and ocular hypertension. *Invest Ophthalmol Vis Sci.* 1981;20:204–212.

Tyler CW, Ernst W, Lyness AL. Photopic flicker sensitivity losses in simplex and multiplex retinitis pigmentosa. *Invest Ophthalmol Vis Sci.* 1984;25:1035–1042.

Ungerleider LG. Functional brain imaging studies of cortical mechanisms for memory. *Science.* 1995;270:769–775.

Vaegan, Taylor D. Critical period for deprivation amblyopia in children. *Trans Ophthalmol Soc UK.* 1980;99:432–439.

Van Essen DC, Andersen CH, Felleman DJ. Information processing in the primate visual system: An integrated systems perspective. *Science.* 1992;255:419–423.

Van Loo JA, Enoch JM. The scotopic Stiles–Crawford effect. *Vision Res.* 1975;15:1005– 1009.

Van Sluyters RC, Atkinson J, Banks MS, et al. The development of vision and visual perception. In: Spillman L, Werner JS, eds. *Visual Perception: The Neurophysiological Foundations.* New York: Academic Press; 1990;349–379.

Varner D, Cook JE, Schneck ME, et al. Tritan discriminations by 1- and 2-month-old human infants. *Vision Res.* 1985;2:821–831.

Verriest G. Les deficiencies de la vision des couleurs. *Bull des Soc d'Ophtalmol.* 1969:19 October:901-927.

Verriest G, Uvijls A. Central and peripheral increment thresholds for white and spectral lights on a white background in different kinds of congenitally defective colour vision. *Atti Fond Giorgio Ronchi.* 1977;32:213–254.

von Melchner L, Pallas SL, Sur M. Visual behaviour mediated by retinal projections directed to auditory pathway. *Nature.* 2000;404:871-876.

Wagner G, Boynton RM. Comparison of four methods of heterochromatic photometry. *J Opt Soc Am*. 1972;62:1508–1515.

Wald G. Human vision and spectrum. *Science*. 1945;101:653–658.

Wallman J, McFadden S. Monkey eyes grow into focus. *Nature Med*. 1995;1:737–739.

Walraven J, Valeton JM. Visual adaptation and response saturation. In Van Doorn AJ, Van de Grind WA, Koenderink JJ, eds. *Limits in Perception*. Utrecht: VNU Science Press; 1984.

Watanabe T, Nanez JE, Sasaki Y. Perceptual learning without perception. *Nature*. 2001; 413:844-848.

Wandell BA. *Foundations of Vision*. Sunderland: Sinauer; 1995.

Wasserman GS, Kong KL. Illusory correlation of brightness enhancement and transients in the nervous system. *Science*. 1974;184:911–913.

Wassle H, Grunert U, Martin PR et al. Immunocytochemical characterization and spatial distribution of midget bipolar cells in the macaque monkey retina. *Vision Res*. 1994; 34:562-579.

Watson JD, Myers R, Frackowiak RSJ, et al. Area V5 of the human brain: Evidence from a combined study using positron emission tomography and magnetic resonance imaging. *Cereb Cortex*. 1993;3:79–94.

Weale RA. Senile cataract: The case against light. *Ophthalmology*. 1983;90:420–423.

Weale RA. *The Senescence of Human Vision*. New York: Oxford University Press; 1992.

Weiskrantz L. *Blindsight. A Case Study and Implications*. Oxford: Oxford University Press; 1986.

Werblin FS, Dowling JE. Organization of the retina of the mudpuppy, *Necturus maculosus*. II. Intracellular recording. *J Neurophysiol*. 1969;32:339–355.

West SK, Rubin GS, Broman, AT, et al. How does visual impairment affect performance on tasks of everyday life? *Arch Ophthalmol*. 2002;120: 774-780.

Westheimer G. The spatial sense of the eye (Proctor lecture). *Invest Ophthalmol Vis Sci*. 1979;18:893–912.

Westheimer G. Is peripheral visual acuity susceptible to perceptual learning in the adult? *Vision Res*. 2001;41:47-52.

White AJR, Sun H, Swanson WH, Lee BB. An examination of physiological mechanisms underlying the frequency-doubling illusion. *Invest Ophthalmol Vis Sci*. 2002;43:3590-3599.

Wiesel TN, Hubel DH. Single-cell responses in striate cortex of kittens deprived of vision in one eye. *J Neurophysiol*. 1963;26:1003–1017.

Wiesel TN, Hubel DH. Spatial and chromatic interactions in the lateral geniculate body of the rhesus monkey. *J Neurophysiol*. 1966;29:1115–1156.

Wiesel TN, Raviola E. Myopia and eye enlargement after neonatal lid fusion in monkeys. *Nature*. 1977;266:66–68.

Wildsoet C, Wallman J. Choroidal and scleral mechanisms of compensation for spectacle lenses in chicks. *Vision Res*. 1995;35:1175–1194.

Williams DR. Seeing through the photoreceptor mosaic. *Trends Neurosci*. 1986;9:193–198.

Wong-Riley MTT. Changes in the visual system of monocularly sutured or enucleated cats demonstrable with cytochrome oxidase histochemistry. *Brain Res*. 1979;171:11–28.

Woo G, Hess R. Contrast sensitivity function and soft contact lenses. *Int Contact Lens Clin*. 1979;6:171–176.

Wood JM, Bullimore MA. Changes in the lower displacement limit for motion with age. *Ophthalmic Physiol Opt*. 1995;15:31–36.

Wright LA, Wormald RP. Stereopsis and ageing. *Eye* 1992;6:473–476.

Wright WD. The sensitivity of the eye to small colour differences. *Proc Physiol Soc Lond*. 1941;53:93–112.

Wright WD. *Researches on Normal and Defective Color Vision.* London: Henry Kimpton; 1946.

Wright WD. The characteristics of tritanopia. *J Opt Soc Am.* 1952;42:509–520.

Wyszecki G, Stiles WS. *Color Science: Concepts and Methods, Quantitative Data and Formulae.* 2nd ed. New York: Wiley; 1982.

Young MP, Scannell JW. Analysis and modelling of the mammalian cerebral cortex. In: Othmer HG, Main RK, Murray JD, eds. *Experimental and Theoretical Advances in Biological Pattern Formation.* New York: Plenum Press; 1993:369–384.

Young RW. Visual cells. *Sci Am.* 1970;223(4):80–91.

Young RW. The renewal of rod and cone outer segments in the rhesus monkey. *J Cell Biol.* 1971;49:303–318.

Young RW. Visual cells, daily rhythms, and vision research. *Vision Res.* 1978;18:573–578.

Young T. On the theory of light and colours. *Philos Trans.* 1802;92:21–71.

Zaidi Q. Simultaneous estimation of illuminance and object colors. *Invest Ophthalmol Vis Sci.* 1997;38(suppl):S476.

Zeki SM. The distribution of wavelength and orientation selective cells in different areas of the monkey visual cortex. *Proc R Soc Lond Biol Sci.* 1983;217:449–470.

Zeki S. *A Vision of the Brain.* Oxford: Blackwell Scientific; 1993.

Zihl J, von Cramon D, Mai N. Selective disturbance of movement vision after bilateral brain damage. *Brain.* 1983;106:313–340.

Index

Page numbers followed by *t* indicate tables; page numbers followed by *f* indicate figures.